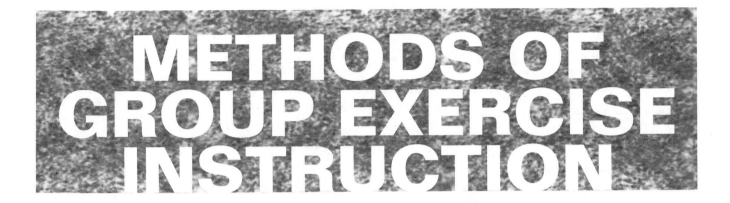

METHODS OF GROUP EXERCISE INSTRUCTION

Carol A. Kennedy, MS
Indiana University, Bloomington, Indiana

Mary M. Yoke, MA, MM
Adelphi University, Garden City, New York

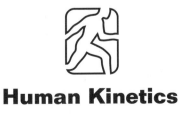

Human Kinetics

Library of Congress Cataloging-in-Publication Data

Kennedy, Carol A., 1958-
  Methods of group exercise instruction / Carol A. Kennedy, Mary M. Yoke.
      p. cm.
  Includes bibliographical references and index.
  ISBN 0-7360-4907-X (soft cover)
  1. Exercise--Study and teaching. 2. Physical education and training--Study and teaching. 3. Exercise
personnel--Certification--United States. I. Yoke, Mary M., 1953- II. Title.
  GV481.K416 2005
  613.7'1--dc22
                                                   2004008300

ISBN-10: 0-7360-4907-X
ISBN-13: 978-0-7360-4907-8

The Web addresses cited in this text were current as of June 28, 2004, unless otherwise noted.

Acquisitions Editor: Judy Patterson Wright, PhD; **Developmental Editor:** Judy Park; **Assistant Editor:** Mandy Eastin; **Copyeditor:** Julie Anderson; **Proofreader:** Kathy Bennett; **Indexer:** Bobbi Swanson; **Permission Manager:** Dalene Reeder; **Graphic Designer:** Nancy Rasmus; **Graphic Artist:** Denise Lowry; **Photo Manager:** Kareema McLendon; **Cover Designer:** Keith Blomberg; **Photographer (cover):** Kelly Huff; **Photographer (interior):** Tom Roberts, unless otherwise noted; **Art Manager:** Kelly Hendren; **Illustrators:** Mic Greenberg and Jason McAlexander/Interactive Composition Corporation; **Printer:** United Graphics

We thank The Student Recreational Sports Center at Indiana University, Bloomington, IN, for assistance in providing the location for the photo shoot for this book.

Printed in the United States of America   10   9   8   7   6   5   4   3

Human Kinetics
Web site: www.HumanKinetics.com

United States: Human Kinetics, P.O. Box 5076, Champaign, IL 61825-5076
800-747-4457
e-mail: humank@hkusa.com

Canada: Human Kinetics, 475 Devonshire Road, Unit 100, Windsor, ON N8Y 2L5
800-465-7301 (in Canada only)
e-mail: orders@hkcanada.com

Europe: Human Kinetics, 107 Bradford Road, Stanningley
Leeds LS28 6AT, United Kingdom
+44 (0) 113 255 5665
e-mail: hk@hkeurope.com

Australia: Human Kinetics, 57A Price Avenue, Lower Mitcham, South Australia 5062
08 8372 0999
e-mail: liaw@hkaustralia.com

New Zealand: Human Kinetics, Division of Sports Distributors NZ Ltd.
P.O. Box 300 226 Albany, North Shore City, Auckland
0064 9 448 1207
e-mail: info@humankinetics.co.nz

CONTENTS

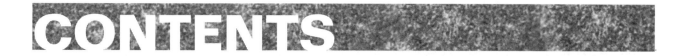

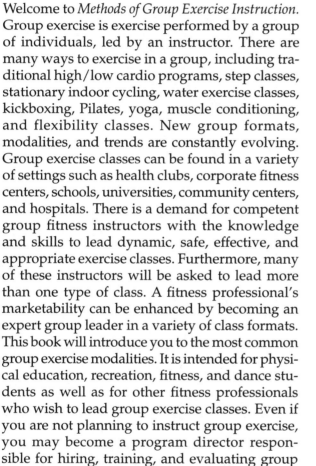

PREFACE

Welcome to *Methods of Group Exercise Instruction*. Group exercise is exercise performed by a group of individuals, led by an instructor. There are many ways to exercise in a group, including traditional high/low cardio programs, step classes, stationary indoor cycling, water exercise classes, kickboxing, Pilates, yoga, muscle conditioning, and flexibility classes. New group formats, modalities, and trends are constantly evolving. Group exercise classes can be found in a variety of settings such as health clubs, corporate fitness centers, schools, universities, community centers, and hospitals. There is a demand for competent group fitness instructors with the knowledge and skills to lead dynamic, safe, effective, and appropriate exercise classes. Furthermore, many of these instructors will be asked to lead more than one type of class. A fitness professional's marketability can be enhanced by becoming an expert group leader in a variety of class formats. This book will introduce you to the most common group exercise modalities. It is intended for physical education, recreation, fitness, and dance students as well as for other fitness professionals who wish to lead group exercise classes. Even if you are not planning to instruct group exercise, you may become a program director responsible for hiring, training, and evaluating group instructors. Knowledge of class format, teaching progressions, and safety considerations will enhance your skills as a group exercise leader or a program director.

We believe that this book fills an important gap in the exercise textbook repertory by providing a research-based text on group exercise that covers a variety of modalities with a strong, how-to, applied focus. We are extremely pleased that Human Kinetics developed the accompanying DVD, thus making it even easier for you to learn the practical skills necessary for effective group instruction. It is nearly impossible to become a competent instructor simply by reading a book; you must practice and experience the leadership skills with your body as well. To that end, we have incorporated numerous practical devices in our book, including several practice drills, given in a logical sequence for optimal learning. In many cases, these drills are shown on the DVD as well, so you can practice right along with the DVD instructor.

A major distinguishing feature of our book is that the information is based on research. Since approximately 1986, a plethora of research has been conducted on group exercise, primarily regarding energy expenditure but also in areas of biomechanics, injury incidence, exercise adherence, and effectiveness of specific exercise programs. Our goal is to present scientific principles and relevant research whenever they are available.

The purpose of this book is to provide you with the practical skills necessary to teach group exercise classes. Numerous other texts address important issues for instructors in the areas of exercise physiology, kinesiology, nutrition, special populations, injury prevention, business matters, behavior modification, and more. Our book focuses on the nuts and bolts: the specific exercises you'll use and the techniques needed for moving to music, designing choreography, and cueing your students. We'll introduce you to the most popular types of fitness classes and provide you with the basic skills required to lead them.

The book has three parts. Part I provides a general overview of the concept of group exercise: its evolution, its advantages, strategies for group cohesion, and the basic components of fitness. We introduce a general group exercise class evaluation form that will be used throughout the book, providing a template for the various modalities covered. Additionally, we introduce basic music structure, communication skills, and programming concepts such as exercise progression.

In part II we offer guidelines for the four major segments of group exercise class: warm-up, cardiorespiratory training, muscular conditioning, and flexibility training. The basic concepts covered here pertain to all class modalities. These concepts include intensity issues, safety concerns, posture and alignment, anatomy, and joint actions. In the muscle conditioning and flexibility chapters, we provide many specific exercises appropriate for group classes, along with important cues and modifications for all major muscle groups.

Part III focuses on the practical teaching skills required for the most common modalities: high/low impact, step exercise, kickboxing, stationary cycling, and water exercise. Basic moves, choreography, and training systems or formats are specifically covered for each type of class. Here's where we really get specific, with drills, routines, and many teaching skills addressed on the accompanying DVD as well as in the text. In many cases, the drills provided in the text are demonstrated by an experienced instructor on the DVD, so you can practice skills such as anticipatory cueing and teaching to a 32-count phrase. Also in part III you'll find a chapter on other group modalities found in some fitness settings, including slide, Latin, hip-hop, yoga, Pilates, t'ai chi, and sport conditioning. We chose to cover these types of group exercise all in one chapter either because they aren't as popular as step or high/low impact, or because an in-depth introduction is simply out of the scope of this text (as in the case of yoga or Pilates).

We have each taught group exercise for approximately 25 years, and in that time we have seen group exercise classes evolve from traditional high-impact aerobics to the broad spectrum of classes available today. We both hold several certifications in group exercise in addition to our graduate degrees in exercise science. We have accumulated certifications and attended countless continuing education workshops for high/low impact programs, step classes, kickboxing, stationary indoor cycling, water exercise, Pilates, yoga, slide, dance, sports conditioning, and cardio, muscular, and flexibility programming. We have presented at numerous fitness conferences around the world to both group exercise leaders and personal trainers, and we continue to teach group exercise classes to the general public, constantly improving our own practical teaching skills. We have each been involved in several research studies, Carol primarily in the area of water exercise and Mary in the area of high/low impact, step exercise, and slide energy expenditures. In fact, we met at an IDEA research symposium many years ago where we had each been asked to speak about our research! We served together for 6 years on the American College of Sports Medicine's Credentialing Committee, working primarily in the area of group exercise. Additionally, we have each authored one other book individually, and we have coauthored another book together. We believe that we bring a unique perspective to this text, because we are both committed to a hands-on, practical approach yet are thoroughly familiar with the demands of academia and the requirements of science.

As with all formal teaching, you become more skilled with practice. Teaching group exercise takes courage, perseverance, and energy. It is a skill that requires continual learning, rehearsal, and discipline. However, the rewards are great because helping others to live more healthful lives by having fun while exercising feels great! There's no better gift to give a person than an improvement in his or her quality of life. Making a difference by educating, caring for, and motivating your students is a gift both to the participant and to yourself. We hope this book helps you to become an agent of change for enhancing healthy lifestyles. We can't think of a better gift to give to yourself and others.

ACKNOWLEDGMENTS

We are very grateful to the many people who have influenced the writing of this book. This book is a tribute to those who have made a difference in our lives. Our parents have inspired us to follow our passion and to work hard to make our passion a reality. Thanks to Joan and Bob Caster (Carol's parents) and James and Margaret Yoke (Mary's parents) for their belief in us and continuous support over the years. To our children, Tony and Jessica Kennedy, Nathaniel Yoke, and Zachary Ripka, thank you for keeping us grounded in the fun of day-to-day living. We love the fact that you kept pulling us away from writing to attend your activities. It helped make this book even better. To Marty Armbruster, thanks for your support and for also providing Carol a quiet place to write. We also acknowledge all the people we have encountered through the years who have influenced our perception of group exercise. Because the accumulation of knowledge makes for a good book, you all have helped to make it happen. Thanks to the following people and organizations for their inspiration and input:

ACSM, ACE, AFAA, AEA, Chris Arterberry, Ken Baldwin, Susan Bane, Jay Blahnik, Penny Black-Steen, Andy Blome, Sharon Bogen, Jane Bradley, Peggy Buchanan, Donna Burch, Can Fit Pro, Sharon Chang, Robyn Deterding, Julie Downing, April Durrett, Ellen Evans, Melinda Flegel, Tere Filer, Bud Getchell, Nancy Gillette, Laura Gladwin, Maureen Hagan, Lisa Hamlin, Cher Harris, Sara Hillard, Shayla Holtkamp, IDEA, Janet Johnson, Gail Johnston, Mindy King, Len Kravitz, Susan Kundrat, Alison Kyle, Abby Landsman, Karen Leatherman, Deb Legel, Deena Luft, Pat Maloney, Patti Mantia, Patti McCord, Colleen McMahon, Michelle Miller, Ghada Muasher, Maria Nardini, Kris Neely, Greg Niederlander, Charlotte Norton, Tony Ordas, Bob Otto, Jacque Pedgrift, Bob Perez, Jim Peterson, Jenny Peterson, Linda Pfeffer, Debi Ban-Pillarella, Janet Reis, Lauri Reimer, Pat Ryan, Mary Sanders, Pearlas Sanborn, Holly Schell, Robert Sherman, Linda Shelton, Siri Sitton, Donna Spears, Dixie Stanforth, Kathy Stevens, Walt Thompson, Kelly Walker-Haley, John Wygand, and Mandy Zulkoski.

Special thanks to the Indiana University Recreational Sports staff for their assistance with the DVD. Utilizing their teaching expertise and the Student Recreational Sports Center equipment made the DVD and still photos possible. The DVD and still photo instructors include: David Auman, Teri Bladen, Erin Brace, Chad Coplen, Lisandra Cuadrado, Ceceila Fortune, Malvika Gulati, Margie Kobow, Tatiana Kolovou, Guo Lei, Evan McDowell, Devin Mcguire, Cherry Merritt-Darriau, Camilla Saulsbury, Misty Schneider, Naima Solomon, Will Thornton, and Mai Tran.

Finally, a great big thanks to the staff at Human Kinetics, especially Judy Patterson Wright, who convinced us to write this book. Special thanks to Doug Fink, Roger Francisco, Mark Herman, and Terry Henricks for their wonderful DVD production. We had a blast taping with you guys! Thanks also to Tom Roberts for his professionalism and high-quality photos. Big thanks to Judy Park, our developmental editor, who was so pleasant to work with.

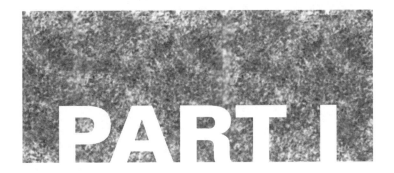

Principles
of Group
Exercise
Instruction

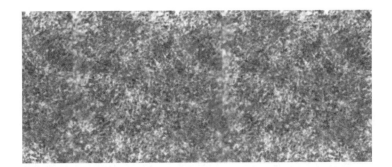

Introduction to Group Exercise

Chapter Objectives

By the end of this chapter, you will

- understand the evolution of group exercise from aerobic dance,

- know the health-related components of fitness and how group exercise relates to them,

- understand the difference between a student-centered versus teacher-centered instructor,

- be able to list the major professional certifications in group fitness instruction, and

- understand group cohesion research in reference to group exercise.

What is the origin of group exercise? A great deal of credit belongs to Jackie Sorensen, who was directly involved with Kenneth Cooper's early work on aerobic capacity (Schuster 1979). Sorenson, a former dancer and cheerleader, was a participant in one of Cooper's experiments, and they discovered that her own aerobic capacity was excellent. With this insight and inspiration, she devised a method of aerobic exercise based on dance. She produced specific dance movements to music that others could copy and teach. The intent of the routines was to elevate the heart rate and keep people moving to music to enhance their fitness.

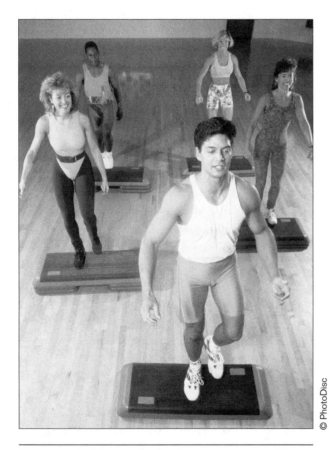

© PhotoDisc

Compared with group exercise instructors today, who focus on health and well-being, aerobic dance instructors in the 1980s typically focused on the quest for the perfect figure.

In the 1980s, aerobic dance provided an outlet for many people, especially women, to exercise in a group. Before this time, "intentional exercise" had not been accepted into the mainstream. The aerobic dance movement brought intentional exercise to the forefront. Aerobic dance became a pop culture phenomenon—in 1982, *Jane Fonda's Workout Book* (Fonda 1981) topped the best-seller lists, followed by her successful high-impact workout video. However, many people's enthusiasm for this new exercise diminished with its increasing injury rates. Injuries to the shins, feet, and knees were particularly common in high-impact aerobics (Mutoh et al. 1988, Richie et al. 1985). Many variations of aerobic dance, such as low-impact aerobics, were then developed to provide more variety and promote a safer way of enjoying exercising to music. One study (Brown and O'Neill 1990) found that 66% of participants in high-impact aerobics had injuries compared with only 9% in low-impact aerobics. Low-impact aerobics was the craze in the late 1980s, and some experts believed it might be a better option than traditional aerobic dance (Koszuta 1986). Less impact produced less jarring on the joints, thus still providing fitness benefits but reducing the risk of injury to the musculoskeletal system. In the late 1980s we started to overcome the "no pain, no gain" experiences that were so prevalent (Francis and Francis 1988).

Kernodle (1992) believed that step aerobics was invented because we don't have the space to engage in large–muscle group activity. He wrote that we have become "pioneers in moving in small spaces." In an aerobic dance class, 20 to 30 people can move effectively in a gym. With steps to go up and down, almost twice as many people can participate.

Bench stepping is another way to maximize space and prevent injury (Francis 1990). In this activity, gravity overloads the body when one steps up on a bench. The injury risk is reduced because the whole body is working against gravity without the impact forces on the lower body of high or low impact aerobics. The step movement in the 1990s led to the development of many different forms of group exercise. Water exercise, indoor cycling, trekking, and many other group exercise activities surfaced. Many classes developed in the 1990s did not require dance skills or even rhythm. Therefore, the term *aerobic dance* was replaced with *group exercise* to better describe the broad scope of activities that had emerged. Eller (1996) noticed that many clubs had dropped the word *dance* entirely from their schedules. He believed that the choreography was becoming too difficult and thus was not helping people get results, so they were looking for other options.

Group exercise has since grown to a diverse offering of exercises, with something for almost every ability and preference (see table 1.1). Many classes include all of the components of fitness in one class. Group exercise classes are the lifelines for many health clubs and fitness centers. These classes generate enthusiasm and fun, and they create the connectedness needed to keep people coming back. Many people first considered group exercise a fad, but it has become clear that group exercise is here to stay. Ryan's (2003) IDEA trend report states that kickboxing, indoor cycling, Pilates, stability ball classes, and yoga all showed growth since IDEA's 1998 survey. In fact, in many clubs, group exercise sessions can actually generate a profit (Nogawa-Wasman 2002) on top of providing health benefits for participants.

Group exercise is an exciting field; although it originated in aerobic dance, current devotees participate in a wide range of activities such as indoor cycling and kickboxing classes. At this point we can ask ourselves, how does group exercise work? Are there common features that we can apply to most sessions? This chapter covers general concepts that guide all group exercise sessions. First, we examine the health benefits of fitness as related to group exercise. Second, we discuss the key teaching skills related to instructing group exercise. Third, we discuss the major certifications available for instructors of group exercise classes, providing a formal educational framework on which all group exercise classes can be evaluated and taught. Fourth, we cover the advantages of group cohesion.

HEALTH-RELATED COMPONENTS OF FITNESS

The purpose of a group exercise class is to enhance health-related components of fitness. These include a participant's cardiorespiratory endurance, muscular strength and endurance, flexibility, and body composition. Our big picture goal is to help people to live happier and healthier lives through exercise. According to Bortz (2003) our nation ultimately will also save money if we are healthy. To help with this cause, we need to understand the guidelines for exercise and healthy living.

The Healthy People initiative is a government-sponsored report that provides a prevention agenda for the United States. In simpler terms, it is a road map to better health for all (Neiman 2003). The *Healthy People 2010* report (U.S. Department of Health and Human Resources 2000) has a major goal of increasing the years of healthy life. Currently, the average baby born can expect to live 77 years, but only 64 of those years will be healthy. Government officials hope that by the year 2010, this number will be raised to 66 years. On another note, obesity continues to increase among U.S. adults and children. The prevalence of overweight is currently 15.5% among 12- to 19-year-olds compared with 10.5% in 1999 (Ogden et al. 2002). The age-adjusted prevalence of obesity was 30.5% in 1999 to 2000 compared with 22.9% in 1988 to 1994 (Flegal et al. 2002). Jakicic and colleagues (2003) found that a 12-month program combining exercise and diet resulted in significant weight loss and improved cardiorespiratory fitness for various durations and intensities of exercise. The study showed a direct relationship between total weekly energy expenditure and

Table 1.1 Possible Group Exercise Class Choices

Choreograph to music	Stretch and strengthen	Mind and body	Coaching and non–beat driven	Combination
High/low impact	Stretching	Yoga	Water exercise	Step crunch
Kickboxing	Abdominal crunch	Pilates	Stationary cycling	Aerostep
Hip-hop	Total muscle conditioning	T'ai chi	Rowing	Step slide
Latin (dance)		NIA	Trekking or rebounding	

Note. NIA = Neuromuscular Integrative Action.

weight loss. Therefore, exercise is an important part of maintaining a healthy body weight. Also, Liemohn and Pariser (2002) state that it is important to strengthen core muscles on a regular basis in order to reduce low back pain.

How does group exercise fit into the national health objectives? A study by Grant et al. (2004) of 26 women in their sixties following a 12-week exercise program revealed that both functional and psychological improvements occurred as a result of a 40-minute group fitness program twice a week. Beginners are often more comfortable getting information about exercise in the group setting. They also like being instructed because it teaches them correct exercise techniques and provides motivation to continue working out. Also important are the socialization and connectedness of the participants. According to Estabrooks (2000), the presence of a highly task-cohesive group had the greatest influence on exercise adherence. For example, many group exercise classes offered at 9 a.m. attract stay-at-home moms who enjoy exercise and sharing stories about their children. Group cohesion can only be accomplished in a group setting. In strength and conditioning rooms, where all participants are on their own machines and performing their own routines, group cohesion is less likely to be formed. Group exercise encourages participants to interact and can enhance emotional as well as physical wellness—especially if the instructor fosters an interactive environment.

As different types of group exercise continue to be created and studied, the American College of Sports Medicine (ACSM) position stand on fitness for healthy adults continues to be updated (ACSM 1998). See table 1.2 for a summary of the 2006 ACSM Position Stand on Fitness for Healthy Adults. The biggest recent change that may affect group exercise is the change in duration. Whereas ACSM previously recommended a cardiorespiratory segment of 20 to 40 min of continuous exercise, ACSM now recommends 20 to 60 continuous minutes OR discontinuous 10-min bouts that accumulate 20 to 60 min total per day. Some experts (Hooker 2003) believe that public health experts and fitness professionals will be collaborating on expanding movement experiences, especially at the community level. We may be bringing the group exercise experience to our parks in the form of outdoor walking classes.

Offering a variety of class times and activities is important for successful fitness programs. Many facilities offering group exercise are finding success with 30-min or shorter classes to help accommodate participants' busy schedules. IDEA is an organization that educates group exercise instructors all over the world. The acronym IDEA used to stand for International Dance Exercise Association. They are now referred to as IDEA, the Association for Fitness Professionals. An IDEA article (Lofshult 2002) stated that the most popular class length was 30 min because of the busy lives of participants. The 1998 ACSM position stand validates what group exercise has offered all along, which is a balanced workout that contains cardiorespiratory training, muscular strength and endurance training, and flexibility training. Finally, the Surgeon General's Report on Physical Activity and Health (Pate et al. 1995) focuses on the importance of activity within daily living like walking the dog or taking the stairs. It states that every U.S. adult should accumulate 30 minutes or more of moderate intensity

Table 1.2   2006 ACSM Position Stand on Fitness for Healthy Adults

Component	Guideline
Frequency	3-5 days/week
Intensity	55-90% of maximum heart rate and 40-85% of $\dot{V}O_2$max, 12-16 RPE
Duration	20-60 continuous minutes or 10-min bouts accumulated throughout the day to equal 20-60 min
Mode	Walk, run, row, group exercise (i.e. dynamic activity of large muscel groups)
Resistance training	2-3 days/week one set of 3-20 repetitions to volitional fatigue (19-20 RPE) or before (16 RPE) 8-10 major muscle groups worked
Flexibility training	2-3 days/week minimum, 5-7 days/week ideal, holding the stretch 15-30 s, repeating the stretch two to four times stretching to tightness (i.e., no pain or bouncing)

physical activity on most, preferably all, days of the week. We cannot assume that people are generally active. Plus, Clapp and Little (1994) studied the physiological effects of participants and instructors while performing three types of group exercise routines (low impact, high impact, and step). They concluded that participants consistently underestimated their level of performance. Guidelines for exercise as well as activities of daily living need to be stressed. For instance, a hip-hop class may involve only moderate movement and may not contain the other class elements. The Surgeon General's report would support the fact that the participants are just moving and not sitting still. The challenge is to apply current research and information from the ACSM Position Stand (see table 1.2) and the Surgeon General's report to develop safe, effective, and highly motivating workouts that make a difference in participants' health and wellness.

Designing an effective class begins with the attitude and atmosphere established by the instructor. A wide range of factors can influence a class environment. We first focus on the professionalism of the group exercise instructor, who needs to be a motivator and an educator (Kennedy and Legel 1992, Claxton and Lacy 1991, Francis 1991).

STUDENT-CENTERED VERSUS TEACHER-CENTERED INSTRUCTION

The motivational and inspirational aspect of instructing includes having new moves, music, and state-of-the-art equipment as well as learning to communicate effectively. The educational part of instructing includes knowing why certain moves are selected, incorporating current research and knowledge within a group exercise session, and making educated choices and decisions about the information given to participants. Let's compare and contrast a teacher-centered instructor with a student-centered instructor. The teacher-centered instructor can often lead to dependence, intimidation, unattainable goals, and a reliance on quick fixes (see table 1.3). The student-centered instructor, on the other hand, strives to establish an atmosphere of independence, encouragement, attainable goals, and reality (see table 1.4). Learning to take responsibility for the health and well-being of participants starts with establishing a positive and professional attitude and atmosphere.

Table 1.3   Teacher-Centered Instructor

Tactic	Example
Dependence	I know the way—do what I do and you'll look like me!
Intimidation	This is an easy exercise: Come on, do 10 more! No wimps in my class!
Unattainable goals	One more week and you'll start to see some changes.
Quick fixes	20 more crunches will flatten those abdominals!

Table 1.4   Student-Centered Instructor

Tactic	Example
Independence	Remember to work at your own pace. I will be teaching an intermediate class but will show modifications. It will be your responsibility to monitor your intensity level accordingly. Here's how to do that . . .
Encouragement	You're doing great! Keep up the good work. Remember that if there is pain, there will be little gain. Stay with it, and you'll achieve your goals.
Attainable goals	Learning to exercise regularly will take time. Adding extra activity outside of class like taking the stairs or mowing your yard will help you reach your goals faster.
Reality	Abdominal exercises will strengthen your abdominal muscles, but you will not be able to spot reduce.

PROFESSIONAL CERTIFICATIONS FOR GROUP EXERCISE INSTRUCTORS

A group exercise class must be built on the foundation of participant safety. An important aspect of safety is becoming certified by a national organization. You do not necessarily have to be certified to teach group exercise, but certification proves that you have content knowledge and are serious about your role as a professional fitness instructor. Malek and colleagues (2002) confirmed that formal education is important. These authors found that a bachelor's degree in exercise science and possession of ACSM or National Strength and Conditioning Association (NSCA) certifications as opposed to other certifications were strong predictors of a personal trainer's knowledge. We suggest that similar credentials might be strong predictors of a group exercise instructor's knowledge. A recent article on ACSM credentialing (Whaley 2003) discussed the importance of formal academic education in creating fitness professionals. We encourage you to continue your formal education especially if you want to manage a fitness center. Many national certifications involve taking written and practical exams that allow an instructor to demonstrate a basic level of skill in exercise leadership and its related components (e.g., anatomy and physiology, heart rate monitoring). We recommend taking nationally recognized certifications because these tests are written by many professionals who agree on pertinent knowledge in the field of exercise instruction. Local or club certifications or training programs are only locally produced. The four nationally recognized certifications that we recommend all require that you have cardiopulmonary resuscitation (CPR) certification before sitting for the exam (see "Fitness Certification Organizations" for contact information).

Many organizations and universities train group exercise leaders, and it is good to experience different kinds of training; however, when it comes to certification, make sure the organizations are credible and the tests are put together in a professional manner. Many fitness professionals have more than one certification depending on what skills will be used. Usually a group-

FITNESS CERTIFICATION ORGANIZATIONS

Aerobics and Fitness Association of America (AFAA)
15250 Ventura Blvd. Suite 200
Sherman Oaks, CA 91403
877-968-7263
www.afaa.com

American College of Sports Medicine (ACSM)
401 W. Michigan St.
Indianapolis, IN 46202-3233
317-637-9200
www.acsm.org

American Council on Exercise (ACE)
4851 Paramount Drive
San Diego, CA 92123
800-825-3636
www.acefitness.org

National Strength & Conditioning Association
1885 Bob Johnson Drive
Colorado Springs, CO 80906
800-815-6826
www.nsca-lift.org

Can-Fit-Pro
2851 John Street
P.O. Box 42011
Markham, ON
L3R 5R7
800-667-5622
www.canfitpro.com

SCW Fitness Education
1618 Orrington Avenue, Suite 202
Evanston, IL 60201
877-SCW-FITT
www.scwfitness.com

World Instructor Training Schools (W.I.T.S.)
206 76th Street
Virginia Beach, VA 23451-1915
888-330-9487
www.witseducation.com

focused certification and a one-on-one certification are good to have. We recommend taking more than one certification exam, because each is a learning experience in itself. We hope that more universities will offer exercise leadership classes so that the certification will simply be a verification of knowledge. We also hope that this book will prompt faculty within universities to provide academic training for group leadership. Currently many academic institutions provide degrees in kinesiology (the study of movement), but often such training does not include a group exercise leadership component. Note that the qualified fitness professional usually has at least one certification through ACSM, which is seen as the gold standard in sports medicine and fitness. ACSM does not have a group certification but does require experience in group leadership in its credentialing of universities. There is a difference between a fitness professional and an instructor who works part time leading fitness classes. The exercise professional often has had formal training and education in exercise prescription and fitness assessments.

Some companies, recreation departments, and health clubs insist that their instructors be nationally certified. Others set up their own training or course work to be completed. Either method is a step toward elevating exercise instruction and also ensures a certain level of knowledge and expertise. But having a certification does not automatically mean that you will be a wonderful instructor. It just means that you are serious and willing to increase your knowledge and experience.

American College of Sports Medicine

ACSM certification is recommended for the professional with a degree in a health-related field who supervises a program in a facility. You need a bachelor's degree to take an ACSM exam. The written exam requires knowledge of exercise science and the practical segment of the exam requires fitness assessment skills and leadership demonstrations.

American Council on Exercise

The American Council on Exercise (ACE) offers a written-only exam for group exercise leaders. You do not need a degree to take this exam. Both ACE and ACSM participate in statistical analysis of their written exams by testing them for reliability and validity. These organizations, along with AFAA, form committees of professionals from all over the country who write test questions, which makes a na-tional exam different than a local training program.

Aerobics and Fitness Association of America

The Aerobics and Fitness Association of America (AFAA), like ACE, does not require a degree to take its exam. This exam includes both a written and a practical component. AFAA offers some of the most specific certifications in the group exercise industry, such as primary group exercise, step, kickboxing, and emergency response. AFAA also offers many continuing education workshops on topics such as Practical Teaching Skills, Prenatal Exercise, Seniors, and Mat Science (yoga and Pilates).

Can-Fit-Pro

Can-Fit-Pro (Canadian Fitness Professionals Inc.) offers a variety of certifications in group exercise, personal training, nutrition, pre- and postnatal, older adult, mind/body, and sport conditioning. Program courses are delivered in person and range from 16 to 25 hours in length. Most certification exams consist of a written theory exam and assessment of practical skills. Can-Fit-Pro courses and exams are delivered by a team of PRO trainers and master trainers nationally.

SCW Fitness Education

SCW certification is a perfect blend of practical, theoretical, and physiological knowledge of successful teaching techniques for group exercise. Emphasis is on class sequencing, warm-up progressions, musical phrasing, proper cueing techniques, choreography development, and all the practical skills required to teach your best class every class. Leave confident in your ability to lead and demonstrate proper teaching skills. Understand cardiovascular training, muscular endurance, and flexibility training techniques. Train with one of the finest leaders in our industry today.

World Instructor Training Schools

W.I.T.S. has neighborhood schools nationwide in colleges and universities to meet the needs of serious students entering the fitness field. Our

6-week courses are 36 hours long and include a final written and practical skills exam. Half of the course is theoretical and the other half is hands-on, practical lab where we "show, tell, and do" everything. Actual group exercise routines will be developed by the students themselves to lead in the final exam. WITS offers a comprehensive course to prepare you for employment.

GROUP COHESION RESEARCH

The major emphasis within group exercise instructor training programs has been on class content. What is lacking is "connecting" the participants so a sense of community is developed. Alan (2003) believes that this connection is often what brings older adults to a group exercise experience. If group classes are taught from a student-centered perspective with an emphasis on developing group cohesion, this can enhance adherence. According to Carron and colleagues (1988), there is a belief that group cohesiveness is related to individual adherence behavior. For example, when participants meet people in class and socialize with them, they are more likely to keep exercising. Carron and colleagues suggest that we examine how to keep groups of participants coming back to enhance the health and wellness of the overall population. Therefore, investing our resources in improving group exercise classes and creating a sense of community within a fitness facility would be a logical step in improving our national health.

Heinzelmann and Bagley (1970) reported that 90% of adult participants in an exercise program preferred to exercise in group settings. Similarly, Stephens and Craig (1990) reported that 65% of participants preferred to exercise in groups rather than alone. Group exercise programs also appear to produce higher rates of exercise maintenance than individual-based programs (Massie and Sheperd 1971). Spink and Carron (1992) found that group cohesion in female exercise participants played a role in adherence behaviors. Finally, Carron and colleagues (1988) had exercise class participants, both dropouts and those who stayed with the program, assess the cohesiveness of their classes. Participants who stayed with the program held higher perceptions of cohesiveness.

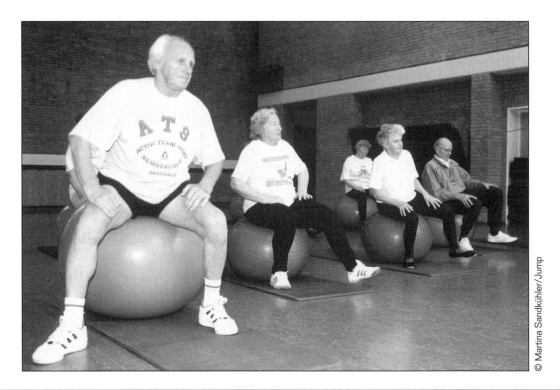

© Martina Sandkühler/Jump

A focus on healthy lifestyles brings many seniors to group exercise classes, where they enjoy the socialization benefits as well.

Spink and Carron (1994) stated that the university setting provides regular exercisers with greater perceptions of task cohesion, whereas in the health club setting, social factors are more related to adherence. For example, when students are graded on attendance, their attendance improves. In clubs, creating social opportunities allows fitness classes to build cohesion.

Seniors also tend to have a better exercise experience when there are social activities outside of the exercise class. Estabrooks and Carron (1999) found that elderly exercisers who have stronger beliefs in the social cohesiveness of their exercise class had more positive attitudes about exercise. In a study by Spink and Carron (1993), one exercise class participated in a team-building intervention program and had significantly fewer dropouts than a similar class where these activities were not performed. Finally, Carron and colleagues (1996) learned that developing a highly cohesive group that is focused on the exercise task and the outcomes it can produce is likely to have a strong effect on compliance.

This research tells us that we need to do more than stand in front of a class and lead exercises. We need to engage in exercise together. We can do this by learning participants' names and having them learn each other's names. Schedule social outings or share personal stories. Interact with class participants and have them introduce themselves to others. If we focus on being student-centered teachers, it can make a difference in the cohesiveness of our classes.

Chapter Wrap-Up

Group exercise can be very powerful if participants feel welcome, learn new things, get to know others, are taught safely, and believe that their time spent is worthwhile. One of the biggest challenges for the group exercise instructor is balancing all of these elements. It is, perhaps, the most difficult skill a fitness professional can master. Once we move beyond emphasizing quantity fitness gains and aesthetics, we will understand that the real power of exercise lies in the experience itself. Group exercise is definitely an experience, and the instructor makes or breaks that experience.

Written Assignment

Observe one group exercise class and evaluate whether the instructor has a student-centered or teacher-centered style of instructing. Give a minimum of three specific examples to support your analysis.

Practical Assignment

Attend a group exercise class and interview the participants about the level of group cohesiveness. Ask whether they have met people through the experience and if that has helped their adherence. Write a one-page paper on your findings.

Evolution of Fitness

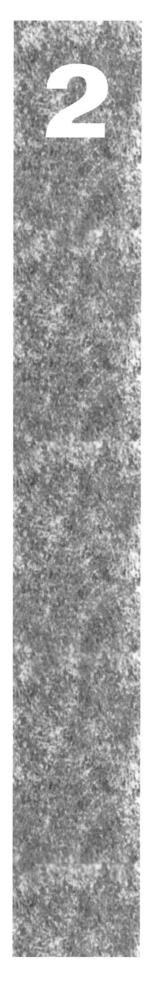

Chapter Objectives

By the end of this chapter, you will

- understand the evolution of fitness from body image to health,

- be able to give some examples of marketing tactics for group exercise,

- understand why group exercise instructors are role models, and

- understand how to create a healthy emotional environment.

The gluteus medius muscle abducts the hip, but why does a participant need to strengthen this muscle, and what exercises work the muscle effectively? During the "aesthetic" movement of the 1970s through 1990s, the main purpose for exercising was to lose weight and look better, and many of us still select exercises based on the cultural influences that dictate what our bodies should look like. You can't turn on a television set without seeing an advertisement about how some group exercise video helped Susie look "like this." Our looks are important, but today we want more out of exercise: We want to feel better. We want to have more energy to enjoy life regardless of our age, and we want to maintain our independence as long as possible by performing daily tasks. As baby boomers age, remaining independent is a life goal, and each of us will fight for our independence in our later years. The baby boomers started the fitness movement, and they continue to dictate its direction. Table 2.1 outlines the effect of the baby boomers on group exercise instruction and how the new functional fitness movement has developed.

Åstrand's (1992) research article titled "Why Exercise?" contained the first hints of the functional training movement. In this article he stated, "If animals are built reasonably, they should build and maintain just enough, but not more, structure than they need to meet functional requirements" (p. 154). In a more recent article, Wolf (2001) stated that "training movements and not muscles may be the paradigm shift needed for today's functional conditioning" (p. 23). Santana (2002) defined functional training as "a specific duty or purpose of a person or thing" (p. 22). In functional training, the muscles are trained and developed to make performance of everyday activities easier, smoother, safer, and more efficient. Functional exercises improve your ability to function independently and perform a

sport more effectively. This fact underlies what is perhaps the most important fitness benefit: Everyday activities become easier, and quality of life improves. Another recent development is that we are studying the impact of body image on women who strength train and we're learning that not only does strength improve with training, but so does body image (Ahmed et al. 2002). Finally, Ginis and colleagues (2003) found that regardless of body image concern, women in mirrored conditions felt worse after exercising than women in the non-mirrored condition. We believe that fitness is moving into a prominent part of people's lives as we find a sense of purpose in our workouts that goes deeper than how we look. We may have started the fitness movement based on appearance, but this is certainly changing.

Also of interest is that the quantum theory of physics is gaining acceptance (Capra 1982). One aspect of this theory is the idea that the world should not be analyzed into independent, isolated elements without considering the whole. For example, somebody may develop arteriosclerosis, a narrowing and hardening of the arteries, as the result of an unhealthy life—improper diet, lack of exercise, excessive smoking. Surgical treatment of a blocked artery may temporarily alleviate pain but will not make the person well. The surgical intervention merely treats a local effect of a systemic disorder that will continue until the underlying problems are identified and resolved. This concept, put into a fitness setting, would be like training individual muscle groups and not training the core that houses those individual muscle groups. We cannot use the strength we gain in individual muscle group training unless we also do some total body strengthening. This is the essence of the new fitness movement. Pilates, yoga, and t'ai chi are some types of group exercise classes that have gained popularity because of this trend.

Table 2.1 Trends in Fitness Have Mirrored the Baby Boomer Generation

Decade	Baby boomers' age	Trend
1970s	20s	High-impact aerobics, running, 10K races
1980s	30s	Low-impact aerobics, walking, 5K races
1990s	40s	Step, slide, water exercise, indoor cycling, yoga
2000s	50s	Functional fitness, merging of medicine and fitness

CULTURAL INFLUENCES ON BODY IMAGE AND EXERCISE

Looking back at the group exercise advertisements for shoes, we can witness this aesthetic movement in action. Many of the ads from athletic shoe companies in the 1970s, 1980s, and 1990s showed a small picture of the shoe and a very large picture of a very fit body (usually a female body). There were two indirect messages. The first message was that if you bought the shoes, you would get "that body." The second message was that participating in group exercise would help you get that body. Several studies (Gaesser 1999, Miller 1999) on exercise and weight loss encouraged a greater emphasis on lifestyle change and less attention to weight loss. Nike was one of the first companies to change its focus. According to Bednarski (1993), who was a marketing executive for Nike at the time, she had a difficult time convincing male managers that women needed a different marketing strategy. Nike finally created an empowering campaign for women that featured ads about how it felt to be fit through sports and exercise. There was more focus on all the things people could do with this newfound energy rather than what they looked like. Many of the ads did not feature any people, and instead the health benefits of exercise were touted. Enhancing self-esteem was seen as more important than changing one's body.

Health clubs and videos also used body image to market programs and products. The "Buns of Steel" video campaign is one example. Naming group exercise sessions by body parts is another example. Classes like Ultimate Abs, Butts and Guts, and Absolute Arms all played on this message. We suggest moving your program into the new functional fitness era by naming your classes in a positive, more educational way. One center uses time to describe classes. An example is calling a class Step 45 instead of Ultimate Step so that participants will know the class lasts 45 min. The more "hard core" the name, the fewer beginners will attend. Although we have come a long way in changing this message, we have a long way to go. A recent article (Kahlkoetter 2002) stated, "women often begin triathlon training for the purpose of losing weight and looking better, rather than for inner satisfactions and health" (p. 48). Hollywood, television, magazines, and movies are often to blame for the unrealistic images put before us. However, in a recent attempt to set things straight, Jamie Lee Curtis exposed her "true self" (Wallace 2002). After being featured in the fitness movie *Perfect,* she admitted to many unhealthy practices in an effort to keep her perfect body. In a *More* magazine article, she posed for a picture with no makeup or body touch-ups so that people could see her true self. This is only one instance, but we hope that the Hollywood myth will continue to be unveiled. Men are not immune to this issue. According to Beals (2003) muscle dysmorphia (a form of body image disturbance in male weightlifters) is on the rise with half of those with this disorder having tried anabolic steroids.

GROUP EXERCISE INSTRUCTORS AS ROLE MODELS

According to Westcott (1991), participants rated knowledge as the most important characteristic of their fitness instructor. He also said that most participants look up to their fitness instructor as a role model. This puts a lot of pressure on instructors: What kind of role models are we? In an article by Evans and Kennedy (1993), results of an informal research study of female fitness instructors showed that their average body fat was 20% (which is quite low, because the average in the United States is 32%), but 46% of the fitness instructors believed they were very or somewhat overweight. A study (Nardini et al. 1999) of 148 female fitness instructors found that 64% of instructors perceived an ideal body as one that was thinner than their current body. Olson and colleagues (1996) also studied female aerobic instructors and found that 40% of the instructors indicated a previous experience with eating disorders. This study found that aerobic dance instructors had Eating Disorder Inventory scores that suggested behavior and attitudes consistent with female athletes whose sports emphasize leanness and comparable to those who have eating disorders such as anorexia and bulimia. A survey at a large water fitness national conference (Evans and Connor 1995) on the body image perceptions of water fitness instructors revealed that 48% of instructors agreed that they constantly worry about being or becoming fat. In another study (Krane et al. 2001) looking at female athletes and regular exercisers, the findings suggested that concern about potential excessive exercise in these women was warranted.

Davis (1994) studied physical activity in the development and maintenance of eating disorders and found that, for a number of anorexic women, sport or exercise is an integral part of the progression toward self-starvation. She suggests that overactivity be viewed as a primary and not secondary symptom of eating disorders. It is important as instructors that we not teach several classes in one day. We will be indirectly telling our participants that over exercising is healthy. We also ought to role model healthy behaviors like taking the stairs to class instead of the elevator, or parking our car farther away from the building and walking in. Modeling daily activities to our participants is as important as modeling healthy intentional exercise patterns.

Freeman (1988) reminded us that body image is independent of physical characteristics. One can feel plain or unattractive when he or she is really attractive. Because body image and self-esteem are perceptions, changing our bodies will not improve our body image or self-esteem unless the physical changes are accompanied by changes in perceptions. Improving body image involves changing how we think about our bodies. Taking charge of our own body image perceptions and educating our participants about body image are important if we are to be positive role models. See "Disordered Eating and Body Image Resources".

DISORDERED EATING AND BODY IMAGE RESOURCES

www.nationaleatingdisorder.org—National Eating Disorder Organization

www.eatright.org—American Dietetics Association

www.4woman.gov—National Women's Health Information Center

CREATING A HEALTHY EXERCISE ENVIRONMENT

Besides being positive role models, we also need to establish a comfortable environment for participants. Education, motivation, and creative class content are not the only factors that keep participants coming back to group exercise. It is necessary to tap into participants' feelings and emotions to affect adherence. Bain and colleagues (1989) performed a research study on overweight women in an organized exercise program. The authors found that 35% of the overweight and only 7% of the normal weight participants dropped out. Although factors such as safety, comfort, and quality of instruction affected the women's exercise behaviors, the most powerful influences seemed to be the social circumstances of the exercise setting, especially concerns about visibility, embarrassment, and judgment by others. It is important to acknowledge all the participants—from the ones you know to the ones who always hide at the back of the room. What we do and say can affect class atmosphere, and a simple hello can make all the difference to a newcomer in group exercise. According to Goleman (1998), having "emotional intelligence" in any group setting dictates the success of the group experience. Goleman believes that "the emotional economy is the sum total of the exchanges of feeling among us. In subtle (or not so subtle) ways, we all make each other feel a bit better (or a lot worse) as part of any contact we have; every encounter can be weighted along a scale from emotionally toxic to nourishing" (p. 165). A specific example of this within a group exercise setting is announcing before class how great it feels to be in a group exercise class to improve overall health and well-being. Contrast this with telling an overeating indulgence story and stating specific intentions to "work it off" during the class. The first statement leaves participants with a health-related sense of purpose for the workout. The second statement can send a message that punishment through exercise is recommended after overindulging. In another study on group dynamics in physical activity, Fox and colleagues (2000) found that enjoyment during physical activity is optimized when a positive and supportive leadership style is coupled with

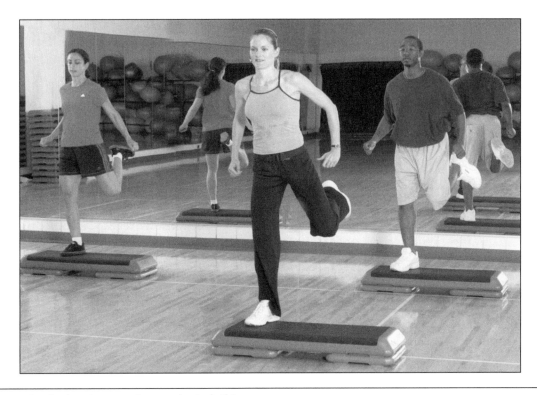

Group exercise instructor wearing modest clothing.

an enriched and supportive group environment. Sending positive health messages throughout the group exercise experience is important for establishing the emotional atmosphere of the workout and serving as a positive role model.

An environment where instructors present a "body beautiful" can also be rather intimidating. Eklund and Crawford (1994) compared like video exercise routines with the instructor wearing a thong-style exercise leotard in one video and the same instructor wearing shorts and a T-shirt in another video. "High physique anxious" participants rated the thong video more unfavorably than the shorts and T-shirt video. Instructors can help participants become more comfortable with their own bodies and keep them exercising by wearing modest exercise clothing. We live in a culture in which a thin and toned body is seen as the ideal. According to Ibbetson (1996), we all accept that thinness is beauty to the point that body image dissatisfaction is remarkably high. Some researchers indicate that body image disturbance is so prevalent that it can be considered a normal part of the female experience (Silberstein et al. 1987). Evans (1993) recommended the following methods for enhancing participant and instructor body image perceptions:

- Wear professional attire that is not too revealing and will make all participants comfortable.

- Display body-image educational materials at strategic locations.

- Use positive motivational strategies. For example, encourage activity outside of class.

- Choose music that sends a positive message.

Chapter Wrap-Up

We can choose either to buy into the media and societal pressures or portray a normal, healthy example to our participants. It is our choice, and it is not something that we can take for granted, knowing that many instructors are affected by their own body image perceptions. Feeling good about oneself and projecting this to participants could be the most important health message that group exercise instructors offer.

Written Assignment

Write your personal exercise and activity story from when you first started exercising and being active until now. Compare and contrast how this has changed for you over the years.

Practical Assignment

Attend a group exercise session and notice the instructor's and participants' attire. Interview three participants about what they believe is appropriate attire. Ask the instructor about his or her attire. Write a one-page paper on your reflections.

Instructing a Group Exercise Class

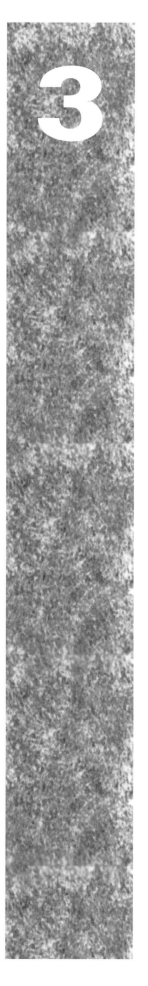

Chapter Objectives

By the end of this chapter, you will

- be able to integrate the components of health into group exercise class design,

- know the principles of preclass organization,

- understand basic health screening for group exercise leaders,

- understand important muscle balance principles,

- comprehend a six-step exercise progression model, and

- understand how music and sound fit into a group exercise class.

Taking the concept of positive attitude and atmosphere into the development of the overall class format is the next challenge. There is no single class format that is appropriate for every type of group exercise class. In a step class, it is very appropriate to warm up using a step; however, in a kickboxing class, it may not be appropriate to use a bench but rather might be acceptable to practice boxing moves during the warm-up segment. In a water exercise class thermoregulation is important, so performing static stretches to enhance flexibility at the end of the workout may not be recommended. It may be appropriate to perform some static stretching in the warm-up and stretching segment of a low-impact class for seniors, but a 15-min abdominal class may not even contain any stretching because the purpose of the class is abdominal strengthening. All are examples of why the same class format may not be suitable for all group exercise classes.

Let's take a closer look at the basic class segments of group exercise:

1. Warm-up
2. Cardiorespiratory activity
3. Muscular conditioning
4. Flexibility and cool-down

These segments apply to all types of group exercise, including high/low impact programs, step classes, water exercise, indoor cycling, and sport conditioning. Typically, most group exercise classes begin with preclass preparation followed by a warm-up, which includes using specific rehearsal moves to prepare for the cardiorespiratory activity. These moves are performed at a low to moderate speed and range of motion; they are designed to specifically warm up the body for activity and increase blood flow to the muscles. A cardiorespiratory segment follows the warm-up and is aimed at improving cardiorespiratory endurance and body composition and keeping the heart rate elevated for 10 to 45 min. After the cardiorespiratory workout, a gradual cool-down returns the heart rate to resting levels and prevents excessive pooling of blood in the lower extremities. A muscular conditioning segment also can be included either before or after the cardiorespiratory segment, depending on the activity. The class then ends with a flexibility and cool-down component that includes stretching and relaxation exercises designed to further

lower heart rate, help prevent muscle soreness, and enhance overall flexibility.

HEALTH-RELATED COMPONENTS OF FITNESS

Notice how the four main components of a group exercise class are aligned with the health-related components of fitness listed in the 2006 ACSM position stand on exercise. When the first ACSM position statement was published in 1978 (ACSM 1978), the statement contained only cardiorespiratory guidelines. At that time there was very little research on strengthening the musculoskeletal system. As clinicians and researchers began to realize that many people suffered from back pain, the research focus turned to the musculoskeletal system. In 1990, when ACSM published its first position stand, muscular strength and endurance were included along with cardiorespiratory fitness but there was no mention of flexibility. As noted in chapter 1, the 2006 ACSM position stand included flexibility as clinicians and researchers learned of the importance of flexible as well as strong muscles. Group exercise classes have long included all components of fitness even though the guidelines for exercise were limited in the past. The current ACSM position stand (ACSM 2006) focuses on all components, which are usually included in a general group exercise class format. With movement in the direction of functional fitness, it is speculated that balance and proprioception soon will be included in the components of fitness, because good balance and proprioception enable us to move efficiently.

The degree to which each of the health-related components of fitness is developed in any particular individual can vary widely. For example, a person may be strong but lack flexibility or may have a good cardiorespiratory endurance but lack muscular strength. It is important that each component of fitness be included in a program.

The ACSM guidelines were briefly reviewed in chapter 1. The emphasis given to each component of fitness will vary depending on the objective of the class as well as the fitness level, age, health, and physical skill of participants. Our overall goal as fitness professionals is to include all components of fitness in our program, although they do not necessarily have to be all in one class. For example, a stretching class will enhance flexibility, and a hip-hop class will provide some cardiorespiratory conditioning. Because our participants have busy schedules, we need to make the most of exercise time by emphasizing the health-related components of fitness in our programming.

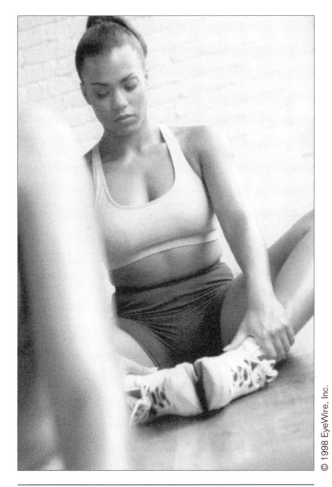

A yoga class may emphasize the flexibility component of fitness.

The points on the group exercise class evaluation form are in appendix A. This form contains all the principles that can be used in most group exercise classes. We review these principles in this chapter. The form also can be used as an evaluation tool when you are observing classes. We hope you can use this evaluation form as an outline or checklist to enhance your teaching and evaluating skills.

Safe, effective, and purposeful class design requires a specific knowledge of fitness so that the appropriate overload is provided to help achieve the desired gains. Therefore, one of the purposes of the group exercise class evaluation form is to help get us all "on the same page" and have a common language with which we discuss class format. We recommend that you use this form to evaluate a class completely and look for the different components of a group exercise class before you attempt to teach. When you complete chapters 4, 5, 6, and 7, you will have a general understanding of the basic concepts. The points on the group exercise class evaluation form are reviewed in later chapters. The preclass organization is outlined in this chapter.

PRECLASS ORGANIZATION

A few common points must be considered in the preclass preparation for any group exercise class. The instructor should know his or her participants and orient new participants, create a positive atmosphere, and begin class on time with equipment ready for use.

Teaching a Mixed-Level Class

Teaching a class with both beginner and advanced participants can be challenging. A mixed class is usually the norm rather than the exception because of time scheduling conflicts. Therefore, describing classes by duration might help a variety of participants find an appropriate level. An example would be having a step class that lasts 30 min, one that lasts 45 min, and another that lasts 1 hr. This gives participants a choice based on their fitness level. The 30-min step classes should contain movements that are less complex to provide beginners with basic cardiorespiratory training and introduce them to basic moves on the step. A recent article (Kennedy 2004) reported that members of a focus group who attended group exercise classes stated that they stayed away from classes that included turbo, ultimate, or extreme in their titles. These names do not always appeal to the beginner. More descriptive names like Step 30, Cycling 45, or Kickboxing 60 may appeal to a broader range of participants and will allow participants to choose their preferred duration. Offering some 20- to 30-min classes of stretching or muscular conditioning only will also help prepare some of the more sedentary participants for the longer classes that contain all the components of fitness. Keep in mind that participants may only need a flexibility or muscular strength and conditioning class, for example, if they walk to work in the morning or engage in other cardio work during the day. Offering different options and not staying with the typical hour-long format that encompasses all components will help meet more people's health goals.

Know Your Participants

How do we individualize programs and protect participants during a group exercise class? By knowing the participants! You must know where they have been and what they want and need in order to lead them successfully. Knowledge of a participant's personal health is an essential part of providing excellent customer service and safety as well as decreasing professional liability.

Although there are many ways of obtaining information, it is ideal for the participant to fill out a written medical history form that you can review before he or she arrives to class. Unfortunately, this situation is often the exception rather than the rule. All of us have been in the situation where our class is just getting underway when a new participant appears. Using a short medical history form can help solve this problem. You can have a new participant fill out the short form upon arrival, after which you quickly review the contents, clarify any vague information, and make a mental note of areas needing emphasis during class.

An example of a completed short history form is included for your reference (see figure 3.1). Short and long health history forms and an informed consent form are located in appendixes B through D. These forms have been adapted

Short Health History and Consent Form

Name: **John Smith**   Date: **8-15-04**

The following information will be kept strictly confidential and will only be utilized to help make the exercise portions of your workout safe. Please check any conditions that may apply to you.

Have you ever been told by a physician that you have or have had:

❏ Heart attack	❏ High cholesterol levels (>200)	❏ Cancer	❏ Arthritis
❏ Seizures	☒ High Blood Pressure	❏ Diabetes	❏ Osteoporosis
❏ Stroke	❏ Abnormal EKG	❏ Lung problems	❏ Gout

If you are currently taking any PRESCRIPTION OR OVER-THE-COUNTER medications, please list:

Beta Blockers

Do you smoke? ❏ Yes ☒ No   Can you swim? ❏ Yes ☒ No (for an aquatics class only)

Do you exercise, aerobically, at least 3–4 times/week? ❏ Yes ☒ No

Do you have any past injuries to, or current problems with, any of the areas listed:

❏ Irregular heart beat	❏ Dizziness	❏ Neck	☒ Low back	❏ Feet
❏ Chest pain	❏ Fainting	❏ Hands	❏ Mid-back	❏ Ankles
❏ Loss of coordination	❏ Cramping	❏ Hips	❏ Shoulders	❏ Knees
❏ Heat intolerance	☒ Shin spints	❏ Calves		

I realize that there are risks to ALL exercise, including injury and possible death. While every effort will be made to decrease any risk of injury, I take full responsibility for my participation in this class. Knowing that I may participate at my own pace, and that I am free to discontinue participation at any time, I will inform the instructor of any problems — immediately.

Signature: **John Smith**   Date: **8-15-04**

Figure 3.1   Short history form.

from many sources and can be changed to fit your specific needs. The format is not really important. What you need is a great deal of information in a small space.

The British Columbia Department of Health designed the Physical Activity Readiness Questionnaire (PAR-Q) to help identify individuals for whom exercise may pose a problem or hazard. The PAR-Q can be used as a short form or conducted verbally. If participants answer yes to any of the questions in the PAR-Q, the developers of the PAR-Q suggest that vigorous exercise or exercise testing may have to be postponed and that medical clearance may be necessary. This form is found in appendix E.

Orient New Participants

Having a health information sheet is the beginning of building a shared responsibility for an exercise class and one way to integrate new participants into your class and orient them. On this form you also can ask participants when their birthday is, what their favorite reward would be, and any other pertinent information that might enhance performance. To further assist them, provide some written information about exercise, the facility schedule, or the program in general.

We also want our participants to immediately feel that they are responsible for their workout and to inform us of their personal physical limitations so we can assist them as much as possible. This can be done by having the participants read and sign an informed consent form. A sample of an informed consent form is in appendix D. The informed consent form ensures an individual's right to know that there are potential risks associated with exercise. Participants also have the right to know how these injuries may manifest themselves, how the risk of injury will be minimized, and what responsibility participants have in avoiding or reducing risk.

You must use some type of medical history or informed consent sheet, which is a critical ingredient in demonstrating care and concern for participants. Also, these forms help establish the foundations of safety, responsibility, and communication, which are necessary elements of the group exercise experience.

Create a Positive Atmosphere

In chapter 2 we discussed many aspects of being a model instructor, from wearing appropriate attire to creating a healthy emotional environment. These points are a very important part of being an effective instructor and therefore need to be part of the evaluation process.

Ways to create a positive atmosphere:

- Introduce yourself to participants and have them introduce themselves to others in the class.
- Wear attire and footwear that fit the population, and tell participants about appropriate gear needed.
- Explain the class format and review what participants can expect.
- Give positive motivational cues, smile, and be energetic with body language cues.

Creating a positive attitude and atmosphere begins with introducing yourself and students before class begins, especially when you are teaching in a facility where different people come to class every week and there is no set class list. This concept helps establish an attitude of, "we're in this together." Also, if participants know your name and the names of other participants in class, they will be more likely to ask questions and talk to one another. New people coming into a group exercise class are often afraid to ask questions and often feel out of place. Understanding this and asking for class communication will create a more open, safe environment for all participants.

The instructor's attire must be appropriate for the specific group exercise class. For example, when you are teaching a senior class it would not be appropriate to wear a midriff spandex outfit, because it might be intimidating. Observe what participants wear to class and try to match their attire so they will feel more comfortable. Ask what attire they prefer. At the same time, balance the comfort level of the class with functional wear. Correct spinal alignment and form should be visible with each movement you demonstrate. Make sure to notice and discuss appropriate footwear and attire for the various group exercise classes. For example, some indoor cycles have special clipless pedals that require a specific type of cycling shoes. In water exercise, a regular swimming suit often does not give the support needed to perform water exercise effectively.

Finally, an overview of the class format should accompany the instructor introduction. With so many different classes being offered and so many unique instructional techniques being used, the participants need to know your class expectations. Tell them about water breaks, expected intensity levels, how to check their heart rate, and any other pertinent information that might help make this a student-centered experience. An example of this introduction might be as follows: "This is a 30-min stretching class. There will not be an aerobic component. The only equipment you will need is a mat. Please leave your shoes on for the class." In some fitness centers a dry erase board is visible on entrance to the class. Before class begins, the instructor writes on the board his or her name, a welcome note, and what equipment will be needed. This informs participants about class expectations if they miss the verbal announcements. After previewing the class format, the instructor should explain to participants their individual responsibilities. One such responsibility is intensity. There is nothing worse than having a participant come to you after class and say, "This class was too easy for me." Intensity is the responsibility of the participant, not the instructor. It is your responsibility to make sure that modifications are given for various intensities to allow participants to make a choice, but you are not responsible for their workout intensity.

FOUR CLASS SEGMENTS IN GROUP EXERCISE

Chapters 4 through 7 review in detail how to implement the health-related components into a group exercise class format. These segments are the warm-up and stretch segment, the cardiorespiratory segment, the muscular conditioning segment, and finally the cool-down and flexibility segment. Before we get into specific class formats, this chapter reviews some common principles that apply to all group exercise classes. Most important, muscle balance principles apply to all aspects of a group exercise class and are important as well in the selection of proper exercise progressions. Later in this chapter, we review the application of music to group exercise classes, because most group exercise classes use music to help make the class fun and motivational.

GENERAL DEFINITIONS FOR MUSCULAR STRENGTH, ENDURANCE, AND FLEXIBILITY TRAINING

The group exercise instructor must understand the definitions of muscular strength and endurance training as well as flexibility training.

Muscular Strength

Muscular strength is the ability of the muscle or muscle group to perform maximal work one time only. For example, how much weight can you lift one time?

Muscular Endurance

Muscular endurance is the ability of the muscles to perform the same amount of work or movement repeatedly. For example, how many curl-ups can you do until you can no longer repeat the movement?

Flexibility

Flexibility is the range of motion around a joint or a set of joints. For example, the range of motion of the hip in abduction for many individuals is approximately 45°. We measure flexibility in degrees.

Muscle Balance

Let's take a moment to review where your major muscles are and what they actually do. Each joint has several muscles around it, and these muscles act in opposition to each other (see figure 3.2). Maintaining a balance of strength and flexibility in the muscles around your joints is an excellent way to help prevent injuries and promote high-level functioning.

You will notice that many of your students already have some typical muscle imbalances attributable to activities of daily living, sedentary lifestyle, obesity, poor posture, or simply the natural tendency to perform activities in a forward direction instead of backward. You need to know what these common muscle imbalances are and how to help correct them by incorporating appropriate strengthening

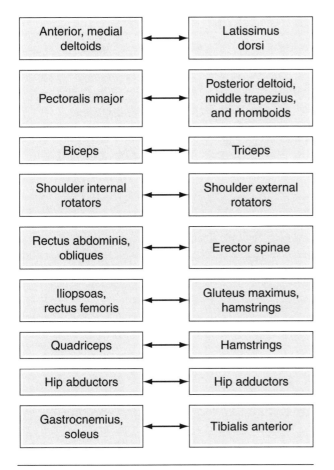

Figure 3.2 Opposing muscle groups.

or stretching exercises into your class. Muscle imbalances, left unchecked, often lead to injury, especially as a participant increases his or her frequency, intensity, or duration of exercise. Table 3.1 lists some of the most common muscle imbalances.

Because most muscle imbalances arise from lack of muscular balance in our daily living activities, we need to keep in mind what participants do when they are not in an exercise class. Then, analyze which muscle groups participants need to develop to counterbalance the muscles they primarily use in daily activities. Think of the group exercise class as an opportunity to balance work from daily living. Stretching and strengthening muscles that are not regularly used can help participants improve overall muscle balance. This approach brings the group fitness instructor's role closer to that of an individualized trainer (Kennedy 1997). For a summary of what muscles generally need strengthening and stretching for improved health, see table 3.2.

This table was created by conceptualizing the muscles we use for routine living. For example, we normally pick an object up using elbow flexion, which works the biceps concentrically (on the up phase). We then put the object down working the

Table 3.1 Common Muscle Imbalances

Muscle	Problem	Typical reason	Correction
Pectoralis major	Tight	Poor posture when sitting and standing	Stretch
Posterior deltoids, middle trapezius, rhomboids	Weak, overstretched	Poor posture when sitting and standing	Strengthen
Shoulder internal rotators	Tight	Poor posture, carrying and holding objects close to body	Stretch
Shoulder external rotators	Weak	Poor posture	Strengthen
Abdominals	Weak	Poor posture, obesity	Strengthen
Erector spinae	Tight (and often weak)	Poor posture, obesity	Stretch (and strengthen)
Hip flexors	Tight	Poor posture, sedentary lifestyle	Stretch
Hamstrings	Tight	Sedentary lifestyle	Stretch
Calves	Tight	Wearing high heels	Stretch
Shin	Weak	Not enough use in daily activities	Strengthen

Table 3.2   Muscle Balance Principles for Functional Training

Muscles that need strengthening	Stabilizers that need strengthening	Muscles that need stretching
Anterior tibialis	Erector spinae	Gastrocnemius and soleus
Quadriceps Hamstrings	Abductors	Quadriceps and iliopsoas
Rhomboids and middle trapezius	Adductors	Upper trapezius
Pectoralis minor and lower trapezius	Abdominals	Pectoralis major
Shoulder external rotators (teres minor and infraspinatus)		Hamstrings
Triceps		Erector spinae
Gluteals		Anterior and medial deltoids
Posterior deltoid		

biceps eccentrically (on the down phase) against gravity. Because of gravity, it's hard to work the triceps a lot in daily living. Keep in mind that the list in table 3.2 is to help enhance functional daily living skills for participants who are exercising for health and fitness. This does not mean that the stronger muscles should not be worked in a group exercise setting; however, focus needs to be on balancing the use of weaker muscle groups and stronger muscle groups especially if our goal is to create workouts that benefit participants in their daily lives.

The basic strategy for dealing with muscle imbalances is this: Strengthen weak, loose, small muscles and stretch tight, short, or strong muscles. For example, if the abdominals are typically weak or loose, it makes sense to regularly include strengthening and shortening exercises such as abdominal crunches in your class. On the other side of the body, the lower back muscles (the erector spinae) are commonly tight and tense, so "feel-good" stretches such as the angry cat stretch on hands and knees help to lengthen and relax the lower back. If this muscle imbalance isn't addressed, the spine will gradually be pulled out of alignment, leading to excessive lordosis, or swayback. Excessive lordosis is a contributing factor in low back pain, a chronic disorder that afflicts 8 of 10 people in developed countries at some point in their lives (Frymoyer and Cats-Baril 1991).

Abdominals can be trained dynamically, through full range of motion as spinal flexors. This is especially important when abdominals are weak and overstretched and are contributing to excessive lordosis. Abdominals also can be trained isometrically, as stabilizers of the spine. In stabilization or core strengthening exercise, a primary focus is contraction of the transverse abdominis, ideally causing a "hollowing" or a sensation of navel to spine. Some practitioners use the term *bracing* when performing hollowing with the spine in neutral. In stabilization exercises, other joints and muscles may be moving, creating the challenge of maintaining a stable, still spine throughout the duration of the exercise. A system of exercise designed primarily to build a strong core is known as Pilates (developed in the 1920s by Joseph Pilates). This type of exercise has become very popular and promotes core strength, endurance, and flexibility. See chapter 13 for more information on Pilates.

Similarly, rounded shoulders and a hunched upper back (known as excessive kyphosis) can become habitual over time, leading to neck, shoulder, and upper back pain. Help your students prevent this problem by providing more posterior deltoid, middle trapezius, and rhomboid exercises than chest exercises and by emphasizing chest and anterior deltoid stretching.

Balancing Strength and Flexibility

Another aspect of balance is the relative balance that exists between the strength and the flexibility of a particular muscle group. If the exerciser has a great deal of flexibility in a particular muscle group, you may need to emphasize strengthening rather than flexibility exercises to avoid injury to joint structures and ligamentous tissues. If the exerciser has greater strength than flexibility in a particular muscle group, you may need to perform flexibility exercises to avoid strains to the muscles and tendons. We often have the misconception that more flexibility and more strengthening are beneficial. In fact, it is the relative balance between flexible and strong muscles that creates a healthy system.

Appropriate emphasis on stretching or strengthening can be applied to both the athlete and the normal adult with back problems. Gymnasts, the epitome of flexibility (especially of the spine), have high rates of back pain and injury. Their back pain can be associated with overly flexible joint structures caused by overstretching of the spinal ligaments as well as the impact forces in dismounting and hyperextending in the spine. Strong muscles may be able to compensate for this hyperflexible condition, but if strengthening exercises are eliminated, pain and injury continue to weaken the spinal structure. The extreme flexibility required in gymnastics means that lifelong back and abdominal strengthening exercises are essential to any gymnast's program. After a gymnast leaves the sport, he or she needs to continue these strengthening exercises to maintain adequate function, because the damage done while participating is very likely irreversible and will continue to be a problem.

People who have suffered an injury from an accident or from repetitive motion injuries of the spine in which the ligaments might be overstretched also have similar problems. As long as they perform their strengthening exercises, they can control pain and maintain a reasonable level of function. When the individual stops back-strengthening exercise, his or her pain increases and reinjury may result. Much of low back pain is caused by improper body mechanics often related to sedentary living. Fitness instructors can make a huge difference by educating clients about proper posture in everyday tasks. A study (Kellett et al. 1991) on the effects of an exercise program on sick leave caused by back pain found that the number of sick leave days attributable to back pain decreased by 50% in the exercising group. Telling someone with back pain to rest may cause even more problems, because the muscle weakness and joint flexibility caused by inactivity are often the reasons for the onset of back pain. Literature on back pain (Cinque 1989) reminds us that a number of physicians recommend getting out of bed and into the gym. In the final analysis, you as the instructor need to recognize what muscle or muscle group is responsible for a specific action and what muscle group works in opposition to that action. You need to consider what exercises you will choose to enable your participants to function optimally during exercise and in their daily lives.

PROGRESSIVE FUNCTIONAL TRAINING CONTINUUM

Used in the traditional sense, progression refers to progressively overloading the body's systems and increasing the training stimulus over time to cause gradually increasing fitness adaptations. In resistance training, depending on the type of training, the muscles gradually become stronger or have more endurance as well as enhanced neuromuscular control, coordination, and balance. This can be achieved by changing the variables of frequency, intensity, duration, and mode of exercise. Our progressive functional training continuum addresses the last variable: mode, or type of exercise. This is very important to group exercise because instructors have to decide what exercises they are going to teach in their classes. The progressive functional training continuum (Kennedy 2003, Yoke and Kennedy 2004) helps instructors make better decisions for their participants. Figure 3.3 outlines the continuum.

"Less skilled" exercises require less balance, stability, proprioceptive activity, and motor control. Such exercises are generally safe for almost everyone and require the least amount of instructor cueing. Many of these exercises are performed

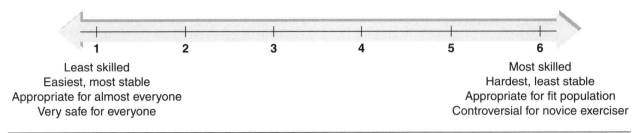

Figure 3.3 Progressive functional exercise continuum.

in a supine or prone position, require isolation movements rather than total body movements, and strengthen individual muscle groups. A few exercise examples include supine triceps extension, prone scapular retraction for the middle trapezius and rhomboids, and prone hip extension for the hamstrings and gluteus maximus. These exercises are low risk, easy to cue, and relatively safe for almost all populations.

At the other end of the continuum are exercises that need a great deal of skill and require an ability to maintain joint integrity, including the spinal joints and those involved in core stability (the ability to maintain ideal alignment in the neck, spine, scapulae, and pelvis no matter how difficult the exercise). These difficult exercises also place a high demand on proprioceptors and on the neuromuscular system for smooth coordination. As a result, the ability to perform challenging exercises safely depends on the exerciser's specific experience and overall fitness level. Many sport-specific exercises are categorized at this end of the continuum. A few examples of difficult and controversial exercises include deadlifts, plyometric lunges, handstand shoulder presses, and V-sits. Although these exercises are considered difficult and higher risk, a very fit person with excellent fitness and core stability might be able to perform them safely and appropriately. As a group exercise leader, you have to choose which exercises will be safe for your whole class. We recommend selecting exercises that allow all participants to be successful. Exercises on the continuum in the 1 to 4 range are most appropriate for group leadership. Exercises in the 5 and 6 portion of the continuum ought to be reserved for advanced classes or personal training. How does the continuum work? The progressive functional training continuum is organized into six levels.

Level 1

Isolate and Educate. Focus on muscle isolation at this level and train participants to selectively contract individual muscle groups, thereby providing confidence and body awareness and increasing the basic levels of muscle function. Exercises shown at this level are often supine or prone, with as much of the body in contact with the floor or bench as possible, lessening the need for stabilizer muscle involvement. As a result, these exercises are generally quite safe; just about everyone can learn to do them effectively with minimal risk of injury. To enhance the participant's muscle awareness and education, gravity is usually the main form of resistance applied. This level is perfect for almost all group exercise classes because all participants would be successful with these choices.

Level 2

Add External Resistance With Weights, Increased Lever Length, or Elastic Bands or Tubes While Keeping Stabilizer Involvement to a Minimum. In many cases, the actual exercise is the same as in level 1. Notice that in both levels 1 and 2, safety and alignment cueing on the part of the instructor is minimized; it's simply easier for exercisers to perform these types of exercises safely and effectively while maintaining proper form because of the decreased stabilizer involvement.

Level 3

Add Functional Training Positions. Select exercises that progress body position to sitting or standing, both of which are more functional for most people. When the participant is sitting or standing, the base of support is reduced and the stabilizer challenge is increased. In most progressions, the targeted muscle group is still isolated as a primary mover with the stabilizers assisting. This is often the stage in which standing dumbbell exercises or standing tubing exercises are introduced.

Level 4

Combine Increased Function With Resistance. Resistance from gravity, external weights, or bands and tubes is maximized and overload is increased on the core stabilizer muscles in functional positions. Most of the exercises in this level are performed in a standing position to use the core stabilizer muscles. These exercises begin the process of overloading the muscles for stresses of daily living.

Level 5

Multiple Muscle Groups With Increased Resistance and Core Challenge. In level 5, multiple muscle groups and joint actions are used simultaneously or in combination with each other. Resistance, balance, coordination, and torso stability are progressed to an even higher level. The emphasis at this level is on challenging the core stabilizers to a greater degree. For example, an overhead press using dumbbells while the participant performs a squat will definitely challenge the core to a greater degree than simply performing a squat or an overhead press independently.

Level 6

Add Balance, Increased Functional Challenge, Speed, and Rotational Movements. Exercises at this level may require balancing on one leg, use of a stability ball, plyometric movements, spinal rotation while lifting, or some other life skill or sport-specific maneuver. For example, training to clean your house requires power and rotation movements, not just single muscle groups. Potentially, risk of injury is increased at this level, so instructors must be cautious and prudent when introducing these exercises to a group. Although including speed and rotation is less safe, it is also how we live. Sensible progression to this level will transition into needed life skills. A sample progression is outlined in figure 3.4.

COMMUNICATION SKILLS

We must not underestimate the participant's overall experience in a group exercise class. How participants are treated and whether they are comfortable can make or break their attendance in your class. Bain and colleagues (1989) compared overweight and regular participants' dropout rates in a structured group exercise class and noted that more overweight participants dropped out. They dropped out not because they did not like the music or routine but rather because they were concerned about being embarrassed and judged by others. Wininger (2002) found that the instructor's ability to communicate was an important aspect of the participant's overall enjoyment. Therefore, how you give your participants feedback is important. Once you have observed improper technique in your group exercise classes, take some action but make sure you are kind. Some instructors find this the most challenging part of instructing because it's often hard to be a strong motivator yet also a soft encourager when a participant needs form correction. See "Examples of Effective Communication" for a few suggestions for cueing the participant on correct position or technique without being threatening or critical, focusing instead on kindness. Figure 3.5 provides cueing examples.

Find ways to make your class a positive experience for all students. Correcting and recommending alignment changes in a polite and nonthreatening way make the exercise experience more comfortable for the participants. If they are comfortable, they will be more likely to come back. If students are ill at ease, they may miss some of the wonderful therapeutic benefits that come from group exercise (Choi et al. 1993, Estivill 1995), such as a positive mood and increased self-esteem. The mental and emotional benefits derived from the group exercise experience can be just as beneficial as the physical gains.

See the DVD practice drill on alignment correction techniques for a stationary lunge.

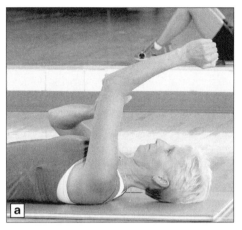
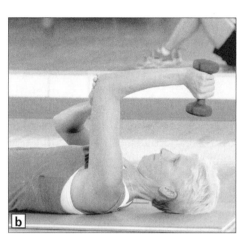
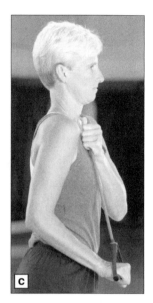
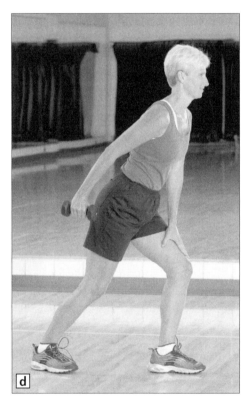
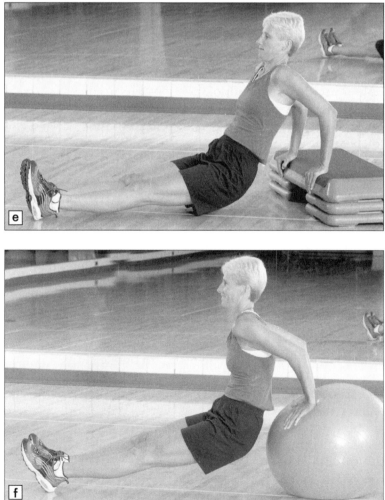

Figure 3.4 A sample progression for triceps: (*a*) supine unilateral triceps extension, (*b*) supine with weights, (*c*) standing press-down with tube, (*d*) triceps kickback, (*e*) dips off a bench, and (*f*) dips off a stability ball.

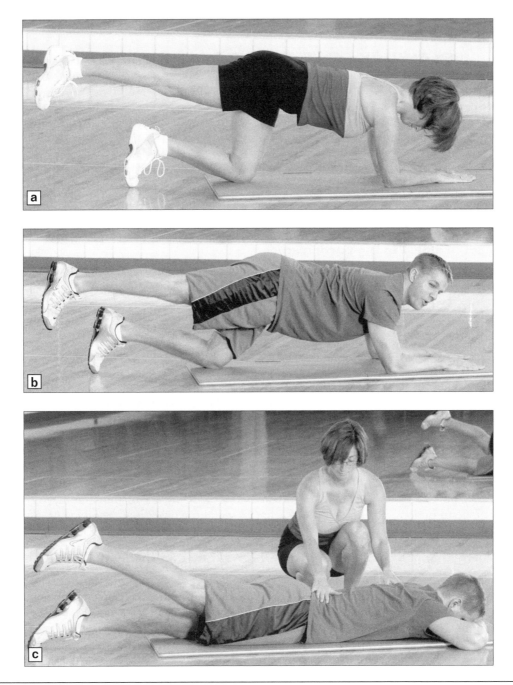

Figure 3.5 Cueing examples: *(a)* good technique, *(b)* poor technique, and *(c)* instructor correction.

MUSIC FOR GROUP EXERCISE

Music is a vital part of almost all group exercise classes. Subjects regularly report that they believe their performance is better with music accompaniment (Kravitz 1994). Music also appears to provide a motivational construct to exercise, positively affecting participants' mental state. In high/low impact programs, step classes, and several other modalities, participants typically time their moves to coincide with the beat of the music. In Pilates, yoga, water exercise, indoor cycling, and some equipment-based classes, however, participants don't necessarily move on the beat, but music helps motivate and makes the movement experience enjoyable. Therefore, music can be used to provide structure to your class or simply to set the mood.

EXAMPLES OF EFFECTIVE COMMUNICATION

1. Deliver general statements to the whole group:

"Stop for just a moment—look at your back foot to see if your toe is facing straight ahead. The toe must be straight ahead to stretch effectively." Or, "I see people having difficulty—let me demonstrate what I want you to do."

2. Make corrections by moving the person into the proper position:

During a wall stretch for the calves, give people having difficulty the following instruction: "I would like to turn your foot so it is straight. Is that OK? Can you feel a difference in the stretch?"

3. Exercise next to the participant:

Stand beside the person having trouble and demonstrate what you want him to do. Perhaps he cannot quite see or hear you well enough to comply. If the person you are correcting is down on the floor, get down next to him to demonstrate. A person on the floor is more vulnerable than the person standing, so you must get down on the same level to instruct in a nonthreatening way.

4. Move around the room:

If you stay at the front of the class, only the people in the front row will be able to observe your technique. If teaching step, put several benches around the room so you can move around during the aerobic segment. Try teaching in the middle of the class instead of the front or regularly move from the front to the back to the side.

5. Catch people doing it right:

Most people respond much better to positive rather than negative reinforcement. If a participant is having difficulty with a movement or series of movements, point out someone performing well in class for her to watch or pair them together. Always demonstrate and instruct good alignment to keep a focus on correct technique.

6. Always appeal to a person's need for safety and give your rationale:

Compare the following statements: "You must have your foot in this position" versus "Place your foot in this position. It will prevent you from falling forward, and will make this exercise easier." Or, "Don't bounce while stretching, that's the wrong technique," versus "If you bounce while stretching you might pull or tear a muscle—I don't want you to get hurt. Try holding the stretch instead." Which statement would you rather hear? The second statements do not differ remarkably; however, they include a rationale and helpful alternatives.

7. Use positive descriptions, rather than labels:

Words such as *good, bad, right,* and *wrong* are emotionally loaded and judgmental. Instead of saying, "Joe, you are doing this movement wrong," try, "Joe, you seem to be having trouble with this movement, let's try this . . . I think it will help."

When teaching most types of group exercise classes, you must understand and work with your music. Especially in a high/low impact class, it simply "feels good" to move on the beat, and your students will feel more successful, positive, and energized when you lead them to

RECOMMENDED BEATS PER MINUTE

Warm-up:	120-136 beats/min
High/low impact cardio:	134-158 beats/min
Step:	118-128 beats/min
Muscle conditioning:	Under 132 beats/min
Flexibility work, yoga, and Pilates:	Under 100 beats/min or music without a strong beat

move with the music. Additionally, because many people innately hear or feel the beat of the music, they unconsciously feel clumsy or uncoordinated when taking a class with an instructor who is "off beat." Participants especially expect the movements to flow with the music in high/low impact and step classes. Also, understanding and using the music structure can reduce the need for constant cueing.

The next sections outline the basic elements of popular music. Practice the suggested drills until hearing the musical components becomes automatic. Most skilled instructors constantly have the beat, the downbeat, the 4-count measure, and the 8- and 32-count phrases in their heads at all times when leading class; hearing the music simply becomes second nature with practice. Note that there are recommended beats per minute for various segments and types of classes of group exercise (see "Recommended Beats per Minute").

Beat

The *beat* is the smallest musical division of a phrase. Each regular rhythmic pulse is a beat, or *count*. Beats are further organized into *downbeats* and *upbeats*. The downbeat is the stronger, more important or emphatic beat. The upbeat is the weaker, less important beat that immediately follows each downbeat. For example, the song "Jingle Bells" in figure 3.6, observe the downbeats (DB) and the upbeats (UB).

The downbeat falls on the most accented part of a word and usually on the most important words in a phrase, whereas the upbeat falls on the unaccented part of a word or the less important words. Also, when you are counting the beats forward in a measure, the downbeats are on the odd numbers (1 and 3) and the upbeats are on the even numbers (2 and 4).

Measure

The measure is the basic organizational unit in music; it contains a series of downbeats and upbeats. In almost all popular music used in step and high/low impact classes, each measure holds 4 beats: downbeat, upbeat, downbeat, upbeat. Such music is said to be in 4/4 metered time, which technically means that there are four quarter notes in each measure. In the example given in figure 3.6, the words *jingle bells* take up one measure.

Phrase

A phrase consists of at least two measures of music. Hence, it is common to speak of an 8-count phrase (two measures), a 16-count phrase (four measures), and a 32-count phrase (eight measures) in step or high/low impact music. A 32-count phrase contains four 8-count phrases grouped together and is ideal for building routines

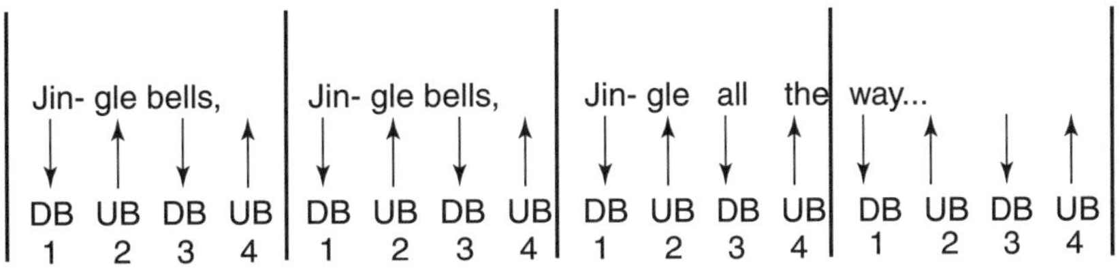

Figure 3.6 Even in simple songs, such as Jingle Bells, the upbeats and downbeats are easily identified.

MUSIC RESOURCE LIST

Aerobic Beat	Los Angeles, CA	800-536-6060
Aerobics With Soul	Minneapolis, MN	800-423-9685
Broadcast Vision	Agoura Hills, CA	800-770-9770
Dynamix	Baltimore, MD	800-843-6499
Hydrophonics	Camarillo, CA	800-794-6626
Kimbo Educational	Long Branch, NJ	800-631-2187
Muscle Mixes Music	Alameda, CA	800-833-1224
Power Productions International	Salt Lake City, UT	800-777-2328
Supreme Audio	Marlborough, NH	800-445-7398
Tune Belt Inc.	Cincinnati, OH	800-860-1175

and choreographic combinations. Participants usually feel more successful and energized when new movement patterns are initiated on the downbeat at the beginning of each 32-count phrase; this is sometimes called the "top of the phrase." Listen for the drum roll or increase in musical momentum at the end of each 32-count phrase (technically the 7th and 8th counts of the last or fourth 8-count phrase), signifying the new 32-count phrase to follow. Furthermore, the 8-count phrases within each 32-count phrase are typically divided into dominant and less dominant phrases, such as the following:

> **See the DVD for the practice drill on counting out the beat (4 counts and 8 counts at 120 beats/min and 132 beats/min).**

- First 8-count phrase: dominant
- Second 8-count phrase: less dominant
- Third 8-count phrase: dominant
- Fourth 8-count phrase: less dominant, but with drum roll or other musical momentum during 7th and 8th final counts

Make this learning process easier on yourself by always selecting music that has a strong, easy-to-hear beat. In addition, commercial music tapes that have been professionally premixed for step, kickboxing, and high/low impact classes will already be blended (metered) into continuous 32-count phrases. This is preferable to music found in music stores, which is not metered for group exercise and will contain extra beats and bridges, making counting, choreography,

and cueing much more difficult. See the "Music Resource List" for contact information.

Half Time and Double Time

When a movement is performed *half time*, it is performed twice as slowly as normal. In other words, a box step (square pattern with your feet) usually takes 4 counts, but when performed half time, it takes 8 counts. *Double time*, then, means to perform a move twice as fast as usual.

■ PRACTICE DRILL ■

Using popular music with a strong beat, listen for the 8-count division within the music. Find the 8-count grouping with the strongest initial downbeat, or emphasis; this is the beginning of the 32-count phrase. To help integrate this information, try this simple drill: (1) leading with your right foot, walk eight steps to the right on the first 8-count phrase; (2) make a sharp 90° turn to your right and walk eight more steps on the second 8-count phrase (always leading right); (3) make another sharp 90° turn to your right and walk eight more steps on the third 8-count phrase; and finally (4) make another sharp 90° turn to your right and walk eight more steps on the fourth 8-count phrase, returning to your starting point. You should have made a large square pattern with your feet. Repeat, or try the same drill to your left, leading always with the left foot. Keep practicing this drill with different speeds and styles of music.

Music Styles

One of the most enjoyable aspects of teaching to music is the availability of so many different styles of music. Adapting the music to your participants' interests and ages will enhance their enjoyment and willingness to keep exercising. Dwyer (1995) found that when participants had a choice of music, they reported higher intrinsic motivation than did the participants who were not asked for input. Ask your participants what they like to listen to. Trying new musical styles can stimulate creative energy and open up new opportunities for choreography. Keep an open mind and have a sense of play when experimenting with these styles:

- Rock, pop, top 40
- House, techno, club
- Oldies, Motown
- Funk, rap
- Latin, salsa
- Reggae
- Big band, swing
- Country

- World beat (Irish, Peruvian, African, Middle Eastern)
- Holiday (Halloween, Valentine's Day, 4th of July)
- Themes (beach, girl power, rainy day music)

PRACTICE DRILL

Listening to any piece of popular music, close your eyes and tap your feet, pat your knee, or clap your hands to the regular continuous beat. Write a list of 20 songs and their beats per minute and describe in which portion of the workout the songs would fit best.

Responsibilities for Exercise Music

The 1976 revision of the Copyright Law, which went into effect in 1978, made clear statements about the responsibilities of exercise and fitness instructors, studios, and fitness centers regarding

RECOMMENDATIONS FOR MUSIC VOLUME IN FITNESS CLASSES

Based on research and volume level safety standards, IDEA, the international association of fitness professionals, makes the following recommendations regarding safe levels for sound volume during group exercise classes (Goodman 1997). These recommendations are based on standards established by the U.S. Occupational Safety and Health Administration (OSHA). Fitness professionals outside the United States are urged to refer to official guidelines established for their countries.

1. Because hearing loss is a slow, cumulative, and usually painless process, group exercise instructors need to be aware that the intensity of their music and accompanying voice may be putting them and their students at risk without causing any apparent symptoms.

2. Health facilities and instructors have an obligation to their members and students to ensure safe music intensity during group exercise classes.

3. Music intensity during group exercise classes should measure no more than 90 decibels (dB).

4. Because the instructor's voice needs to be about 10 dB louder than the music in order to be heard, the instructor's voice should measure no more than 100 dB.

5. Fitness facilities are urged to place a Class C sound level meter (available from many electronics stores for less than $100) on a stand near the front middle of the group exercise room to get a continuous measure of sound levels during classes. Instructors or other staff members should regularly check the meter. The volume control on the music amplifier is not an accurate means of measuring sound level.

the music they use. Tested throughout the judicial system and upheld by the U.S. Supreme Court, the law states that the copyright owner has the right to charge a fee for the use of his or her music in a "public performance."

A public performance is defined as a place open to the public or any place where a substantial number of persons outside a normal circle of a family and its social acquaintances are gathered.

All exercise and fitness classes—whether they take place in a private club, public hall, exercise gym, or corporate fitness center—fall into the category of public performance. Because music is a copyrighted entity, corporations, studios, fitness centers, and instructors who use music during their exercise classes place themselves in jeopardy of violating the Copyright Law if they do not pay royalties to the people who write, publish, and distribute the music.

The American Society of Composers, Authors and Publishers (ASCAP) and Broadcast Music, Inc. (BMI) are the two organizations in the United States that represent all of the artists and performers who record the music used in group exercise classes. A combined total of more than 80,000 composers, lyricists, and publishers are represented by these two organizations. These performing rights societies see to it that their members get their fair share of royalties and that the Copyright Law is enforced. Violators and potential violators of the Copyright Law are vigorously pursued by both ACSAP and BMI. The American Council on Exercise (2000) recommends that most clubs and studios obtain a blanket license for their instructors. The license fees for the clubs are determined by the number of students who attend classes each week, by the number of speakers used in the club, or by whether the club has a single or multi-floor layout. For more specific information on what it costs and for clarification of rules pertaining to the copyright laws, check out their Web sites at www.bmi.com and www.ascap.com.

Sound System Fundamentals

A good sound system is essential in most group exercise classes. A basic sound system consists of one or more sources (microphones, tape, CD, radio, cassette) connected to an amplifier and speakers. All systems, whether they are portable systems or fixed, studio-type systems, contain these basic elements.

The more self-contained systems (portables and ministereo systems) have no capacity for adding extra speakers or other source devices, like wireless microphones (Goodman 1997). These systems also have no provisions for mixing sounds from more than one source, such as a wireless microphone and a CD. More accessible systems—karaoke systems, keyboard amplifier and speaker systems, and professional portable sound systems—provide connections that allow you to add external sound sources and speakers. The "Music Resource List" gives vendor names for products. The products change so quickly that we are unable to give a specific recommendation for a sound system. However, it is worth your time to research a product that will sound good and also be easy to maintain. Call other organizations to see what they use and have had success with.

According to Long and colleagues' (1998) study on voice problems with aerobic instructors, 44% of instructors surveyed experienced partial or complete voice loss during and after instructing. They also had increased episodes of voice loss, hoarseness, and sore throat unrelated to illness since they began instructing. Heidel and Torgerson (1993) also found that instructors experienced a higher prevalence of vocal problems compared with individuals participating in group exercise. If you are instructing on a regular basis, a microphone will be essential to your health (see "Recommendations for Music Volume").

The technology of sound systems advances as quickly as computer technology, because they go hand in hand. The bottom line is that you must get a good sound system, a microphone with a headset and receiver, and good quality speakers. These products will create a big difference in the quality of your group exercise instruction. After all, music is often one of the main reasons participants venture into the group exercise setting versus exercising alone on a stepper or elliptical machine. Monroe (1999) stated that music (along with the creative use of silence) is still the heart of movement. She said, "If you love your music and have a passion for it, it will move you—and it will move the people you teach" (p. 37).

Chapter Wrap-Up

The general components outlined in this chapter are important for all group exercise classes. We need to integrate the health components of fitness into our classes, have preclass introductions and screenings, apply muscle balance principles to group exercise, and learn proper progression of exercises. We also must strive to make exercise fun by using quality music played on good sound systems to enhance the health and well-being of our participants.

Written Assignment

Interview an instructor at your facility and see if the facility pays ASCAP and BMI for the rights to use music. Observe an instructor getting ready to teach a class. Write down all the steps she or he takes to set up the music and microphone, how participants are greeted, and how equipment is set up. Research the Web or contact one vendor from the music resource list and create a price list of a complete sound system for use in a group exercise setting. Write a one-page summary of your findings.

Practical Assignment

Using the group exercise class evaluation form (appendix A), fill in the preclass organization segment with the specifics of what you intend to do. Using a song from a pre-mixed group exercise tape, practice hearing the 32-count phrases and moving in a large square pattern, turning every 8 beats, as described in the practice drill.

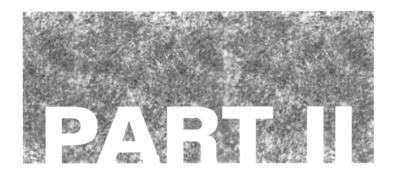

PART II

Guidelines for Group Exercise Class Segments

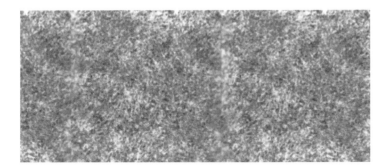

Warm-Up

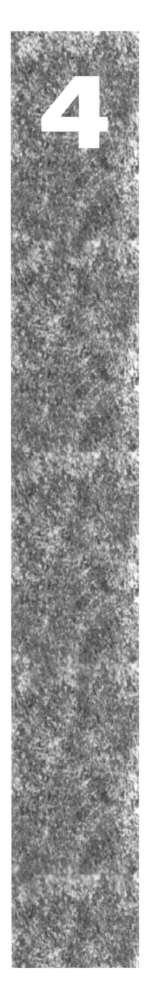

Chapter Objectives

By the end of this chapter, you will

- ■ be able to prepare a warm-up and stretching segment,

- ■ know how to create rehearsal moves for a warm-up, and

- ■ understand how stretching fits into the warm-up segment.

An effective group exercise class starts with a warm-up and stretching segment (figure 4.1). If you are using music, the first song sets the tone for your class and gets people ready to begin moving. During the first portion of the warm-up, movements should be dynamic with large muscle groups predominantly used. The second portion builds on the first and should permit a combination of warming up and stretching if appropriate. A class tends to flow better if the second portion is more upbeat and if the stretching portion (if used) is performed standing so that you can move right into the cardiorespiratory segment. In this section we review the components listed in the group exercise class evaluation form (found in appendix A).

1. Includes appropriate amount of dynamic movement ❏

2. Provides rehearsal moves ❏

3. Stretches major muscle groups in a biomechanically sound manner with appropriate instructions ❏

4. Gives clear cues and verbal directions ❏

5. Uses an appropriate music tempo ❏

Figure 4.1 General guidelines for warm-up and stretching.

DYNAMIC MOVEMENT

One of the purposes of the warm-up is to prepare the body for the more rigorous demands of the cardiorespiratory and muscular strength and conditioning segments by raising the internal temperature. For each degree of temperature elevation, the metabolic rate of cells increases by about 13% (Åstrand and Rodahl 1977). In addition, at higher body temperatures, blood flow to the working muscles increases, as does the release of oxygen to the muscles. Because these effects allow more efficient energy production to fuel muscle contraction, the goal of an effective warm-up should be to elevate internal tempera-

tures 1 or 2° F, and you may notice that sweating occurs. Increasing body temperature has other effects that are beneficial for exercisers as well. The potential physiological benefits of warming up are listed in figure 4.2.

Potential physiological benefits of warming up are as follows:

- Increased metabolic rate
- Higher rate of oxygen exchange between blood and muscles
- More oxygen released within muscles
- Faster nerve impulse transmission
- Gradual redistribution of blood flow to working muscles
- Decreased muscle relaxation time following contraction
- Increased speed and force of muscle contraction
- Increased muscle elasticity
- Increased flexibility of tendons and ligaments
- Gradual increase in energy production, which limits lactic acid buildup
- Reduced risk of abnormal electrocardiogram
- Joint lubrication

Figure 4.2 Physiological benefits of the warm-up.

Many of the physiological effects listed in figure 4.2 may reduce the risk of injury because they have the potential to increase neuromuscular coordination, delay fatigue, and make the tissues less susceptible to damage (Alter 1996). Therefore, the overall focus in the warm-up period should be on dynamic movements that increase core body temperature.

Remember that the diaphragm, the major muscle involved in breathing, is like any other muscle group and needs time to shift gears. A rapid increase in breathing without time to warm up properly can result in side aches and hyperventilation (rapid, shallow, breathing). Sudden increases in breathing mean that the transition into the cardiorespiratory segment was not gradual enough.

REHEARSAL MOVES

Rehearsal moves are a less intense version of the movement patterns that participants will perform during the cardiorespiratory portion of class. These moves make up the majority of the warm-up, preparing participants mentally and physically for the challenges of the workout (Anderson 2000). Blahnik and Anderson (1996) defined rehearsal moves as "movements that are identical to, but less intense than, the movements your students will execute during the workout phase" (p. 50). Examples of rehearsal moves for various group exercise class formats can be found in the following sidebar. The concept of rehearsal moves relates to the principle of specificity of training. This principle states that the body adapts specifically to whatever demands are placed on it. Some researchers believe that specificity applies not only to energy systems and muscle groups but also to movement patterns (ACSM 1998). Because motor units used during training demonstrate the majority of physiological alterations, move-

ment patterns also must be specifically trained. In a group exercise class, one of the main reasons participants become frustrated is that they are not able to perform the movements effectively. Introducing these movement patterns in the warm-up will help wake up associated motor units.

Using rehearsal moves in the warm-up not only specifically warms up the body for the movement ahead but also can be a time to set down some neuromuscular patterns by introducing new skills not yet used. For example, in a high/low impact class where a grapevine movement (R, L, R, tap; L, R, L, tap) is used, use the warm-up to break down the move, identify the directional landmarks in the room, and name the specific move. If this is done, when a grapevine is referred to in the cardiorespiratory segment, the class participants will know what to do. The same idea applies to a complex choreography movement in a step class. Practice this type of movement slowly in the warm-up when maintaining a higher level of intensity is not the main focus. When this movement comes up in the routine, it will have been rehearsed, and this will make it easier for participants to maintain their cardiorespiratory intensity level. Rehearsal moves, therefore, should make up a large part of the warm-up.

REHEARSAL MOVE SUGGESTIONS FOR VARIOUS GROUP EXERCISE FORMATS

These suggested movements preview actions that will be used in the cardio segment following the warm-up.

- Step: Use the bench during the warm-up.

- Indoor cycling: Teach participants how to climb a hill properly.

- Water exercise: Practice an interval segment (30 s rest, 30 s work) using a cross-country skier movement.

- Muscle conditioning: Use muscle-specific movements in the warm-up, such as biceps curls, triceps kickbacks, and squats.

- Kickboxing: Use shuffles, kicks, and punches.

- High/low impact class: Review a 32-count series.

- Sport conditioning: Use the ladders and walk through the movement.

MAJOR MUSCLE GROUPS STRETCHED

Whether to stretch during the warm-up is a debated issue, one on which the literature has not yet come to complete agreement. Taylor and colleagues (1990) found that gains in flexibility were most significant when a stretch was held for 12 to 18 s and repeated four times per muscle group. Another study (Walter et al. 1995) found that stretching the hamstrings for 30 s produced significantly greater flexibility than stretching for 10 s. If these two studies were the complete story, we would probably recommend not stretching in a group exercise warm-up, because it is impossible to stretch a muscle group four times and hold it for 30 s and still accomplish the goals of increasing the heart rate and core temperature. Another study (Girouard and Hurley 1995) of strength and flexibility training in older adults found that stretching before and after training did not increase flexibility. Convincing research on runners (Lally 1994, Shrier 1999, Van Mechelen et al. 1993) demonstrated that static stretches performed during the warm-up did not prevent injury. These studies encourage injury prevention through dynamic warm-up. The 1998 ACSM position stand on exercise included flexibility for the first time. This position stand states, "The inclusion of recommendations for flexibility exercise in this position stand is based on growing evidence of its multiple benefits including: improving joint range of motion and function and in enhancing muscular performance" (p. 980). Finally, Shrier and Gossal (2000) reviewed the stretching literature and found that one static stretch of 15 to 30 s per day was sufficient to enhance flexibility. It is generally agreed that flexibility exercises are beneficial, but questions remain about where to put them in the class format for group exercise.

Most prominent exercise education textbooks (Baechle and Earle 2003, McArdle et al. 2001, Neiman 2003, Wilmore and Costill 1999) and stretching books (Alter 1996) recommend an active warm-up with rehearsal moves followed by brief stretching; these books recommend that the majority of flexibility work be done during the cool-down portion of the workout. However, these books are written with the individual and, often, the athlete in mind, and they are not nec-essarily about working with a group. Generally though, they include some stretching within the warm-up and they all advocate that a warm-up precede any stretching. According to Neiman (2003), a warm-up will enhance the activity of enzymes in the working muscle, reduce the viscosity of muscle, improve the mechanical efficiency and power of the moving muscles, facilitate the transmission speed of nervous impulses augmenting coordination, increase muscle blood flow and thus improve delivery of necessary fuel substrates, increase the level of free fatty acids in the blood, help prevent injuries to the muscles and various supporting connective tissues, and allow the heart muscle to adequately prepare itself for aerobic exercise. There is no conclusive evidence showing any inherent benefit to stretching during the warm-up, but few studies suggest that it might be dangerous. Thus, the dynamic warm-up should contain mostly warm-up movements with some static stretches held briefly if this is the only place flexibility is included in the format. Many participants avoid stretching, so including it in the warm-up is a good strategy to ensure that all components of fitness are addressed.

In terms of organizing a group exercise class format for the warm-up segment, it's best to focus on rehearsal movements; if static stretches are included, try to focus on active movement as well. For example, while performing a standing calf or hamstring stretch, keep the upper body moving with arms moving up and down to stay warm (figure 4.3).

See the DVD for a warm-up example in a high/low impact group exercise class.

In a cycling class, keep the legs pedaling and perform some upper body stretches. When you are teaching a 30-min class, it might be better to save the stretching for the end when it will be most beneficial in enhancing flexibility. In this situation, it might not be appropriate to do static stretching in the beginning at all. When you are teaching a group of seniors, you might find that they prefer warming up and performing several minutes of static stretching. For seniors, balance is also an issue. After they have warmed up, they can hold a stretch for increased flexibility and balance. By the end of the class, fatigue may prevent them from performing static stretches appropriately.

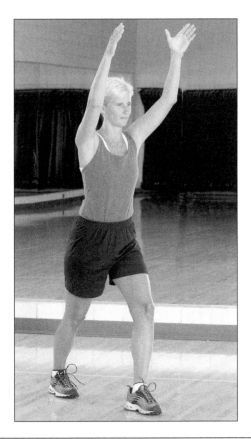

Figure 4.3 A static stretch with an active movement: performing a standing hamstrings stretch with deltoids moving to keep the upper body warm. This may be performed with one arm while the opposite hand rests on the thigh, providing support for the low back.

Only instructors who know their participants well know what the most appropriate warm-up and stretching format are for them. How to go about warming up and stretching is an individual decision. There is controversy over what is most effective in this component. However, all group exercise classes ought to include a warm-up and stretching segment. What we definitely know is that flexibility is a health-related component of fitness, that it needs to be included in the overall workout, and that warming up and performing rehearsal moves before any static stretching is performed are important no matter what group exercise format is being taught. This segment should be included in all group exercise classes.

Chapter Wrap-Up

Written Assignment

Attend the beginning of a group exercise class and notice how the instructor sets the atmosphere for the class. Write down everything the instructor does in the preclass organization and warm-up segment using the group exercise class evaluation form.

Practical Assignment

Create a 4-min group warm-up (for four to five individuals) integrating the concepts discussed in this chapter. Focus on developing demonstration skills and leadership confidence.

Cardiorespiratory Training

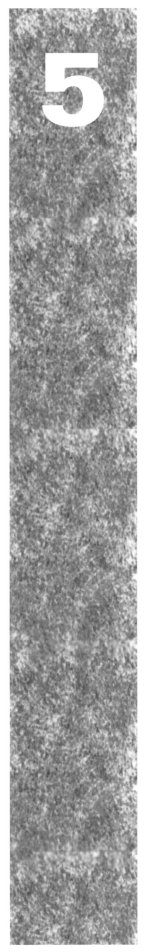

Chapter Objectives

By the end of this chapter, you will be able to

- explain the importance of appropriate beginning intensity,

- understand the principles of muscle balance in cardiorespiratory programming,

- give movement options and verbal cues,

- understand the importance of participant interaction,

- explain the importance of postcardio cool-down, and

- demonstrate two methods for monitoring intensity in the cardio segment.

A few common principles apply to the cardiorespiratory segment of most group exercise classes. These principles are listed on the group exercise class evaluation form (appendix A) under the cardio segment and repeated here (see figure 5.1). During the cardiorespiratory segment of a group exercise class, it is also critical that you monitor exercise intensity. Important details for learning and teaching these techniques are discussed at the end of this section.

1. Gradually increases intensity ☐

2. Uses a variety of muscle groups and minimizes repetitive movements ☐

3. Promotes participant interaction and encourages fun ☐

4. Demonstrates movement options and gives clear verbal cues and directions ☐

5. Gradually decreases intensity during postcardio cool-down ☐

6. Uses music appropriately ☐

Figure 5.1 Cardiorespiratory segment general guidelines.

BEGINNING INTENSITY

Even though the human body adapts to exercise very efficiently, gradually increasing intensity is necessary for many reasons:

- Blood flow is redistributed from internal organs to the working muscles.

- The heart muscle gradually adapts to the change from a resting to a working level.

- Respiratory rate gradually increases.

The most dangerous times for changes in the heart's rhythm are in the transitions from resting to high-intensity work and from high-intensity activity back to resting levels. At rest, the cardiorespiratory system circulates about 5 L of blood per minute. Imagine the contents of 2 1/2 2-L soda pop containers circulating through the body every minute. At maximal strenuous exercise, the increase in workload requires as much as 25 L/min to accommodate working muscles—that's 12 1/2 pop containers per minute!

To gradually increase intensity within a group exercise setting, start with moves that use small range of motion, short lever length, and limited traveling. Keep moves less intense at first by not using propulsion-type moves in a step class. In a water exercise class, use moves that have a smaller range of motion or shorter lever length. Finally, in an indoor cycling class, keep the flywheel tension set at a lower resistance for the first few minutes.

MUSCLE BALANCE

Instructors often have base moves (a series of movements that appear over and over again in their routine) within the cardiorespiratory segment. These base moves often involve the use of the quadriceps and hip flexor muscle groups. Examples include the basic march in place, the basic step, the cross-country skier in water exercise, and a flat road medium resistance in cycling. Many participants use these muscle groups primarily in daily living activities; therefore, continuing to use the quadriceps and hip flexors repeatedly during exercise is problematic. Striving to balance daily flexion with other movements is important. Although it is impossible to individualize within a group exercise setting, understanding how the body functions in daily movement can help instructors determine which muscles are stronger and which muscles need to be focused on within group exercise. For example, walking forward works the hip flexors. Focusing on movement selection that uses the buttocks and the hamstrings (the opposing muscle groups to the hip flexors) would help with muscle balance. The abductors are important stabilizer muscles for the hips. Incorporating some abductor moves within the cardiorespiratory segment is also recommended (figure 5.2).

In water exercise, muscle balance is automatically achieved because there is no gravity. If we flex the hip in water, the iliopsoas and rectus femoris perform the work. When the hip is extended in the water, the hamstrings and buttocks perform the work. On land, this movement

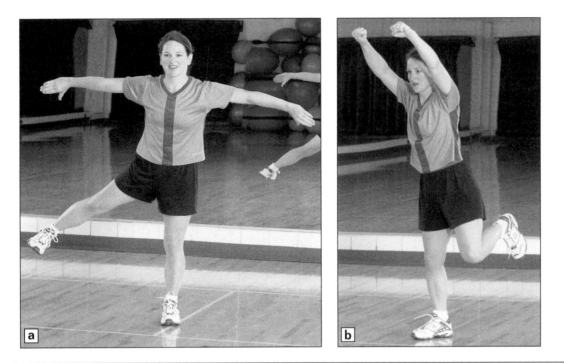

Figure 5.2   Opposing muscle groups for balance: *(a)* abductors and *(b)* hamstrings.

would be performed by an eccentric contraction of the quadriceps. With the exception of water exercise, it is important to analyze what movements work which muscle group and vary the selection to promote overall muscle balance as well as minimize repetitive movements.

Finally, make the most of your floor space to minimize repetitive movements and use the muscle groups in a different way. Use different geometric configurations during the aerobic segment in a floor group exercise class to help increase safety and interest. Performing figure eights, walking in circles, walking around the step, and making letters like an A or a T either on the floor or on a step all help create more interest and variety in your cardio segment.

See the DVD for an example of a high/low impact routine using space, intensity options, and good verbal cueing.

MOVEMENT OPTIONS AND VERBAL CUES

Instructors are often selected because excellent form is something they naturally have. For exam-ple, potential high/low impact or step instructors are often picked from among the front row participants who regularly attend class. Cyclists often instruct indoor cycling classes. However, having the skill and teaching the skill are two different things. Instructors who have good form may need instruction on teaching good cueing for the skills they naturally have, whereas those who need instruction on good form may learn more readily how to explain what good form looks like. Avid participants who become instructors are most challenged by giving intensity and movement options, especially for beginners. This is similar to the challenge faced by personal trainers, who also have to avoid giving their own workouts to their clients. Giving good movement options is one of the most difficult skills to acquire yet also one of the most important.

Whether you are leading a high/low impact class or teaching a treadmill, circuit, or cycle class, it is impossible to be everywhere or help everyone simultaneously. Each participant is working at a different fitness level and has different goals. Ideally, all classes would be organized according to intensity and duration options. The reality is that many participants come to a class because the time is convenient, not necessarily because the class length or intensity level is suitable. If participants try to exercise at the instructor's level or at another participant's level, they may work too hard and sustain an injury or they may not work hard enough to meet their goals. A few ways to help promote self-responsibility are to encourage participants to work at their own pace, demonstrate heart rate (HR) monitoring or rating of perceived exertion (RPE) checks, and inform participants how they should feel through common examples. For example, during the peak portion of the cardiorespiratory segment, tell participants that they should feel out of breath but still be able to talk. During the postcardio cool-down, tell them that they should feel their HRs slowing down. Be as descriptive as possible concerning perceived exertion throughout the workout. Demonstrate high, medium, and low intensity and impact options in order to reach the participants at various levels.

Help participants achieve the level of effort they need to reach, and continually remind them that reaching this point is their responsibility. You cannot be responsible for participants' exercise intensity. Pointing out participants who work at higher or lower levels also can help. We recommend that you maintain a medium intensity most of the time but also present other options and intensities as the need arises. Mastering this concept is the true art of group exercise instruction and the reason why group exercise can be more difficult to teach than one-on-one instruction.

MONITORING EXERCISE INTENSITY

Understanding the use of HR, RPE, and the talk test is the first step in monitoring exercise intensity. One method is not advocated over another, because all have applications depending on the type of activities participants will perform during the group exercise class. However, research (Parker et al. 1989) on group exercise has determined that HRs taken during high/low impact group exercise reflect a lower relative exercise intensity ($\dot{V}O_2$max) than HRs taken during running. Other research (Roach et al. 1994) on different forms of group exercise (step, interval high/low impact, and progressive treadmill training) concluded that HR may not be an appropriate

predictor of exercise intensity and that RPE is the preferred method. Finally, research (Frangolias and Rhodes 1995) suggests that using land HRs in water exercise when the chest is submerged is not an appropriate technique. There is no one test that works for all group exercise participants (see "Application of Intensity Monitoring to the Group Exercise Setting"). Many group exercise instructors have stopped using manual HR monitoring because it disrupts the flow of the class, although using a HR monitor is always an option. There are no hard and fast rules for monitoring intensity other than that it is an important responsibility of the group fitness instructor. Monitoring intensity or giving constant intensity monitoring gauges shows empathy for the participants. A summary of how to use target HR, RPE, and the talk test is given next.

Heart Rate Method

Exercise intensity within the cardiorespiratory segment must be monitored. Participants need to know the purpose of monitoring HR during exercise and information on how to obtain a pulse rate. Proper instruction on how to take a HR is the first step to monitoring intensity effectively.

The following are the recommended sites for taking HR (see figure 5.3):

- Carotid pulse site. This pulse is taken from the carotid artery just to the side of the larynx using light pressure from the fingertips of the first two fingers, not the thumb. Never palpate both carotid arteries at the same time, and always press lightly.

- Radial pulse site. This pulse is taken from the radial artery at the wrist, in line with the thumb, using the fingertips of the first two or three fingers.

Heart Rate Reserve Method

The main method recommended for determining target HR (THR) range is the HR reserve method, commonly known as the Karvonen formula (see figure 5.4). The recommended intensities for the HR reserve method (50-85%) corresponds to similar recommended percentages of maximal oxygen uptake. The HR reserve method takes into account resting heart rate when determin-

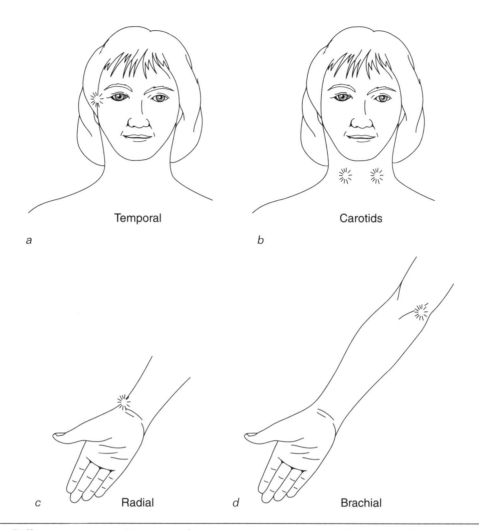

Figure 5.3 Different anatomical locations for measuring heart rate: (a) temporal, (b) carotids, (c) radial, and (d) brachial.

ing THR. It is estimated that 220 beats/min minus the age is maximal heart rate. Several new studies are challenging this, but we do not have enough data to verify the change and make new recommendations. Keep in mind that 220 minus age is only an estimate of maximal heart rate and may not be accurate for everyone. A maximal heart rate measured during a stress test must be used in this method when the participant is taking prescribed medications that alter HR. The key to this method is to take a percentage of the difference between maximal HR and resting HR and then add the resting HR to identify the THR.

Rate of Perceived Exertion

RPE is another common method of determining exercise intensity. By observing subjective perceptions of intensity, participants rate the level of steady-state work, using the 6 to 20 RPE scale or the 0 to 10 RPE scale developed by Borg (1982). Interestingly, RPE is both valid and reliable (Dunbar et al. 1992, Robertson et al. 1990) and is closely associated with increases in most cardiorespiratory parameters, including work, maximal oxygen uptake, and HR. In a group exercise setting, RPE can be used independent of, or in combination with, HR to monitor relative exercise intensity of most participants. Participants taking medication that alters HR can use the RPE scale to monitor relative exercise intensity. The verbal description that reflects the intensity of work is important when using either numerical RPE scale (see table 5.1). For example, a rating of 6 to 7 could represent the intensity of standing still, 11 could

Example: A 40-year-old participant with a resting HR of 60 beats/min who wants to exercise at 50-85% of HR reserve

Step 1: Find estimated maximal HR

- Estimated maximal HR = 220 – age
- Estimated maximal HR = 220 – 40
- Estimated maximal HR = 180 beats/min

Step 2: Find HR reserve

- HR reserve = Estimated maximal HR – resting HR
- HR reserve = 180 – 60
- HR reserve = 120 beats/min

Step 3: Find 50% of HR reserve

- 50% of HR reserve = HR reserve × 50%
- 50% of HR reserve = 120 × 50%
- 50% of HR reserve = 60 beats/min

Step 4: Find target HR range (low end of range at 50%)

- Target HR range = % of HR reserve + **resting** HR
- Target HR range = 60 + 60
- Target HR range = 120 beats/min

To find the high end of range, repeat steps 3 and 4 using the higher percentage.

Figure 5.4 Using the HR reserve method to determine target HR.

Table 5.1 Borg RPE Scale

6	No exertion at all
7	
8	Extremely light
9	Very light
10	
11	Light
12	
13	Somewhat hard
14	
15	Hard (heavy)
16	
17	Very hard
18	
19	Extremely hard
20	Maximal exertion

Borg RPE scale
© Gunnar Borg, 1970, 1985, 1994, 1998

be walking to the store, 13 could be breathing hard during an activity, and 15 could be chasing the dog down the street. Relating real tasks in life to RPE helps participants understand how they should feel.

Talk Test

The talk test is another subjective method of gauging exercise intensity and can be used as an adjunct to HR and RPE. When participants exercise, it is highly recommended that breathing be rhythmic and comfortable. Particularly for newer clients, talking while exercising can indicate whether an appropriate intensity is being achieved. If the participant is winded and needs to gasp for breath between words when conversing, then the exercise intensity is too high and should be reduced. As higher intensity activities are performed, it is expected that breathing

APPLICATION OF INTENSITY MONITORING TO THE GROUP EXERCISE SETTING

Whether you are using target HR, RPE, or the talk test to monitor exercise intensity, there are a few practical application points to remember and share within a group exercise setting. Several of these points are listed in the group exercise class evaluation form (appendix A).

- If using music and measuring HR, turn off the music so the beats do not influence the counting of HRs.
- Radial pulse is encouraged over the use of the carotid pulse: If you are using the carotid pulse, cue to press lightly to avoid reducing blood flow to the brain.
- Check intensity toward the middle of the workout so it can be modified if necessary.
- Keep participants moving to prevent blood from pooling in the lower extremities when checking intensity.
- Use a 10-s pulse count if using target HRs and start with 1.
- Give modifications based on results and encourage participants to work at their own levels.

rate will become faster and shallower. For higher fitness levels, the use of the talk test may not be appropriate.

PARTICIPANT INTERACTION AND ENJOYMENT

One reason people like to exercise in a group is because they enjoy interacting with other people. Promote participant interaction in your classes so that participants will get to know each other and reap the social benefits of exercise. Keep in mind the research quoted in chapter 1 on group cohesion—people who adhered to a program had higher levels of group cohesiveness. Group cohesiveness does not just occur but needs to be fostered with your leadership skills. Many participants derive a great deal of satisfaction and a feeling of belonging from interacting with other class members. This increase in self-esteem, through exercise and social contact, is as important as the physical changes that take place. In fact, Ornish (1998) believes that interpersonal interaction might be the single most important concept that breeds a loving and accepting environment in your program. It may be extremely important to the whole exercise experience in terms of making a difference in participants' health. Figure 5.5 outlines some suggestions for increasing interaction in your classes.

- Talk to people and call them by name.
- Introduce new people to other members of the class.
- Post your name where it's visible.
- Have people choose partners and perform hand slap activities while moving or have people introduce themselves to one another.
- Use holidays for musical themes and special activities.
- Have social gatherings before or after class.
- Keep records of birthdays. Have participants do as many seconds of a sprint on the bikes as the participant's age.
- Use partner exercises in muscle conditioning.
- Use circuit classes where participants work together in small groups.
- Use circles with participants showing or leading their favorite move.

Figure 5.5 Ideas for promoting participant interaction.

Involving your participants in this process lets them feel good about exercise and your class in general. This camaraderie makes up for the hard work of exercise. Although techniques like these are challenging and require some motivation on your part, they can make you an extraordinary instructor and help keep people coming back. If you believe in yourself and the power of exercise, it will be very easy for you to project fun and enthusiasm to all who attend your class.

POSTCARDIO COOL-DOWN

The last few minutes of any group exercise session that contains cardiorespiratory work should be less intense to allow the cardiorespiratory system to recover. Lack of a postcardio cool-down is also correlated with an increased risk of heart arrhythmias (American Council on Exercise 2000). Because metabolic waste products get trapped inside the muscle cells, many people experience increased cramping and stiffness if they do not cool down gradually. Cooling down enables waste products to disperse and the body to return to resting levels without injury. Participants also should cool down to prevent blood from pooling in the lower extremities and to allow the cardiovascular system to make the transition to more gradual workloads. This is especially important if some type of muscle work will follow the cardiorespiratory segment. During the cool-down, encourage participants to relax, slow down, keep arms below the level of the heart, and put less effort into the movements. Use less intense music, change your tone of voice, and verbalize the transition to the participants to help create this atmosphere.

Chapter Wrap-Up

Outlined in this chapter are the variables that are common to cardiorespiratory segments of most group exercise classes. Whether you are teaching a cycling, water, step, or high/low impact class, you should gradually increase intensity, vary muscle groups used, give movement options, interact with participants, monitor intensity, and lead a postcardio cool-down. We refer to these principles in the following chapters on various group exercise classes.

Written Assignment

Attend a group exercise class of your choice that contains a cardiorespiratory segment. Observe how the instructor monitors intensity. Write a reaction paper on what you observe.

Practical Assignment

Attend a group exercise class of your choice that contains a cardiorespiratory segment. Monitor your intensity every 5 min, switching between HR and RPE. Which method worked better? Why?

Muscular Conditioning

Chapter Objectives

By the end of this chapter, you will

- ■ understand basic muscle anatomy and joint actions,

- ■ be able to show exercise progressions and multiple muscle group modifications,

- ■ know a variety of muscle-conditioning exercises appropriate for the group setting,

- ■ be familiar with equipment used in group muscle conditioning,

- ■ understand basic safety issues in muscle conditioning,

- ■ be able to demonstrate exercises with proper form and alignment, and

- ■ be able to cue muscle-conditioning exercises using a variety of cues.

The development of muscle strength and endurance is essential for overall fitness and is an integral part of any group fitness program (see "Benefits of Resistance Training"). To be a competent muscle-conditioning instructor, you will need to understand basic anatomy, kinesiology (joint actions), safety and equipment issues, and appropriate cueing. You will also need to know a large variety of exercises. A few common principles guide the muscular conditioning segment of most group exercise classes. The main points on the group exercise class evaluation form (appendix A) under the muscular strength and endurance segment are found in figure 6.1.

1. Gives verbal cues on posture and alignment ❏

2. Encourages and demonstrates good body mechanics ❏

3. Observes participants' form and suggests modifications for injuries or special needs and progressions for advanced participants ❏

4. Gives clear verbal directions and uses appropriate music volume ❏

5. Uses appropriate music tempo for biomechanical movement ❏

Figure 6.1 Muscular conditioning segment of the group exercise class evaluation form.

BENEFITS OF RESISTANCE TRAINING

- Easier performance of daily activities
- Increased lean body (muscle) mass
- Increased metabolism due to increased lean body mass
- Stronger muscles, tendons, and ligaments
- Stronger bones
- Decreased risk of injury
- Decreased risk of low back pain

POSTURE AND ALIGNMENT

Because 8 of 10 Americans will have back problems during their lifetime (Frymoyer and Cats-Baril 1991), it is essential to give verbal cues on posture and spinal alignment in each segment of the class, but especially in the muscular conditioning and stretching segment. Here are some points to remember when teaching posture in a standing position (the numbers correspond to those in figure 6.2).

In the standing position:

1. Head should be suspended (not pushed back or dropped forward) with ears in line with shoulders, shoulders over hips, hips over backs of knees, and knees over ankles.

2. Arms should be relaxed and hang from the shoulder with the palms facing the sides. Have participants circle the shoulders back and down. Shoulder blades should be in a neutral position (depressed, slightly retracted).

3. Maintain the four natural curves of the spine. A decrease or increase in the low back curve changes the amount of compression forces on the spine.

4. Lightly compress the abdominal muscles to help support the spinal column, especially when lifting. Abdominal compression helps to distribute weight over the entire torso, not just the low back. Extreme abdominal compression, however, restricts breathing.

5. Pelvis may be tucked slightly for swayback individuals, pregnant women, and participants with a large protruding abdomen. Otherwise, the pelvis should be in its neutral position (neither anteriorly or posteriorly tilted).

6. Knees should be unlocked or soft. Hyperextended knees shift the pelvis anteriorly, contributing to an increased low back curve and back strain. Hyperextended knees can also gradually overstretch the knee ligaments, leading to knee joint instability.

7. Feet should be shoulder-width apart with the weight evenly distributed. Participants

who roll their feet to the inner or outer edges need to concentrate on keeping their weight over the entire bottom surface of each foot.

8. An imaginary plumb line dropped from the head should pass through the cervical and lumbar vertebrae, hips, backs of knees, and ankles.

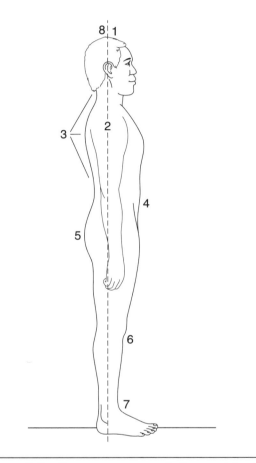

Figure 6.2 Proper posture and alignment for the back.

Giving appropriate postural and alignment cues is one of the most important aspects of the muscular conditioning portion of your class. When giving alignment cues, focus on joints: neck, spine, pelvis, scapulae, shoulders, wrists, elbows, hips, knees, and ankles. As a general rule, in most exercises, stabilizer muscles will be engaged. Give several posture cues before giving instruction on the specific muscle group to be worked. For example, when performing a latissimus dorsi strengthening exercise using exercise tubing, cue participants to soften the knees, get a good base of support with the feet apart comfortably, and contract the abdominals while keeping the spine in neutral position. Then cue the movement for the latissimus dorsi.

Encourage and Demonstrate Good Body Mechanics

It is imperative that you perform exercises correctly when giving verbal cues. If an instructor says to keep a leg movement at 45° range of motion but the instructor is lifting higher than that, this confuses the participants. Whatever instructions you give need to be duplicated in your movement example. Practice is the key to becoming an effective visual demonstrator. Work constantly on your own form and alignment so that you can be an inspiration for your class.

These are just a few ways to give participants feedback on form. Note what style of communication comes easiest to you—verbal, visual, or physical—and work on the area that is most difficult for you. Feedback is another way to learn and grow. Those of you who give a lot of feedback and regularly ask participants for feedback are providing good customer service. Practice student-centered learning as opposed to teacher-centered learning, especially in the area of verbal cues.

Observe Participants' Form and Suggest Modifications for Special Needs

A big difference between the teacher-centered instructor and the student-centered instructor is that the student-centered instructor helps individual participants to make exercise safe and less painful or problematic. To facilitate this, you must observe your participants and understand their problems and limitations.

In addition to knowing the basic exercises, skilled instructors are familiar with a wide variety of modifications, enabling them to give appropriate exercises for every person in their class. If a participant complains that his knee, shoulder, back, or any other body part hurts in an exercise, you need to either modify the exercise so he'll be more comfortable or give him a completely different exercise for the same muscle group. For example, a student tells you her wrists hurt when she does push-ups. You can suggest that she try the push-up either up on her fists or fingers or with her hands curled around sturdy dumbbells, all of which help to keep her wrists in a straight line and may alleviate the problem. Or you might suggest she try push-ups on the wall, where she has to lift less of her body weight. If none of these options relieves the pain, suggest an alternative exercise, such as a bench press, which still targets the chest muscles. As always, if her wrists still hurt and if she hasn't sought medical help, recommend that she see her physician.

In the functional training continuum, discussed in chapter 3, exercises for a particular muscle group are ordered from easiest to hardest. As a participant continually improves his strength and endurance, harder and harder exercises can be selected. Or, conversely, if you are giving an exercise from the more difficult end of the continuum and you notice that a participant is having trouble performing the exercise correctly, you simply move back down the continuum toward the easier end, helping the participant to find either a modification or a different exercise that she can do safely with good form.

We encourage all group exercise instructors to get out on the floor to observe and assist. Demonstrate a move, perform a few repetitions, and then begin watching participants or move around the room while demonstrating. When you stay in one place, this only gives your participants one frame of reference. Plus, coaching participants is a large part of the group exercise experience: When the instructor is nearby and observing, participants listen and perform more effectively. Coaching skill is important to all segments of the class and needs to be evaluated throughout the class. Allow participants to see that you have empathy as well as the knowledge to modify problematic exercises.

INTENSITY

Most group exercise instructors include some form of muscle strength and endurance training and flexibility training in their classes. To promote total fitness, you must include exercises for maintaining muscular strength, endurance, and tone as well as exercises for flexibility and cardiorespiratory fitness. The ACSM (1998) position

stand on the recommended quantity and quality of exercise for developing muscular strength and endurance in adults is as follows:

Resistance Training should be progressive in nature, individualized, and provide a stimulus to all the major muscle groups. One set of 8-10 exercises that conditions the major muscle groups 2-3 days per week is recommended. Mutiple-set regimens may provide greater benefits if time allows. Most persons should complete 8-12 repetitions of each exercise; however, for older and more frail persons (appropriately 50-60 years of age or above), 10-15 repetitions may be more appropriate.

According to Feigenbaum and Pollock (1997), single-set programs performed a minimum of two times per week are recommended over multiple-set programs because they are less time-consuming, are more cost-efficient, and produce most of the health and fitness benefits. The National Strength and Conditioning Association (NSCA) adds that training should occur at least 3 days/week, with a minimum of 24 hr rest between training sessions (Pearson et al. 2000). Westcott (2000) found that subjects who trained once and twice a week showed 73% as much strength gain as those who trained 3 days per week. The bottom line is that strength training is an important health-related component of fitness and needs to be included in group exercise instruction. This is not always easy to do in the group setting, because you may not have access to heavier weights.

Students in the group setting often ask the following question: "How many sit-ups (curl-ups, leg lifts) should I do?" The answer is, "It depends." You want to do as many as you can with good form and alignment until you reach the point of fatigue (not total muscle failure). The exact number varies from exercise to exercise and from person to person. Also, the harder the exercise, and the harder you push yourself during the exercise, the more quickly you'll reach the point of fatigue. (For example, the intensity in an abdominal curl-up can be varied by changing the lever length: Holding the arms at the sides while curling up is biomechanically easier than placing the arms overhead.) This means you'll do fewer repetitions than someone performing an easier modification or someone who is not pushing him- or herself.

How is intensity increased in the group exercise setting? There are at least three ways:

1. In group exercise, the intensity can be increased by having your students focus on conscious muscle contraction with each repetition. This is similar to the tension that can be created when one is isometrically contracting a muscle. Most people, if asked, can "squeeze" their biceps while holding their elbow at a fixed angle. Imagine continuing to squeeze the biceps muscle (hard!) while moving the elbow through its full range of motion. This is what we mean by conscious muscle contraction, and it's a great technique to teach your students. In addition to helping increase the intensity, conscious muscle contractions promote increased body awareness and better alignment.

2. Various resistance devices are also used to increase intensity and provide overload. These include dumbbells, Body Bars, barbells, elastic tubing, and elastic bands. Steps can be inclined or declined to increase the resistance, depending on the exercise. Stability balls can significantly increase the potential for overload in a wide variety of exercises as well. Resistance in water exercise can be increased with aquatic gloves, dumbbells, barbells, paddles, fins, elastic bands and tubes, and buoyancy boots. Because it is impractical to supply a wide range of dumbbells or weight plates in the group setting, most facilities stock dumbbells for groups only up to 8 or 10 lb. This means that you must be more creative to provide sufficient overload for more advanced participants.

3. Another important option for overload is to change the mode (Yoke and Kennedy 2004). In group resistance training, this means progressing from easier exercises to harder (compound) exercises. To do this you need a comprehensive knowledge of a wide variety of exercise choices for all major muscle groups, and you must be able to evaluate whether an exercise is appropriate for someone who is deconditioned or whether it is appropriate only for the very fit. Many exercises, such as the push-up, have several variations. For example, push-up modifications from easiest to hardest include wall push-up, hands and knees (tabletop) push-up, knee push-up with hands on step, knee push-up with hands on floor, knee push-up with knees elevated on step, full body push-up with hands on step, full body push-up with hands on floor, and full body push-up with feet on step. A competent instructor will be able to show these modifications and help participants determine which one is right for them.

Another alternative that instructors commonly use is to increase the duration or to encourage more repetitions. Although this may be appropriate in some classes, we advise you to be cautious with this approach. It's hard to adequately challenge 8 to 10 major muscle groups in a 1-hr class with a cardio component if large numbers of repetitions are given for each exercise.

We often stretch a muscle group immediately after strengthening to promote relative balance between flexibility and strength for a particular group of muscles. For specific flexibility exercises by muscle group, see chapter 7. Coupling a strengthening and endurance exercise with a stretching exercise ensures that you have included both aspects in your class format and promotes the optimal benefit of each.

See the DVD for muscular conditioning progression options and instructor cueing on the following exercises: squats, bent-over row, push-ups, and abdominal exercises on a stability ball and a Bosu.

SAFETY ISSUES

Safety should be a major concern when you are leading a group fitness class. In general, you need to be more cautious and conservative in your muscle conditioning programming than would a personal trainer. Responsible personal trainers take thorough health histories on all their clients, require physicians' clearances when appropriate, and create individualized programs that account for each client's unique musculoskeletal needs and peculiarities. Group leaders, in contrast, usually don't have the luxury of individually assessing each participant in their class and creating programs specifically for each. Ideally, each exercise that is given in a class is safe for everyone in that class, including beginners or deconditioned members. Modifications can be shown for more fit students, although after demonstrating an advanced modification, you should return to the variation of the exercise that best fits the majority of your participants and continue to

KEY DEFINITIONS

Stress Adaptation

Increasing the intensity of the workout by increasing the number of repetitions or the amount resistance should be gradual and progressive. Sudden increases in intensity (e.g., doubling the number of repetitions or resistance) could result in muscle damage. Cue and instruct your participants so that musculoskeletal stress adaptation can occur: "Add 1 to 2 lb if you are able to perform 15 or more repetitions." "Go to the next thickness of rubber band and decrease your number of repetitions."

Rebuilding Time

When a muscle is stressed beyond its normal limitations, time is needed for repair, recovery, and positive physiological change. Generally, 1 to 2 days (24-48 hr) is required, so resistance and particularly strength training should be performed every other day. Training can occur daily, but different muscle groups need to be emphasized, especially if intensity is high.

Controlled Speed of Movement

Slow, smooth, and controlled movement ensures consistent application of force throughout the range of motion. Keep in mind that the use of faster music tempos (≥130 beats/min) increases momentum and the risk of injury. Slower music tempos (~116 beats/min) demand control and strength. If you want to progress a class, use slower music tempos as the class session proceeds.

Full Range of Motion

Use the full range of motion of the muscle and joint structure to help preserve flexibility. Training the muscles and tendons through a greater range of motion enables more muscle fibers to perform work. "Pulsing" (or performing only a limited range of motion) is discouraged unless limited range of motion is your goal, as in some abdominal work. Limited range of motion may be appropriate for rehabilitation or to avoid injury: for example, perform partial range of motion during weight training to help an injured rotator cuff to heal.

Training Specificity

To increase muscle endurance, train with less resistance and more repetitions. If you want to increase muscle strength, emphasize weight or resistance and decrease repetitions. Individuals who need equal amounts of strength and endurance (triathletes) may have a difficult time training to meet and maintain both of these demands.

demonstrate that variation. The reason for this is that most students will try to copy whatever the instructor is demonstrating, even though that particular variation may be inappropriate for them. (Participants will also unconsciously copy your form and alignment, so always demonstrate all exercises with excellent alignment.)

Here are some injury prevention basics:

1. The major cause of exercise-related injury is too much, too soon. Students must progress gradually to harder, more intense exercises and longer durations. Your exercise choices must be appropriate for the students in your class. This means that you must be prepared to alter your class plan on a moment's notice, depending on the fitness levels and skills of the participants who have shown up. Experienced instructors have a large repertoire of exercises and exercise modifications that can be used to reformat or even individualize a class on the spot.

2. Follow the tenets of good technique and correct alignment. These include avoiding

- hyperextended knees or elbows,
- excessive use of momentum,
- inappropriate torque (a rotational, twisting force applied to a joint), and
- hyperflexing the knee (bending past 90°) in a weight-bearing position.

Also, always maintain a neutral spine, pelvis, neck, scapulae, and wrists.

3. Avoid risky moves and follow industry guidelines with regard to high-risk exercises to protect your students and yourself. Moves that have been considered higher risk include

- deep squats (hips drop below knees),
- extreme lumbar hyperextension,
- cervical spinal hyperextension,
- unsupported forward flexion of the lumbar spine,
- unsupported forward flexion with rotation,
- unsupported lateral spinal flexion,
- hurdler's stretch,
- full sit-ups,
- double-leg raises,
- deadlifts, and
- good mornings (Yoke 2001).

For the average class participant interested in health-related fitness, the risk of performing these exercises outweighs any potential benefit. Always consider the risk to benefit ratio.

4. Encourage your participants to listen to their bodies, noting twinges or slight annoyances, which can be warning signals of future injury. Most participants have heard the saying, "No pain, no gain" and often think that if they don't hurt after an exercise session, it wasn't a good workout. No pain, no gain may be appropriate for athletes during competition but is completely inappropriate in a group health and fitness setting. Educate your students about the difference between muscle soreness and joint pain. Muscle soreness usually disappears after 24 to 48 hr and may be acceptable for some of your students who want to challenge themselves. Joint pain, however, is never OK and is a sign that something is wrong. Teach your students to distinguish the difference and stop whatever exercise or activity is causing joint pain. Remember, if there is pain, there is little gain!

MUSCLE-CONDITIONING EXERCISES

In this section we examine the major muscles, joint by joint, and include strengthening exercises with verbal cues for each. We have also included tables in appendix F listing the specific muscles for each area and their actions.

Shoulder Joint

Table 6.1 lists some muscles of the shoulder joint, the actions of those muscles, activities that use those muscles, and strengthening exercises. Figure 6.3 shows the major shoulder joint muscles, and figures 6.4 through 6.19 demonstrate exercises for the shoulder joint.

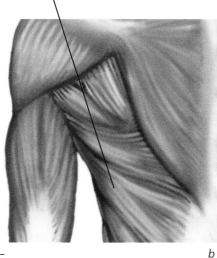
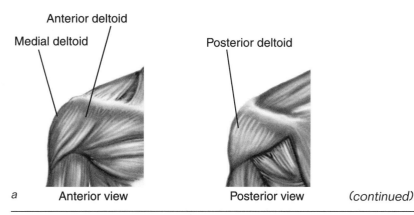

a   Anterior view   Posterior view   *(continued)*

b

Figure 6.3   Shoulder joint muscles: *(a)* anterior, medial, and posterior deltoids; *(b)* latissimus dorsi;

Adapted, by permission, NSCA, 2000, The biomechanics of resistance exercise. In *NSCA's essentials of strength training and conditioning*, edited by T. Baechle and R. Earle (Champaign, IL: Human Kinetics), 29.

Shoulder Joint

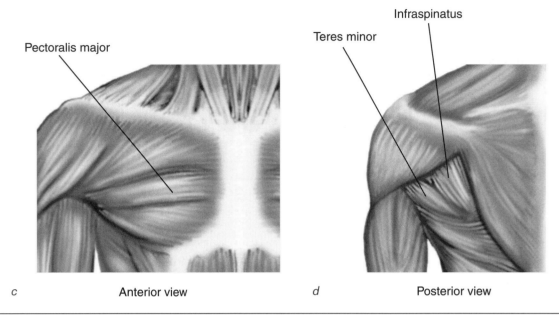

c	Anterior view	d	Posterior view

Figure 6.3 Shoulder joint muscles *(continued)*: *(c)* pectoralis major; and *(d)* external rotator cuff.

Adapted, by permission, NSCA, 2000, The biomechanics of resistance exercise. In *NSCA's essentials of strength training and conditioning*, edited by T. Baechle and R. Earle (Champaign, IL: Human Kinetics), 29.

Table 6.1 Shoulder Joint Muscles

Muscle	Joint actions	Daily activities	Exercises for groups
Anterior and medial deltoid	Shoulder: flexion, abduction, horizontal adduction	Lifting and carrying, pushing items up overhead	Front raise, lateral raise, overhead press, upright row
Latissimus dorsi	Shoulder: extension, adduction	Pulling items toward you, lifting	Bent-over low row, bent-over shoulder extension, seated low row, unilateral adduction with tube
Pectoralis major	Shoulder: horizontal adduction, flexion	Pushing items in front of you, lifting, throwing	Push-up, bench press, dumbbell fly, standing chest press with tube
Posterior deltoid (works with scapular retractors)	Shoulder: horizontal abduction, extension	Pulling items toward you, lifting	Bent-over high row, reverse fly, prone dorsal lifts, seated high row
Four rotator cuff muscles (supraspinatus, subscapularis, infraspinatus, teres minor)	Shoulder: internal and external rotation, abduction	Opening and closing doors, stabilizes the shoulder joint	Side-lying external shoulder rotation, supine internal rotation, standing rotation with tube

See appendix F, table F.1 for a complete list of shoulder joint muscles and their joint actions.

FRONT RAISE

Anterior deltoid, clavicular pectoralis major (shoulder flexion)

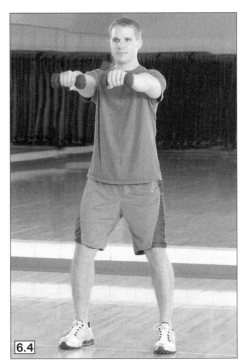

Cues: Stand (or sit on a step or stability ball). Feet are shoulder-width apart, knees slightly bent, and neck, spine, and pelvis in neutral. Elbows are straight but not hyperextended. Shoulder blades are down and slightly retracted (neutral position). Wrists are straight throughout. Palms are down (pronated). Keep torso stable while flexing shoulders to about shoulder height (90°). Avoid momentum.

FYI: Consider limiting the use of this exercise in a group. The reason is that the anterior muscles are much more frequently challenged by everyday activities (and in high/low and step classes) than the posterior muscles. Dumbbells, barbell, or tubing may be used. This exercise may be performed bilaterally or unilaterally, with the unilateral version being safer for the back.

LATERAL RAISE

Medial deltoid, supraspinatus (shoulder abduction)

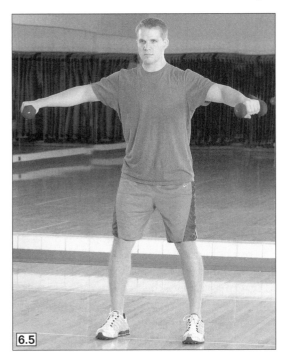

Cues: Stand (or sit on step or stability ball). Feet are shoulder-width apart with the knees slightly flexed. Maintain the neck, spine, and pelvis in neutral. In addition, the scapulae should be in neutral (down and slightly retracted). Wrists should also be neutral (neither flexed nor extended). Elbows may be bent at 90° for a short lever variation or held nearly straight (flexed at about 15°) for the more traditional long lever version (long lever is more difficult). Palms face the sides (midpronated position) at the start of the exercise and maintain this position throughout, thumbs facing straight ahead. As the shoulders abduct, stay in partial shoulder internal rotation, lifting to no more than 90°. At the end of the movement, the shoulders should be slightly higher than the elbows, which should be slightly higher than the wrists.

FYI: It is particularly important to avoid momentum and to avoid bringing the arms higher than the shoulders (they should not abduct any higher than 90°). Both of these actions can cause shoulder impingement. Lateral raises can be performed with dumbbells or tubing.

Shoulder Joint

OVERHEAD PRESS

Medial and anterior deltoids, supraspinatus, triceps (shoulder abduction, elbow extension)

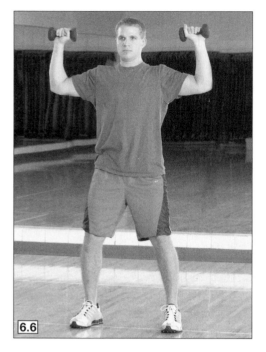

6.6

Cues: Stand (or sit on bench or stability ball). Feet are shoulder-width apart for stability, knees are soft, and spine, neck, and pelvis are in neutral. Shoulder girdle is down and slightly retracted (neutral). Start in the down position with the palms facing forward (pronated) and the hands slightly wider than the shoulders. When pressing up, make sure the elbows straighten without locking (hyperextending). Keep the chest lifted and avoid leaning backward.

FYI: This exercise can be performed with dumbbells, barbell, or tubing. The press should be performed in front of the head to minimize injury to the shoulder joint. (The behind-the-neck press has become controversial because of the vulnerable shoulder position of external rotation behind the frontal plane and the increased risk of injury.) This exercise may be performed unilaterally or bilaterally.

UPRIGHT ROW

Medial and anterior deltoids, supraspinatus, biceps brachii (shoulder abduction, elbow flexion)

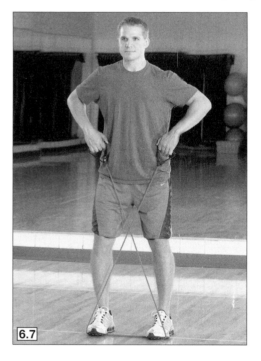

6.7

Optional: upper trapezius, rhomboids, and levator scapulae; scapular elevation

Cues: Stand with feet shoulder-width apart, knees flexed, and spine, neck, and pelvis in neutral. Hands are pronated (overhand grip) and about 6 to 8 in. apart. Lead with the elbows (not the wrists), and do not lift elbows above shoulders. Wrists stay as neutral as possible (watch for the tendency to flex wrists, increasing the risk of wrist and elbow injuries). Avoid momentum.

FYI: The upright row has become somewhat controversial because of concerns about shoulder joint injury. Because the exercise is performed while the shoulders are internally rotated, it is very important that the elbows do not come higher than the shoulders (no more than 90° of abduction) because of the risk of shoulder joint impingement. Even though the traditional weight room variation of the upright row includes shoulder girdle elevation, we do not recommend this for the general public or for group exercise. From a functional perspective, most fitness and health exercisers need to strengthen the muscles required to keep the scapulae down, not up. Therefore, scapular elevation can be considered an optional movement in an upright row. This exercise may be performed with dumbbells, barbell, or tubing.

BENT-OVER ROW

Latissimus dorsi, teres major, posterior deltoid, biceps brachii
(shoulder extension, elbow flexion)

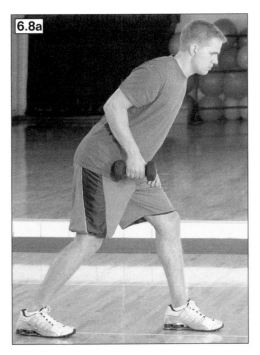

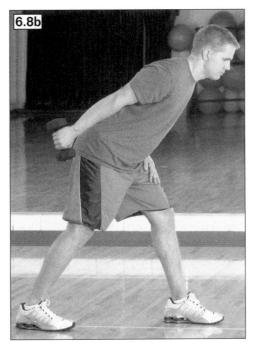

Note: Middle trapezius and rhomboids are strong stabilizers because of the antigravity position. If the exercise is performed bilaterally, the erector spinae and abdominals are very important stabilizers of the spine.

Cues: Stand with feet staggered and the nonworking hand placed on the front thigh (front knee bent) for support. All joints face the same direction, with the hips and shoulders evenly squared and level. Ideally, one long line is created from the back heel to the top of the head. The spine is in neutral, with no rounding or hunching of the upper back. The neck continues the line of the spine with no ducking toward the weight. The arm starts in a hanging position with the elbow straight down, perpendicular to the floor, then moves into the up position shown in figure 6.8a. Keep scapulae stabilized in neutral; do not protract or retract with the exercise. The only moving joints are the working-side shoulder and elbow during the row; all else is kept still. The moving arm brushes against the rib cage. Avoid rotating the spine when lifting the weight. Keep shoulders level throughout (see the concentric phase in figure 6.8a).

FYI: This exercise is one of the best choices for lat work in group exercise. However, we recommend performing it unilaterally. Although the bilateral version is an excellent exercise, it is quite unlikely that every student in a group class will be able to correctly stabilize the spine and maintain proper alignment. This exercise may be performed with dumbbells or tubing or, for advanced participants, both dumbbells and tubing. Another variation is *long lever shoulder extension* (elbow held straight through the movement), the up, or concentric, phase of which is shown in figure 6.8b.

Shoulder Joint

SEATED LOW ROW

Latissimus dorsi, teres major, sternal pectoralis major, posterior deltoid, biceps brachii
(shoulder extension, elbow flexion)

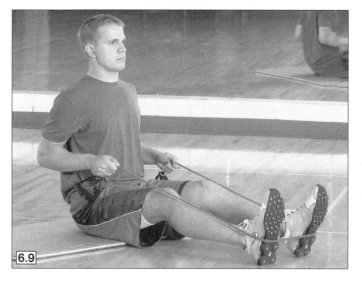

Cues: Sitting on the floor (or step), bend knees slightly to help ensure that the pelvis and spine are aligned directly over the "sitting bones" (ischial tuberosities). Hold the spine erect and tall, maintaining neutral alignment throughout. Keep neck in line with the spine, scapulae down and away from the ears. Move the arms through the sagittal plane, keeping the upper arms close to the rib cage. Hold the handles of the tubing in a midpronated position (palms face each other). Move only the shoulders and elbows, keeping the lower back still.

UNILATERAL LAT PULL-DOWN

Latissimus dorsi, teres major, sternal pectoralis major, biceps brachii
(shoulder adduction, elbow flexion)

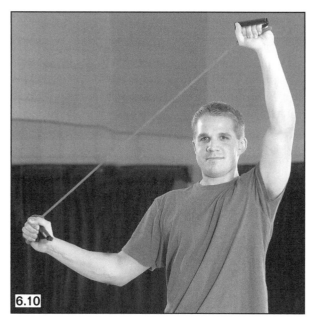

Cues: Stand with feet shoulder-width apart for stability. Spine, neck, and pelvis are in neutral. Grasp the tubing or band with one hand, keeping it anchored overhead. Perform the pull-down with the other hand, keeping the shoulder blades down and the head high. Release the tubing or band upward slowly, with control.

FYI: Without a high pulley (found in most weight rooms), the only way to make this exercise effective in the group setting is to use elastic resistance. Although some instructors try to duplicate the pull-down exercise with dumbbells, the muscles actually resisting gravity's pull when holding free weights are the deltoids, not the lats.

CHEST FLY

Pectoralis major, anterior deltoid (shoulder horizontal adduction)

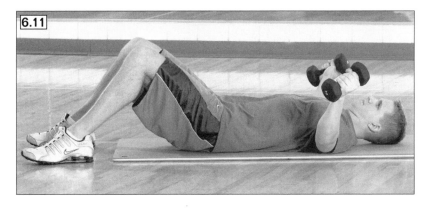

6.11

Cues: Lie supine, with feet flat on floor or bench and knees bent. Keep the neck, spine, and pelvis in neutral alignment. Start in the up position, with elbows just slightly flexed. Palms can be either pronated or midpronated (facing each other). Moving only the shoulder joints, stabilize the elbows, wrists, scapulae, spine, and pelvis. Lower until the upper arms are parallel with the chest, being especially careful not to exceed the appropriate end range of motion, which can lead to shoulder injury.

FYI: This exercise is performed with dumbbells and can be inclined or declined on a step. Another variation is the short lever fly, or pec dec, in which the elbows are flexed at a 90° angle.

BENCH/CHEST PRESS

Pectoralis major, anterior deltoid, triceps (shoulder horizontal adduction, elbow extension)

Cues: Lie supine on floor or bench with knees bent and feet on floor. Keep spine, neck, and pelvis in neutral, abdominals engaged. Use a wide, pronated grip. Stabilize all joints, including the scapulae, wrists, and spine while the shoulders and elbows move. Upper arm is angled 80° to 90° out from torso, and forearms are perpendicular to the floor. Keep the movement slow and controlled, avoiding a sudden descent. If on a step, avoid letting the elbows drop too far below the bench, to decrease shoulder joint stress. Avoid rolling the wrist, arching the back, and hyperextending the elbows.

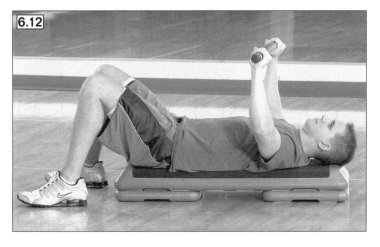

6.12

FYI: The more narrow the grip, the more the triceps are involved and the less the chest is involved. This exercise can be performed with dumbbells or a bar and may be inclined or declined on a step. If the bench press is performed while the participant is lying supine on the floor, note that the floor interferes with full range of motion.

Shoulder Joint

PUSH-UP

Pectoralis major, anterior deltoid, triceps (shoulder horizontal adduction, elbow extension)

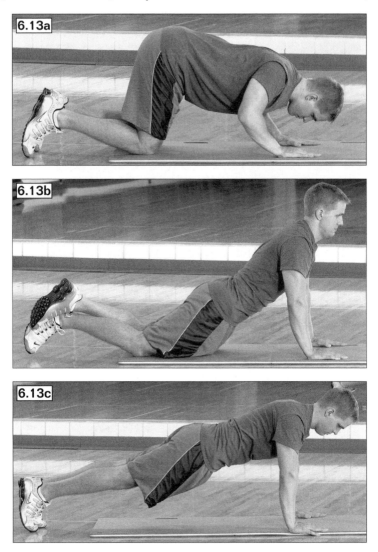

6.13a

6.13b

6.13c

Note: There are several important stabilizers—abdominals, erector spinae, gluteus maximus, trapezius, rhomboids, serratus anterior, and pectoralis minor.

Cues: Keep head, neck, spine, and pelvis in neutral. Head and neck continue the line of the spine. In all positions except tabletop, the hips are in neutral as well (in tabletop, the hips are flexed at 90°). Fingers point straight ahead to minimize wrist stress; hands are slightly wider than shoulders with upper arms perpendicular to torso (in the horizontal plane). The only moving joints are the shoulders and elbows; all other joints are stabilized. This is very important for injury prevention. Avoid sagging through the back, hyperextending the elbows, or hyperextending the cervical vertebrae. Exhale on the way up.

FYI: Push-ups are a good option for chest work in the group setting. Always show at least three variations to accommodate varying ability levels. Here are a few variations, listed from easiest to hardest: wall push-up, tabletop push-up (figure 6.13a), knee (intermediate) push-up with hands on step, knee push-up with hands on floor (figure 6.13b), knee push-up with knees on step and hands on floor (decline), full body push-up with hands on step, full body push-up with hands on floor (figure 6.13c), full body push-up with feet on step, and full body push-up on one leg. The closer the elbows are to the ribs, the more the exercise becomes a triceps push-up and the less it challenges the chest muscles.

STANDING CHEST PRESS

Pectoralis major, anterior deltoid, triceps (shoulder horizontal adduction, elbow extension)

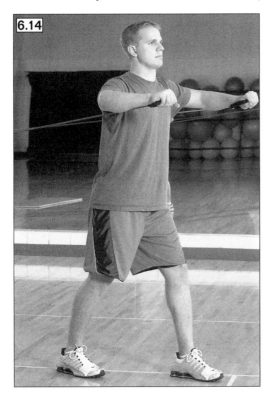

Cues: Stand with feet either parallel and shoulder-width apart or staggered and hip-width apart. Loop tube or band around a ballet barre or hook and face away from the barre, grasping ends of the tube or band in the hands with the elastic under the arms. Place spine, neck, pelvis, scapulae, and wrists in neutral; contract abdominals. Moving only the shoulders and elbows, exhale and perform a pressing motion directly away from the anchor point. Stabilize the entire torso throughout.

FYI: For an ideal line of pull and optimal muscle recruitment, the tube or band must be anchored behind the body on a stationary object; wrapping the elastic behind the back reduces the exercise effectiveness. Traditional standing chest exercises with dumbbells are not an effective choice because gravity's pull is not directly opposing the muscle action. (The muscles holding the arms up against gravity in these exercises are the deltoids; the chest muscles actually do very little work.)

SCAPULAR RETRACTION PRONE (DORSAL LIFTS)

**Middle trapezius, rhomboids, posterior deltoids
(scapular retraction, shoulder horizontal abduction)**

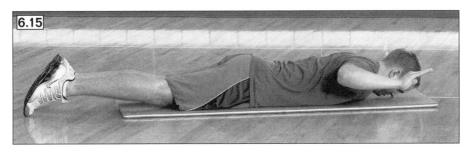

Cues: Lie prone on the floor (or on a step), with the forehead down and the neck in line with the spine. Place arms on the floor with the upper arms at a 90° angle to the torso and the elbows flexed at 90°. Place palms down on the floor. Retract the scapulae together, pulling the shoulder blades toward each other. Keep your forehead on the floor and your neck and spine in neutral. Be sure to lift your elbows up toward the ceiling, not back toward your hips.

FYI: This exercise requires no equipment other than a mat and can make a great superset when alternated with sets of push-ups. Most participants will have a small range of motion in this position and will be unable to lift much more than the weight of their arms. Even so, prone scapular retraction is an excellent exercise for posture correction and education.

Shoulder Joint

SEATED HIGH (HORIZONTAL) ROW

**Middle trapezius, rhomboids, posterior deltoids, biceps brachii
(scapular retraction, shoulder horizontal abduction, elbow flexion)**

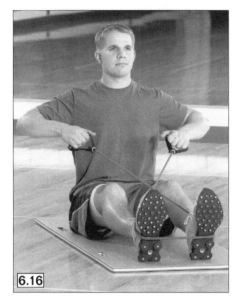

6.16

Cues: Sit on the floor with the hips flexed at 90° and spine and neck in neutral. Keep knees slightly bent to help keep torso aligned over the sitting bones. Wrap the tubing around your feet and grasp the handles with your palms down (pronated). Start with your elbows extended and arms in the horizontal plane in front of your chest. Row your elbows back (keeping them in the horizontal plane, parallel to the floor) and consciously retract your shoulder blades together. Keep wrists straight and avoid rocking the lower spine.

FYI: Do not confuse this exercise with a low row, which targets the latissimus dorsi. In a high row, the arms are held up in the horizontal plane just slightly below the shoulders. A standard row can be performed, or, for variety, try a 4-count row: pull back on 1, retract the shoulder blades on 2, release the shoulder blades on 3, and release the row on 4; use a tube or band.

REVERSE FLY

**Middle trapezius, rhomboids, posterior deltoid
(scapular retraction, shoulder horizontal abduction)**

6.17

Cues: Choose whichever standing bent-over position feels the most comfortable: feet shoulder-width apart and parallel with one hand on thigh, or feet staggered with one hand on the front thigh. Square the hips and shoulders and place the spine and neck in neutral alignment, with shoulders and shoulder girdle pressed down, away from the ears. With working arm perpendicular to torso, lift backward toward ceiling, finishing the move with the scapula moving toward the spine (retraction). Only the scapula and shoulder joint move; the spine, neck, hips, elbow, and wrist remain perfectly still. Consciously contract the rear deltoid, middle trapezius, and rhomboids.

FYI: May be performed with dumbbells, band, or tube. Bilateral (both arms moving) bent-over reverse flys are not recommended for most group exercise classes. Most participants are unable to properly stabilize the torso and maintain strongly contracted abdominal and erector spinae muscles. Bent-over movements performed unilaterally with one hand on the thigh (supporting the spine) are much less risky. This exercise may also be performed in the half-kneeling position or prone on a step.

BENT-OVER HIGH ROW

**Middle trapezius, rhomboids, posterior deltoid, biceps brachii
(scapular retraction, shoulder horizontal abduction, elbow flexion)**

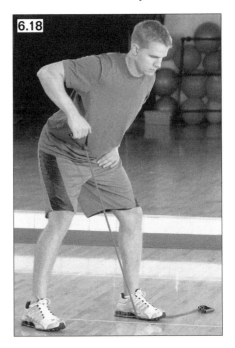

6.18

Cues: Choose whichever standing bent-over position feels the most comfortable: feet shoulder-width apart and parallel with one hand on thigh, or feet staggered with one hand on the front thigh. Square the hips and shoulders and place the spine and neck in neutral alignment, with the shoulders and shoulder girdle pressed down, away from the ears. With working arm perpendicular to torso, lift elbow backward toward ceiling, finishing the move with the scapula moving toward the spine (retraction). Only the scapula, shoulder joint, and elbow move; the spine, neck, hips, and wrist remain perfectly still. Consciously contract the rear deltoid, middle trapezius, and rhomboids.

FYI: This exercise may be performed with dumbbells, barbell, band, or tubing. Do not confuse this exercise with a low row, which targets the latissimus dorsi. In a high row, the arms are held in the horizontal plane just slightly below the shoulders. For variety, try a 4-count row: pull back on 1, retract the shoulder blade on 2, release the shoulder blade on 3, release the row and return to start on 4. As discussed in the reverse fly, be very cautious with bilateral bent-over high rows in the group setting.

STANDING SHOULDER EXTERNAL ROTATION

Infraspinatus, teres minor (shoulder external rotation)

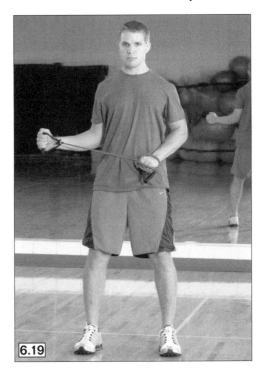

6.19

Cues: Stand with feet shoulder-width apart; place spine, neck, and pelvis in neutral alignment. Keep shoulder blades down and slightly retracted (neutral scapulae). Anchor the tube by holding it on the opposite hip with the nonworking hand. Flex the elbow on the working side at 90° and grasp the tube or band. Hold the upper arm close to the side of the body and move the forearm to the side, externally rotating the shoulder joint (as if you were opening a door). Keep your forearm parallel to the floor and maintain a neutral wrist. Move slowly and with control.

FYI: External rotator cuff strengthening is important to counteract the large forces generated by the powerful internal rotator muscles of the shoulder. These muscles include the subscapularis, teres major, pectoralis major, anterior deltoids, latissimus dorsi, and biceps brachii. Strong external rotator muscles help to maintain proper function of the shoulder joint and decrease the risk of injury. We recommend occasionally incorporating this exercise into your class.

Shoulder Girdle Joint

Key shoulder girdle muscles are also worked in the prone scapular retraction exercise, seated high row, reverse fly, and bent-over high rows just described. Keeping these muscles strong is very important for good posture. Additionally, scapular shrugs and dips may be used to train the muscles responsible for shoulder girdle elevation and depression (with depression exercise having the most importance functionally of the two). Figure 6.20 illustrates some muscles of the shoulder girdle. Table 6.2 lists some muscles of the shoulder girdle, the actions of those muscles, activities that use those muscles, and strengthening exercises.

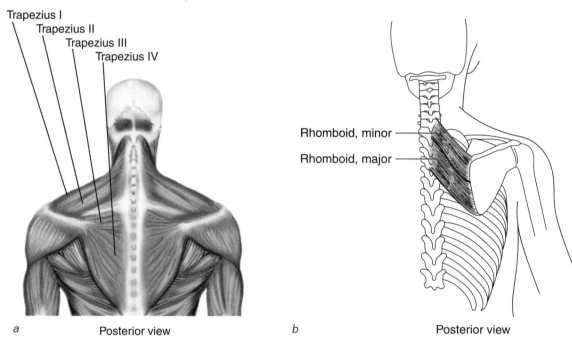

Trapezius I
Trapezius II
Trapezius III
Trapezius IV

a   Posterior view

Rhomboid, minor
Rhomboid, major

b   Posterior view

Figure 6.20   Important shoulder girdle muscles: *(a)* posterior view including trapezius I, II, III, and IV and *(b)* rhomboids.

Adapted, by permission, NSCA, 2000, The biomechanics of resistance exercise. In *NSCA's essentials of strength training and conditioning*, edited by T. Baechle and R. Earle (Champaign, IL: Human Kinetics), 29.

Table 6.2   Shoulder Girdle (Scapulothoracic) Joint Muscles

Muscle	Joint actions	Daily activities	Exercises
Trapezius I and II	Scapular elevation	Holding phone to ear	Shrugs
Trapezius III and rhomboids	Scapular retraction	Posture stabilizer	High rows, reverse flys, prone dorsal lifts, seated high row
Trapezius IV	Scapular depression	Stabilizer when pushing out of a chair	Resisted depression in a dip position

See appendix F, table F.2 for a complete list of shoulder girdle muscles and their joint actions.

Elbow Joint

The major muscles of the elbow joint are illustrated in figure 6.21. Figures 6.22 through 6.28 demonstrate exercises for the elbow joint. Table 6.3 lists the major muscles of the elbow joint, the actions of those muscles, activities that use those muscles, and strengthening exercises.

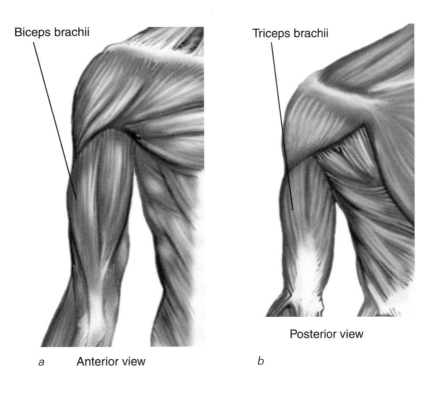

Biceps brachii

Triceps brachii

a   Anterior view   *b*   Posterior view

Figure 6.21   Elbow joint muscles: *(a)* biceps brachii and *(b)* triceps brachii.

Adapted, by permission, NSCA, 2000, The biomechanics of resistance exercise. In *NSCA's essentials of strength training and conditioning,* edited by T. Baechle and R. Earle (Champaign, IL: Human Kinetics), 29.

Table 6.3   Elbow Joint Muscles

Muscle	Joint actions	Daily activities	Exercises
Biceps brachii, brachialis, brachioradialis	Elbow flexion	Carrying, lifting	Biceps curls, concentration curls, hammer curls, reverse curls
Triceps brachii	Elbow extension	Getting in and out of chairs, throwing balls	Dips, kickbacks, press-downs with tube, supine elbow extensions

See appendix F, table F.3 for a complete list of elbow and radioulnar joint muscles and their actions.

Elbow Joint

ALTERNATE DUMBBELL BICEPS CURL

Biceps brachii, brachialis, brachioradialis, optional supinator (elbow flexion, optional radioulnar joint supination)

6.22

Cues: Stand with feet shoulder-width apart, knees flexed, and the spine, neck, and pelvis in neutral. Press the shoulders down and slightly back (neutral scapulae). Hold upper arms close to the ribs (shoulder joints are neutral), palms facing outer thighs. Curl first one arm and then the other, smoothly supinating the palms (palms face up) at the end range of motion. Keep hands as relaxed as possible, maintaining tension in the biceps. Wrists stay in complete neutral (no active wrist flexion or extension). Control the movement on the way down, avoiding elbow hyperextension and returning the palms to the mid-pronated position (facing the thighs).

FYI: This exercise may be performed standing or seated on a step. Dumbbells or tubing may be used. Supinating the wrist (palm facing upward at the end of the range of motion) is optional. Other variations include maintaining supination throughout and holding tubing, dumbbells, or a barbell and performing the exercise bilaterally, without alternation. Hammer curls (palms stay in midpronated position throughout) or reverse curls (palms are pronated and facing down throughout) are additional exercises that challenge the biceps, brachialis, and brachioradialis.

CONCENTRATION CURL

Biceps brachii, brachialis, brachioradialis (elbow flexion)

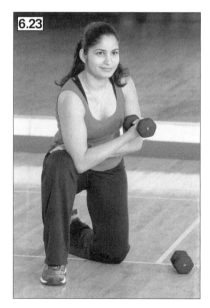
6.23

Cues: Half-kneel with one knee on the floor and the other foot on the floor, knee bent at 90°. Place the elbow of the working arm slightly inside the thigh while placing the opposite hand behind the elbow for support. Hinge forward from the hips, maintaining a neutral spine and neck, with shoulders down. Flex the elbow, moving the weight diagonally across the body, keeping the wrist neutral. Slowly return, keeping the elbow from locking (hyperextending).

FYI: This exercise may also be performed seated on a step with a dumbbell.

SUPINE TRICEPS EXTENSION

Triceps (elbow extension)

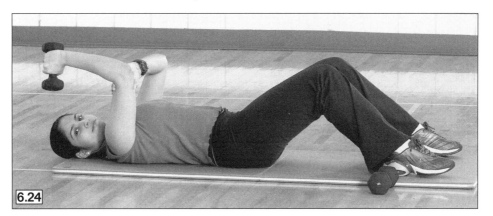

6.24

Cues: Lie supine on the floor or on a step. Keep knees bent with the spine and neck in neutral and abdominals contracted. Flexing the shoulder of the working arm, point the elbow straight up to the ceiling with the hand near the side of the head. Smoothly extend the elbow, contracting the triceps. Without flaring the elbow, carefully lower the dumbbell back to starting position. Keep upper arm still throughout.

FYI: This exercise may be performed unilaterally (one arm), which is the easiest variation; bilaterally holding a dumbbell in each hand or holding a single heavier dumbbell in both hands; or bilaterally holding a barbell (hardest variation).

TRICEPS PRESS-DOWN WITH TUBE

Triceps (elbow extension)

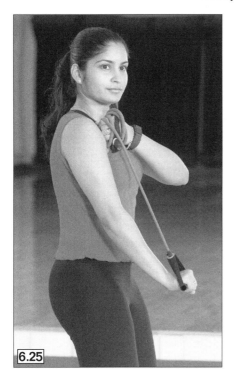

6.25

Cues: Stand with feet shoulder-width apart and spine, pelvis, and neck in neutral. Contract abdominals and press shoulders down. Holding the end of the tube or band in the working-side hand, use the other hand to anchor the tube or band to the working-side shoulder. Extend the elbow so that the working arm presses straight down. Straighten the elbow without hyperextending it, and keep the wrists as neutral as possible. Control the motion on the way up (eccentric phase), maintaining a conscious muscle contraction.

Elbow Joint

TRICEPS KICKBACK

Triceps (elbow extension)

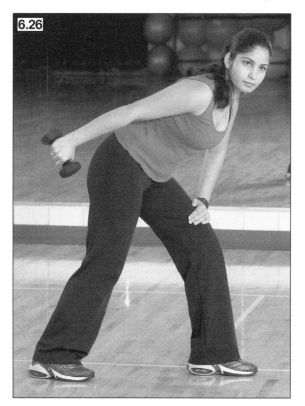

Cues: Stand in a bent over position with feet staggered and all joints pointing in the same direction; keep hips and shoulders squared. Place the nonworking hand on the same-side thigh for low back support. Place the spine and neck in neutral with abdominals in; be sure the shoulders are pressed down with scapulae neutral. Bring the working arm up so that the upper arm is parallel to the floor (shoulder stays down). With control and conscious muscle contraction, straighten the elbow without hyperextending it. Maintain a neutral wrist.

FYI: Although this exercise may be performed bilaterally, we don't recommend its use in the average group fitness class. Most students are unable to assume the proper bent-over position with a neutral spine and correct alignment; in addition, sufficient core stability is critical for low back protection. Performing the exercise unilaterally makes a fine modification for almost everyone. In addition to the bent-over position, kickbacks can be performed in the half-kneeling position. Common mistakes include rotating the spine, hunching the shoulders, locking the elbow, and using momentum.

FRENCH PRESS (OVERHEAD PRESS FOR TRICEPS)

Triceps (elbow extension)

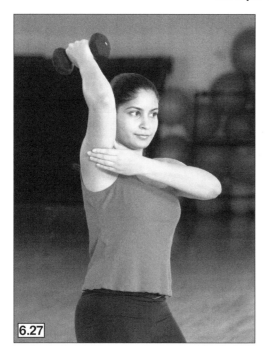

Cues: Stand (or sit on step) with knees soft; pelvis, spine, and neck in neutral; and abdominals contracted. Point the working elbow straight up to the ceiling with the lower arm behind the head. Support the upper arm with the opposite hand. Smoothly, with control, move the weight straight up toward the ceiling and carefully lower it back behind your head. Hold your head high and maintain a perfectly neutral neck throughout, keeping your elbow next to your head.

FYI: This exercise is difficult for participants with tight shoulder muscles or kyphosis. If proper alignment is difficult or impossible, suggest a different triceps exercise (such as a press-down or kickback) that participants can more safely perform. The French press also may be performed bilaterally, but this is especially inappropriate for those with poor upper body flexibility.

TRICEPS DIP

Triceps (elbow extension)

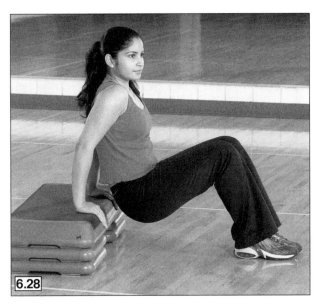

Cues: Place your hands on the floor or step with the fingers pointed forward. Suspend your buttocks off the floor or step, supporting your body weight on your hands. Press the shoulder blades down and away from the ears, lengthening the neck. Stabilize the lower body, and avoid moving the legs and hips. The elbow joint should be the only moving joint. Straighten and flex the elbows, keeping them close to the sides of the body and avoiding hyperextension as you straighten.

FYI: This is an advanced exercise. Even the beginner version (seated with hands behind buttocks) demands heightened body awareness. Avoid flexing the elbows greater than 90° and extending the shoulder joint too far back (avoid dips that are too deep), because this increases the risk of shoulder joint injury. A dip progression from easiest to hardest is as follows: dip seated on floor, dip on floor with buttocks lifted, dip with hands on step, dip with hands on step and feet on another step, and dip with hands on a stability ball.

Spinal Joints

Figure 6.29 shows the major spinal muscles, and figures 6.30 through 6.36 show exercises for the spinal joint muscles. Table 6.4 lists some muscles of the spinal joints, the actions of those muscles, activities that use those muscles, and strengthening exercises.

Rectus abdominis

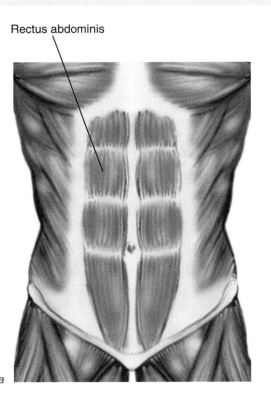

(continued)

Figure 6.29 Spinal muscles: *(a)* rectus abdominis,

Adapted, by permission, NSCA, 2000, The biomechanics of resistance exercise. In *NSCA's essentials of strength training and conditioning*, edited by T. Baechle and R. Earle (Champaign, IL: Human Kinetics), 29.

a

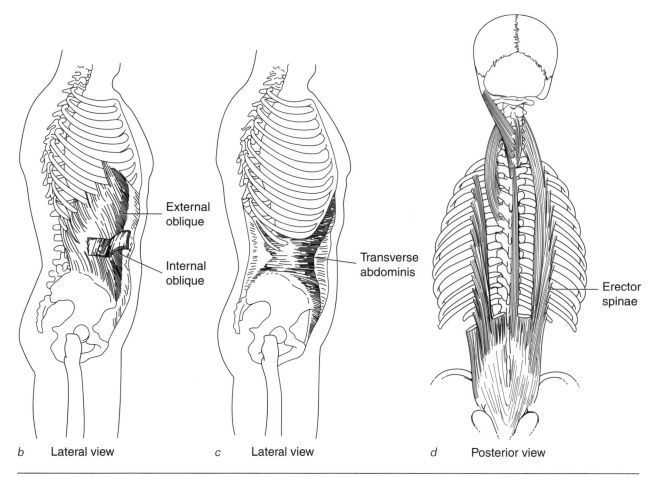

b Lateral view *c* Lateral view *d* Posterior view

Figure 6.29 *(continued)*, *(b)* internal and external obliques, *(c)* transverse abdominis, and *(d)* erector spinae.

Table 6.4 Spinal Joint Muscles

Muscle	Joint actions	Daily activities	Exercises
Rectus abdominis	Spinal flexion	Getting out of bed, posture maintenance	Crunches, pelvic tilts, hip lifts
Internal and external obliques	Spinal flexion with rotation, lateral flexion	Bending sideways to pick something up, maintaining posture	Diagonal twist crunch
Transverse abdominis	None; provides abdominal compression, vigorous exhalation	Laughing, coughing, maintaining posture	"Hollowing" in planks, crunches, Pilates exercises, quadrupeds
Erector spinae	Spinal extension	Bending forward to pick something up, maintaining posture	Prone extensions, quadrupeds

See appendix F, table F.4 for a complete list of spinal joint muscles and their joint actions.

PELVIC TILT FOR ABDOMINALS

Rectus abdominis, transverse abdominis
(spinal flexion and posterior pelvic tilt, abdominal compression)

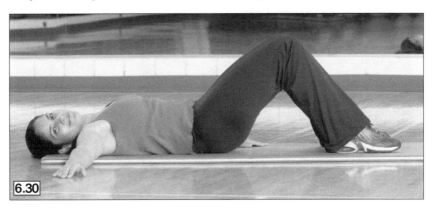

Cues: Lie supine with knees bent, upper body relaxed on the floor, and spine in neutral. Using a diaphragmatic or abdominal breath, exhale and firmly contract the abdominals, allowing them to posteriorly tilt the pelvis. Because the focus of this exercise is the abdominals, avoid allowing the buttocks muscles to participate. Work to isolate the abdominals, feeling a tug on the pubic bone attachment. Keep the movement small; more is not better. Avoid arching the lower back on the return; simply go back to the neutral spine.

FYI: This is an excellent exercise to teach abdominal awareness and proper diaphragmatic breathing. Here's a progression from easiest to hardest: feet flat on floor with knees bent, legs semi-straight with heels on floor, supine on a slanted bench with pelvis below head, and pelvis hanging off a stability ball. In all variations, try to perform lumbar spinal flexion and posterior pelvic tilt, using the abdominals but not the buttocks.

BASIC CURL-UP OR CRUNCH

Rectus abdominis (spinal flexion and posterior pelvic tilt)

Cues: Lie supine with knees bent and spine and neck in neutral. Perform a correct diaphragmatic breath, exhale, and flex your spine, pulling ribs toward hips. Keep the neck in neutral; it has no independent movement of its own (it just goes along for the ride). Avoid performing "neck-ups" or hyperextending the neck. Bring the shoulder blades up off the floor, and avoid arching the low back on the descent, returning only to neutral.

FYI: There are many variations of this exercise. Upper body arm variations from easiest to hardest include arms at sides, arms crossed on chest, hands behind ears, hands on forehead, arms crossed behind head, and arms extended overhead. Lower body variations from easiest to hardest include feet supported on wall or bench (great for those with low back problems), supine on an inclined step (hips below head) with knees bent, supine flat with feet on floor and knees bent, supine flat with legs elevated and knees bent, supine flat with legs elevated and knees straight, supine on declined step (head below hips), supine on a stability ball (may be inclined, flat, or declined), and supine with a medicine ball toss. For variety and increased difficulty, combine the upper body curl-up with a hip lift and pelvic tilt.

Spinal Joints

ABDOMINAL HIP LIFT

Rectus abdominis (spinal flexion and posterior pelvic tilt)

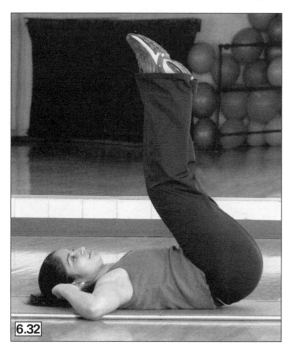
6.32

Cues: Lie supine and elevate the legs with the knees slightly bent. Stabilize the knees and the hips at one joint angle. Keep this angle (or position) constant, exhale, and contract the abdominals firmly, posteriorly tilting the pelvis. (The movement will be small.) Avoid active hip flexion or swinging and rocking the legs.

FYI: This exercise is the more difficult version of the pelvic tilt described earlier. Before progressing to the hip lift, make certain your participants can perform a correct pelvic tilt with coordinated abdominal breathing. Knees may be bent or straight, depending on hamstring flexibility and low back status. Using a declined step or slant board with the hips below the head increases the difficulty, as does the addition of an upper body crunch (full spinal flexion). For variety, try this 4-count variation of a hip lift: tilt the pelvis (legs are in the air) on 1, curl the upper body up on 2, curl the upper body down on 3, and untilt the pelvis on 4.

DIAGONAL TWIST CRUNCH

External and internal obliques (spinal flexion and rotation)

Cues: Lie supine with one knee bent, foot on floor. Place your other foot on your thigh. Place one hand on the floor, with the other hand behind your head. Exhaling, crunch diagonally the left ribs toward the right hip. Keep your neck in neutral (apple-sized space between chin and chest) and bring the left shoulder blade off the floor. Keep the movement slow and controlled, avoiding momentum.

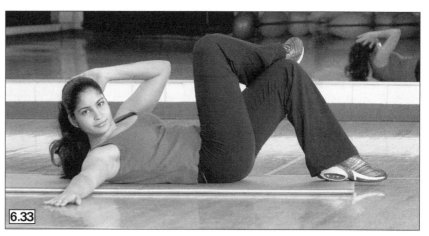
6.33

FYI: Many variations exist for this exercise. Upper body variations may be performed unilaterally and bilaterally and include, from easiest to hardest, arms at sides, arms crossed on chest, hands behind ears, arms crossed behind head, and arms stretched overhead. Lower body variations include both feet on floor (knees bent), both legs in the air (knees bent or straight), and one foot on the floor with the other leg extended in the air. In addition, a slanted step or a stability ball may be used for additional overload.

SINGLE-LEG CIRCLES

Iliopsoas, rectus femoris, transverse abdominis (hip circumduction, abdominal compression)

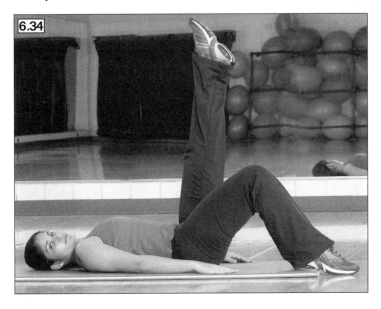

Cues: Lie supine with one leg extended on the floor and the other leg extended toward the ceiling, toes pointed.

Firmly anchor the torso by hollowing the abdominals and pulling the navel toward the spine, all the while staying in neutral spinal alignment with the four natural curves of the spine maintained.

Press both hips and shoulders evenly into the floor. Make small circles in the air with the perpendicular leg, first clockwise and then counterclockwise. Increase the size of the circles when the pelvis can be kept level and absolutely still. Repeat on other side.

FYI: In this Pilates exercise, the hip flexors act as the prime movers; the rectus abdominis, obliques, transverse abdominis, and erector spinae muscles stabilize the spine. Adequate hamstring flexibility is required to perform the exercise as described; keeping the bottom knee bent is an acceptable modification.

QUADRUPED

**Erector spinae, transverse abdominis, gluteus maximus, hamstrings, deltoids
(maintenance of neutral spine, abdominal compression, hip extension, shoulder flexion)**

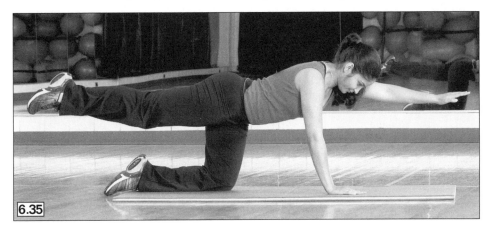

Cues: Kneel on all fours with the hands directly under the shoulders and the knees directly under the hips. Place the pelvis, spine, neck, and scapulae securely in neutral alignment. Slowly extend one arm and the opposite leg, maintaining level hips and shoulders and the neutral spine and neck. Hold. Return slowly to all fours without disturbing your alignment and repeat on the other side.

FYI: This exercise may be performed either statically (holding 5-30 s per side) or dynamically (smoothly alternating back and forth between sides). The purpose of both variations is to promote torso stability and to challenge both the erector spinae and the abdominals as stabilizers.

PRONE SPINAL EXTENSIONS

Erector spinae (spinal extension)

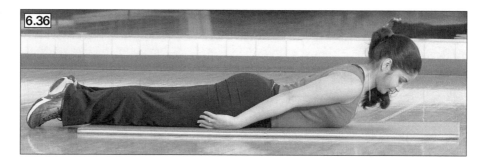

Cues: Lie prone with your forehead on the mat and your neck in neutral, hips pressed into the floor, arms at sides. Lengthening the spine, slowly lift the upper body, maintaining a neutral neck (chin will remain slightly tucked). Lower smoothly and repeat.

FYI: Active lumbar extension or hyperextension can be problematic for some participants. Always ask your participants how they feel and give them options for modifications. Tell them to stop if they feel any pain. The most conservative approach is to perform isometric extension only and encourage students to work with their physicians. Other variations from easiest to hardest include extension with arms at 90°, extension with arms overhead, extension with opposite arm and leg, and extension performed on a stability ball.

Hip and Knee Joint

Since so many lower body exercises use these two joints simultaneously, we will combine the exercises for hip and knee joints in this section. Figures 6.37 and 6.38 show hip and knee joint muscles, and figures 6.39 through 6.45 demonstrate exercises for the hip and knee joints. Table 6.5 lists the major muscles of the hip joint, the actions of those muscles, activities that use those muscles, and strengthening exercises. Table 6.6 gives the same information for the muscles of the knee joint.

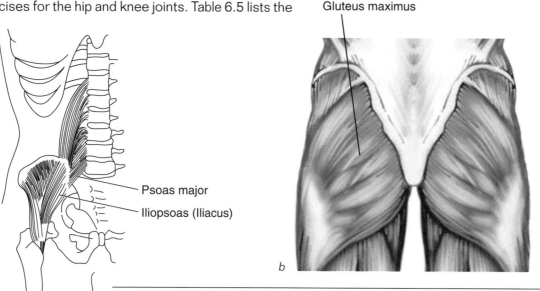

b   *(continued)*

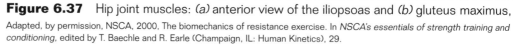

Figure 6.37 Hip joint muscles: *(a)* anterior view of the iliopsoas and *(b)* gluteus maximus,

a   Anterior view

Adapted, by permission, NSCA, 2000, The biomechanics of resistance exercise. In *NSCA's essentials of strength training and conditioning*, edited by T. Baechle and R. Earle (Champaign, IL: Human Kinetics), 29.

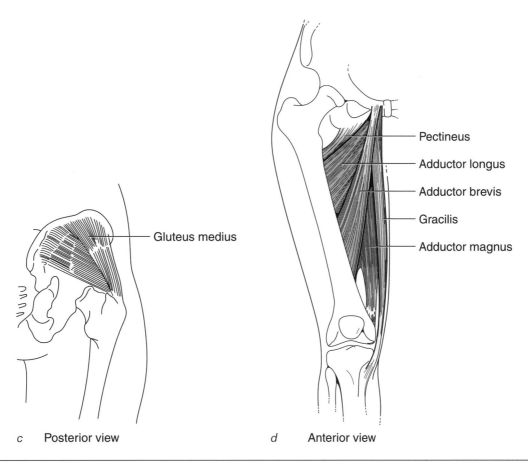

c   Posterior view   *d*   Anterior view

Figure 6.37   *(continued), (c)* posterior view of the gluteus medius, and *(d)* anterior view of the hip adductors.

Table 6.5   Hip Joint Muscles

Muscle	Joint actions	Daily activities	Exercises
Iliopsoas and rectus femoris	Hip flexion	Climbing stairs, walking, getting in a car, kicking a ball	Standing and supine leg lifts (hip flexion)
Gluteus maximus, hamstrings	Hip extension	Climbing stairs, running, walking uphill	Squats, lunges, leg lifts in the all-fours position, pelvic tilts
Gluteus medius	Hip abduction	Hip stabilizer when walking, balancing	Side-lying leg lifts, standing abduction
Hip adductors	Hip adduction	Hip stabilizer when walking, horseback riding	Side-lying leg lifts, supine adduction

See appendix F, table F.5 for a complete list of hip joint muscles and their actions.

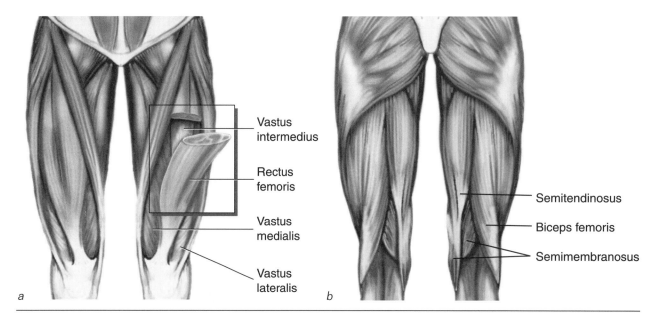

Figure 6.38 Knee joint muscles: (a) quadriceps and (b) hamstrings.

Adapted, by permission, NSCA, 2000, The biomechanics of resistance exercise. In *NSCA's essentials of strength training and conditioning,* edited by T. Baechle and R. Earle (Champaign, IL: Human Kinetics), 29.

Table 6.6   Knee Joint Muscles

Muscle	Joint actions	Daily activities	Exercises
Quadriceps	Knee extension	Walking, cycling, stair climbing, sitting down, standing up	Squats, lunges, knee extensions, pliés
Hamstrings	Knee flexion	Swimming, running	Prone knee curls, knee curls on all fours

See appendix F, table F.6 for a complete list of knee joint muscles and their actions.

SUPINE LEG LIFTS AND KNEE EXTENSIONS

Iliopsoas, quadriceps (hip flexion, knee extension)

Cues: Lie supine with spine in neutral and abdominals firmly anchored. Place one foot on the floor with the knee bent, and straighten the other knee and raise it to a 45° angle from the floor. Using a controlled, smooth motion, bend and straighten the elevated knee; alternate with hip flexion, if desired.

FYI: Knee extension and hip flexion can be performed supine, supine propped on elbows, or standing, with supine being the easiest. In addition, knee extension can include quad sets (isometric-type contractions of the quadriceps that "tighten" the patella) and terminal knee extensions (moving the knee joint through only the last few degrees of motion). These varia-

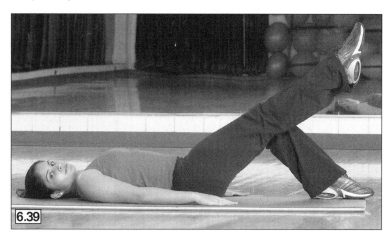

6.39

tions help to correct potential muscle imbalances around the knee joint. Bands or ankle weights can be added for additional overload.

SQUATS

Quadriceps, gluteus maximus, hamstrings (knee extension, hip extension)

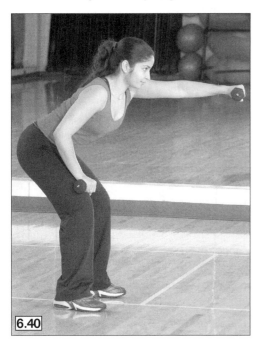

Cues: Stand with feet shoulder-width apart and toes straight ahead or slightly rotated out (in the same direction as the knees). Spine, neck, and pelvis are in neutral, and abdominals are pulled up and in. Bending the knees, press the tailbone and the middle third of the body back. Keeping the torso erect, chest lifted, and head in line with the spine, lower until the thighs are almost parallel to the floor or until the lumbar curve becomes excessive. Do not allow your hips to drop below your knees; avoid overshooting the toes or lifting the heels off the floor. Keep the abdominals contracted and the spine stable and still throughout. Keep one hand on your thigh for low back safety and allow the other arm to flex forward, providing a counterbalance.

FYI: Almost everyone can benefit from learning to squat properly. This very functional exercise helps students have better mechanics in lifting, getting in and out of chairs, and other daily activities. Variations from easiest to hardest include squat supported by a ballet barre, squat holding a Body Bar vertically placed in front, squat with hands on thighs, squat with one hand on thigh, squat with dumbbells held at sides, back squat with barbell, and front squat with barbell (the last three variations pose a greater risk for the low back).

PLIÉS

Quadriceps, gluteus maximus, hamstrings, adductors (knee extension, hip extension, hip adduction)

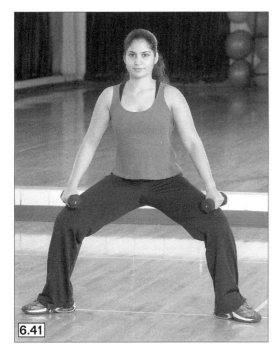

Cues: Stand with feet wide apart and toes angled away from the midline. Turning out from the hips, make sure that knees are aligned in the same direction as the toes (if this isn't possible, adjust the feet so that toes and knees are in the same line). Pelvis is in neutral with the tailbone pointing straight down. Spine is in neutral with the shoulders level and chest lifted. Maintaining this lifted, turned-out alignment, bend the knees to no more than a 90° angle (thighs will be parallel to the floor). Straighten the knees and return to the starting position, consciously contracting the buttocks and inner thighs.

FYI: This exercise may be performed with dumbbells or barbell; upper body exercises can be combined with the plié once good alignment has been mastered. A plié is really just a modified squat. Some students may find it easier than a squat because the pelvis is kept neutral and the spine is kept upright. Other students may find it more difficult because of the amount of "turnout" required. Although the quadriceps are the prime movers, the gluteus maximus isometrically contracts to maintain external hip rotation, and the adductors can be recruited during the lifting phase of the movement (although there is no resistance against gravity).

Hip and Knee Joint

LUNGES

**Quadriceps, gluteus maximus, hamstrings, hip abductors, hip adductors
(knee extension, hip extension, stabilization of hips)**

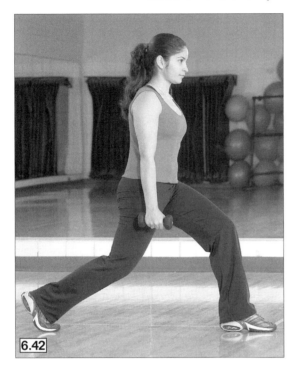

6.42

Cues: For a stationary lunge, stand with the feet staggered at least 3 ft apart (even farther apart if you have long legs). Raise up onto the ball of the back foot. Place the pelvis in neutral, tailbone down, and the spine and neck in neutral, abdominals contracted. Hips and shoulders are level. Bending both knees, slowly lower. Go only low enough that the front knee bends to a right angle (90°) and the front thigh is parallel to the floor.

Avoid dropping the hips below the knee or letting the back knee touch the floor. Keep the pelvis and spine upright; avoid leaning forward. Return to the starting position, keeping the back heel elevated. For a front lunge, start in a standing position with the feet shoulder-width apart and the spine, pelvis, and neck in neutral. Step forward and land on heel, ball, and then toe. Slowly lower and bend front knee to no more than 90°. Keep the front knee behind the toes (avoid overshooting). Torso remains completely upright (requiring hip flexor flexibility). The heel of the back foot is off the floor. Push off with the front foot and return back to standing. (For a long lunge with the back leg straight, it may be necessary to "stutter step" back with the front foot—this more advanced method uses two or three smaller steps).

FYI: In general, lunges are a more advanced exercise. To perform a proper lunge, students need to have lower body strength, flexible hip flexors, stable torsos, balance, and coordination. There are many variations of the lunge exercise including the front, back, side, and crane lunges. All of these types of lunges can be performed with stationary, dynamic, or walking or traveling variations. Front, back, and crane lunges can be performed with the back leg bent or straight (straight leg being more difficult and requiring much more flexibility). The lunge exercise can be an excellent lower body strengthener, but care must be taken to maintain strict form (especially with regard to the knees) to avoid injury.

ALL-FOURS BUTTOCKS AND HAMSTRINGS EXERCISE

Gluteus maximus, hamstrings (hip extension, knee flexion)

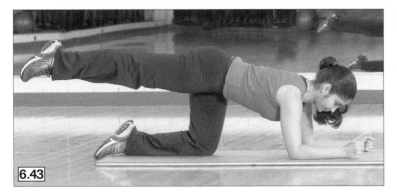

6.43

Cues: In the all-fours position, place hands directly under the shoulders with knees directly under the hips, forming a "tabletop" with the spine, neck, and head. Lift abdominals, placing the spine in neutral with the head and making the neck a natural extension of the spine. Hips and shoulders are level. Keeping your torso absolutely still, slowly raise one leg on 1, flex the knee on 2, straighten the knee on 3, and lower the leg on 4, consciously squeezing the buttocks and hamstring muscles.

FYI: Hip extensions and knee curls can be performed prone, on all fours, or even standing. Hip extension can be performed alone and knee flexion can be performed alone, or the two moves can be combined, as described previously. The prone position is the most stable and appropriate for beginners, although the range of motion at the hip joint is small. Both the all-fours and standing positions are more difficult to stabilize, and both challenge the abdominal and low back muscles isometrically. Avoid momentum in this position, because performing the movements too quickly can lead to back hyperextension and potential injury. Performing the exercise on elbows and knees (versus hands and knees) is an excellent alternative; range of motion may be increased without as much risk of back hyperextension.

ABDUCTION EXERCISES

Gluteus medius (hip abduction)

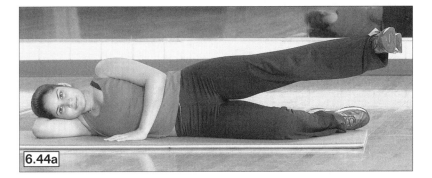

6.44a

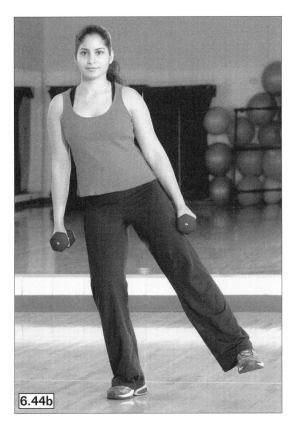

6.44b

Cues: For side-lying hip abduction: Lie on your side with your head resting on your arm. Maintain a neutral neck and spine (do not place your head on your hand, as this can place undue stress on the neck), and keep your hips stacked. Both kneecaps face forward (helping to avoid external hip rotation and flexion and the subsequent use of muscles other than the hip abductors) if the goal is to isolate the outer thigh muscles. Consciously contracting the abductors, slowly raise and lower the leg. If standing, make certain that the standing knee is bent slightly, allowing the pelvis and spine to maintain a neutral position. Keep your hips level; keep the moving kneecap facing forward, and maintain a stable torso as the leg abducts and returns.

FYI: Effective isolation-type exercises for the abductors may be performed in either the side-lying or the standing position, with the side-lying position being the safest and arguably the most effective choice, because of its stability and direct resistance against gravity. Several variations exist, including top leg straight, top leg bent, top leg in line with the body, top leg at 45° of hip flexion, and numerous rhythm variations. Bands or ankle weights may be added for additional overload.

Hip and Knee Joint

ADDUCTION EXERCISES

Adductor longus, adductor brevis, adductor magnus, gracilis, pectineus (hip adduction)

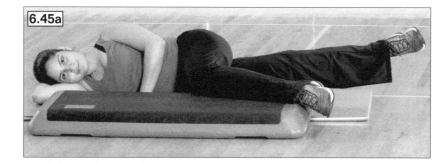

6.45a

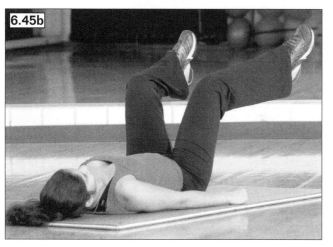

6.45b

Cues: In the side-lying position, lie on the side with your head resting on your arm. Keep hips stacked and spine and neck in neutral (do not place head in hand because this takes the neck out of alignment). Bottom (moving) leg is in line with the body, and the top leg is in front of the body with the inside edge of the foot resting on the floor. Unless students have long thigh bones and narrow hips, the top knee should be held in a slightly elevated position to help ensure that the hips remain

stacked. (Unstacked hips lead to a greater reliance on muscles other than the hip adductors and to potential stresses on the back.) Using conscious muscle contraction, slowly raise and lower the bottom leg. In the supine position, lie supine with the legs elevated in the air. Participants with tight hamstrings should bend their knees to ensure that the weight of the legs is over the torso and not over the floor. Anchor the abdominals to help maintain torso stability. Open and close the legs together, consciously tightening the inner thigh muscles.

FYI: Isolation-type exercises for the adductors may be performed in the side-lying or the supine positions, with the side-lying position being the most effective because of the more optimal resistance against gravity's pull. The exercises may be varied by using short or long levers, adding rhythm variations, and using bands or weights. To help maintain the slight elevation of the top knee in the side-lying position, use a step, towel, or small ball.

Ankle Joint

Ankle Joint

Figure 6.46 shows ankle joint muscles and figures 6.47 and 6.48 demonstrate exercises for the ankle joint. Table 6.7 lists some muscles of the ankle joint, the actions of those muscles, activities that use those muscles, and strengthening exercises.

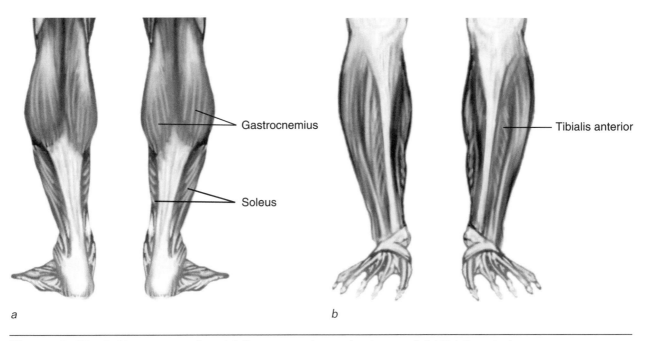

Figure 6.46 Ankle joint muscles: *(a)* Gastrocnemius and soleus and *(b)* tibialis anterior.

Adapted, by permission, NSCA, 2000, The biomechanics of resistance exercise. In *NSCA's essentials of strength training and conditioning*, edited by T. Baechle and R. Earle (Champaign, IL: Human Kinetics), 29.

Table 6.7   Ankle Joint Muscles

Muscle	Joint actions	Daily activities	Exercises
Tibialis anterior	Ankle dorsiflexion	Walking uphill, toe tapping	Toe lifts
Gastrocnemius, soleus	Ankle plantar flexion	Walking, running, jumping	Heel raises

See appendix F, table F.7 for a complete list of ankle joint muscles and their actions.

SHIN EXERCISE

Anterior tibialis (ankle dorsiflexion)

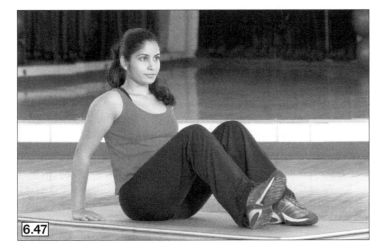

Cues: Sit in good alignment with weight over sitting bones and spine and neck in neutral. Keeping knees slightly bent, point and flex each foot one at a time. Move through full range of motion, allowing each foot to fully point and then lift as far toward the shin as possible, consciously contracting the shin muscles.

Ankle Joint

CALF EXERCISE

Gastrocnemius and soleus (ankle plantar flexion)

Cues: Stand with proper alignment; knees soft; pelvis, spine, and neck in neutral; abdominals contracted; and feet hip-width apart. Lift both heels off floor, rising up onto the balls of the feet as high as possible. Lower to floor.

FYI: To achieve full range of motion for the calf muscles, stand on the edge of a step, lowering heels as far off the step as possible and then returning.

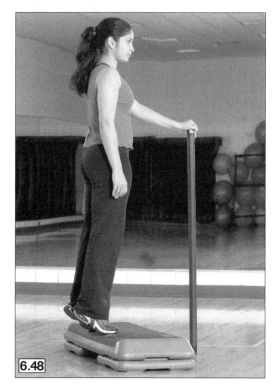

6.48

▓ **PRACTICE DRILL** ▓

Practice each of the preceding exercises with a partner, each taking a turn. Study the pictures, cues, and information given and give your partner cues while they are performing the exercise.

MUSCLE CONDITIONING EQUIPMENT

A wide variety of equipment can be used in group exercise muscle conditioning. Dumbbells, tubes, and resistance bands are standard in most fitness facilities, but many clubs also stock weighted bars, bars with plates, stability balls, Bosus, medicine balls, foam rollers, core boards, wobble boards, fitness circles, and more for participants. We next discuss training issues for some of equipment options.

Dumbbells

Most health clubs and fitness centers supply several sets of dumbbells from 1 to 10 lb for group exercise class use. Dumbbells provide a practical and convenient way to overload the musculoskeletal system and can be used in a wide variety of exercises. Here are some recommendations for the safe and effective use of dumbbells:

1. Participants should not use weights until they can perform muscle conditioning exercises with proper form and technique using gravity first; this includes the ability to consciously contract the targeted muscle throughout the entire range of motion. The eccentric or lengthening phase of the muscle action (the movement where the weights are lowered) always should be performed with awareness and care. An uncontrolled eccentric action is a primary mechanism of musculoskeletal injury (see "Common Mistakes in Weight Training").

2. Teach participants to hold the weights with a relaxed grip: in other words, no tight fists, because this may inadvertently raise blood pressure. Many participants also hold their breath and strain when clenching their fists. This action, called the Valsalva maneuver, can be potentially dangerous for cardiac patients, people with high blood pressure,

and pregnant women. The Valsalva maneuver increases the possibility of fainting, light-headedness, and irregular heart rhythms. Consistently remind your students to breathe!

3. Make sure participants maintain a neutral wrist throughout all exercises, especially when holding hand weights, tubes, or bands. Holding weights or tubes while repeatedly flexing or extending the wrists may increase the likelihood of developing carpal tunnel syndrome or tennis elbow.

4. Encourage participants to select a weight load that allows them to move with proper form yet still fatigues the targeted muscle group after several repetitions.

COMMON MISTAKES IN WEIGHT TRAINING

- Using weights that are too heavy to maintain good form
- Lack of core stabilization (pelvis, spine, and scapulae)
- Breath holding (Valsalva maneuver)
- Excessive speed or momentum, especially on eccentric phase
- Range of motion problems (too little or too much)

Caution should be used if hand weights are used during the cardio segment of class. Studies have shown that 1- to 2-lb weights do not significantly increase the caloric expenditure or oxygen uptake (Blessing et al. 1987, Kravitz et al. 1997, Stanforth et al. 1993, Yoke et al. 1988). Although local muscle endurance may be improved, the risk-to-benefit ratio should be considered; rapidly moving 1- to 2-lb hand weights (or higher) while performing complex lower body patterns offers questionable benefit while increasing the risk of injury, especially to the vulnerable shoulder joint. Upper body form may be compromised because the attention and focus are on the footwork. We encourage you to reserve the use of weights for the time when they can have the most benefit—the muscle conditioning portion of your class.

☑ TECHNIQUE AND SAFETY CHECK

Teach participants how to pick up and put down their weights correctly without jeopardizing their low backs:

- ❑ Face the dumbbells with the feet shoulder-width apart. Placing one hand on the front of the thigh for support, reach for a dumbbell with the other hand.
- ❑ Pick up the dumbbell and transfer it to the hand that is resting on the thigh. (Just hold the dumbbell against the thigh, continuing to lean on the thigh for support.)
- ❑ Pick up the other dumbbell with your free hand. Holding this dumbbell against your other thigh, press up to standing.
- ❑ To put the dumbbells back on the floor, reverse this process. The idea is to teach your students to always keep one hand on the thigh for support and perform a one-handed lift. This is a great habit to protect the spine; whenever possible, pick objects up with one hand while supporting your back by keeping the other hand on the thigh.

Barbells and Weighted Bars

Some facilities have invested in sets of barbells and weight plates for group exercise. These can provide an excellent option for those participants who are more fit. Many of the specific exercises that are performed bilaterally with barbells, however, are more challenging because of the increased need for core stabilization and therefore may be troublesome in a mixed-level class that includes beginners and intermediates. Instructors must provide several modifications and be wary of continually demonstrating and exercising with barbells while in front of the group. (Even when the instructor gives an easier variation, if she or he continues to demonstrate the more advanced version, participants tend to copy that variation although it may not be appropriate for them.) Examples of exercises typically done with a barbell that are not appropriate for many participants include weight room–style back or front squats, bent-over bilateral lat rows, bent-over bilateral high (horizontal) rows, upright rows, and deadlifts. All of these exercises require a high degree of core stability and body awareness for safe execution.

Additionally, participants need to be able to perform a weight room–style squat with proper form to safely pick the barbell up from the floor. We encourage you to reserve most group barbell work for classes clearly labeled as advanced.

Elastic Resistance

Elastic bands and tubes are another option for overloading the muscular system. Many facilities stock tubing and bands in different strengths and thicknesses, allowing participants to progressively overload. Elastic resistance is different from most weighted exercise in that tension is less at the starting position and greatest at the end of the range of motion. For instance, in a biceps curl with the tubing anchored under the foot, the tension is greatest at the top of the curl—the end range of motion (Miller et al. 2001). In contrast, when a biceps curl is performed with a dumbbell, the tension is greatest at the *sticking point*, the point where the elbow is at approximately 90° of flexion and where maximum force against gravity is present. Providing a variety of exercises with both free weights and elastic resistance is an optimal way to provide overload and stimulate improvement throughout a muscle's entire range of motion.

Following are recommendations for safe and effective band and tubing use:

1. When exercising with elastic resistance, always match the line of pull with the direction of the tubing or bands. In other words, the tubing or bands must fall in the same plane as the muscle action of the exercise. In a biceps curl, for example, the tubing must fall straight down from the forearm; the anchor point should be directly below, behind, or even in front of the moving arm. If the anchor point is off to the side (not in the same plane), the exercise is both less effective and less safe; a rotary force, or torque, is applied to the moving joints and ligaments and may lead to injury.

2. Adjust the resistance or intensity by choosing different thicknesses of bands or tubing, or by "choking up" or "re-gripping" the tubing in such a way as to shorten it. Multiple pieces of thin tubing also may be used to increase the resistance. This method has the potential advantage of allowing for multiple lines of pull within the plane of motion. For example, tubing can be anchored both anterior and posterior to the elbow joint in a standing biceps curl.

3. Make certain participants maintain a neutral wrist when holding tubes or bands. Have participants check with a physician before using a band or tubing if they have had carpal tunnel syndrome.

4. Maintain a relaxed grip whenever possible so as not to elevate blood pressure. Using tubing with handles makes it easier to avoid a clenched fist and keep the hands relaxed.

5. Teach your participants to control the eccentric (negative) phase of the exercise. Avoid the "rebound" effect and joint stress that occur when students suddenly stop consciously contracting the working muscle at the point of greatest resistance, thus letting the elastic rapidly "pull" the joint back to its starting point.

6. Regularly inspect the tubing or bands for cracks and tears.

7. When placing tubing under a step, use tubing especially designed for that purpose (usually there is a nylon strip that prevents excessive rubbing and deterioration of the tubing as it contacts the step).

8. Place tubes and bands over clothing whenever possible to avoid pinching or rubbing skin and pulling body hair.

9. Look away from the band (especially in upper body resistance work) to protect the face in the event that the band might break.

Steps and Benches

Steps or benches can be used to increase or decrease the amount of resistance in a given exercise and to change the muscle group focus. If you place the steps on risers only at one end, participants can be inclined or declined, and the exercise can be gravity assisted or gravity resisted. For example, if participants are inclined (head is higher than the hips) when performing an abdominal curl-up, the exercise becomes easier than if they were lying flat (supine). The exercise is gravity assisted. If participants are declined (head is lower than the hips), the curl-up is harder than if they were supine and the gravitational resistance is greater (gravity resisted).

The muscle group focus also can be altered by inclining or declining an exercise. A classic example is the bench press, an exercise that, in the supine position, targets the majority of the pectoralis major muscle fibers as well as the anterior deltoids. If a bench press is performed in an inclined position, there will be increased anterior deltoid and clavicular pectoral involvement and less sternal pectoral fiber recruitment. When a bench press is performed in a declined position, the reverse is true: There is increased sternal pectoral and latissimus dorsi involvement and less anterior deltoid and clavicular pectoral recruitment.

Steps are also useful props for lower body conditioning. Lunges, squats, and one-leg step-ups all can be performed with a step as well as flat on the floor. The use of steps or benches during the muscle-conditioning portion of class adds variety and increases your potential for individualizing and appropriately overloading your students.

Stability Balls

These large, resilient balls (also known as Swiss balls) have been used for years by physical therapists for both strength and flexibility training. Stability balls are an extremely effective prop for training the core muscles (abdominals and lower back) to stabilize the trunk and spine (Hahn et al. 1998) (figure 6.49). Other muscle groups can also be effectively strengthened using the ball through a variety of exercises. In general, exercises performed using stability balls are more advanced than those performed without balls because of the increased balance challenge, which results in more stabilizer muscles being recruited (Cosio-Lima et al. 2001). The ball, of course, provides an unstable surface and improves balance by improving muscle reflex, proprioception, and small muscle involvement. We recommend that participants develop basic muscle strength and endurance before progressing to stability ball

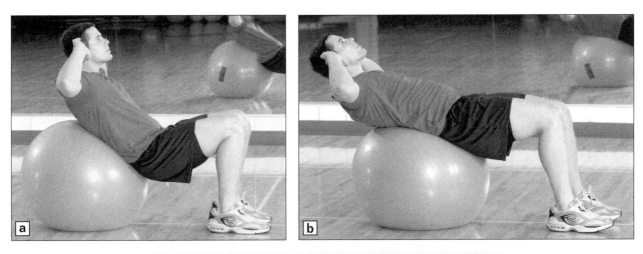

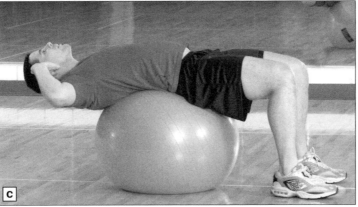

Figure 6.49 Curl-ups performed on stability ball (a) inclined (gravity assisted), (b) parallel to floor, and (c) declined (gravity resisted).

exercises. Stability balls should be sized according to participant's height or leg length and should always feel firm and be inflated to the designated amount (see table 6.8).

Table 6.8 Stability Ball Size Recommendations

Participant height	Ball size, cm (in.)
<5 ft	45 (18)
5 ft to 5 ft 7 in.	55 (22)
5 ft 8 in. to 6 ft 2 in.	65 (26)
>6 ft 2 in.	75 (30)

Note. Knees and hips should both form 90° angles when the participant sits on the ball.

Following are some of the more common exercises using the stability ball:

1. Seated knee extensions with a band: quadriceps (see figure 6.50). Sitting with good posture on the ball, with the band around both ankles, smoothly extend one knee. Maintain level hips and shoulders; keep abdominals contracted.

2. Seated overhead press: deltoids, triceps. Sit on ball with good alignment, spine neutral, and abdominals contracted. Press arms overhead, keeping scapulae down. For additional challenge, lift one leg (see figure 6.50).

3. Supine buttocks squeezes (hip extension): buttocks and hamstrings (see figure 6.51). Lying supine with feet on ball, contract buttocks and smoothly press up into a planklike position, abdominals contracted.

4. Standing wall squat: quadriceps, buttocks, hamstrings. Stand with ball against the wall and pressed into lower back. Place feet far enough away from wall that when you are squatting the knees form a 90° angle and shins are vertical. Toes, knees, hips, and shoulders all face same direction (see figure 6.51).

5. Side-lying abduction: gluteus medius (see figure 6.52). Lying on one side over the ball, maintain proper alignment with hips and shoulders stacked and neck continuing the line of the spine. Bottom leg may either have the knee down or, for greater challenge, keep knee straight with feet stacked on top of each other. Perform hip abduction with top leg.

6. Side-lying adduction: hip adductors, gracilis, pectineus (see figure 6.53). Lie on side with top leg resting on ball, ball resting on bottom leg, hips stacked, and spine and neck in neutral. Moving both legs and ball upward, adduct bottom leg.

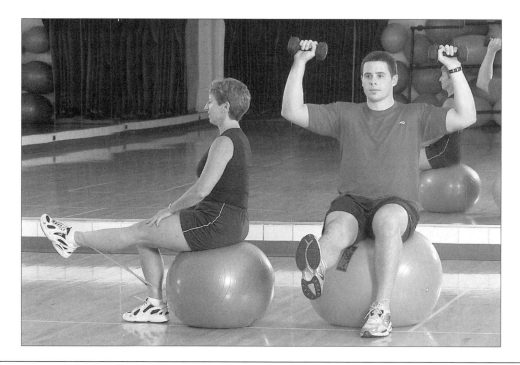

Figure 6.50 Seated knee extension with band and seated overhead press with dumbbells.

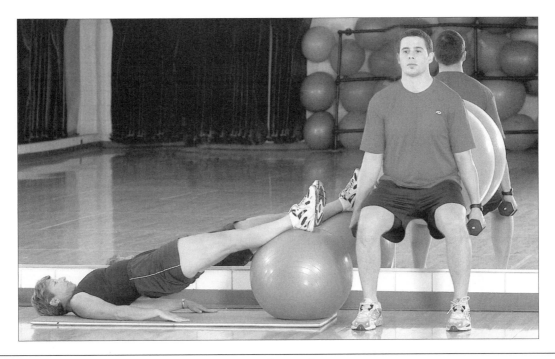

Figure 6.51 Supine buttocks squeezes and standing wall squat.

7. Prone push-up: pectoralis major, anterior deltoids, triceps (see figure 6.54). With ball under hips, walk hands away from ball, maintaining plank position with abdominals securely contracted and neck in line with spine. The closer the ball is to the feet, the more difficult the push-up. (Try balancing on one leg for a difficult challenge!)

8. Prone reverse fly: middle trapezius, rhomboids, posterior deltoids (see figure 6.55). Lie prone with ball under lower ribs and arms perpendicular to torso, elbows slightly flexed, wrists neutral, and neck in line with spine. Horizontally abduct arms toward ceiling, retracting scapulae.

9. Prone shoulder extensions: latissimus dorsi, posterior deltoids (see figure 6.56). Lie prone with

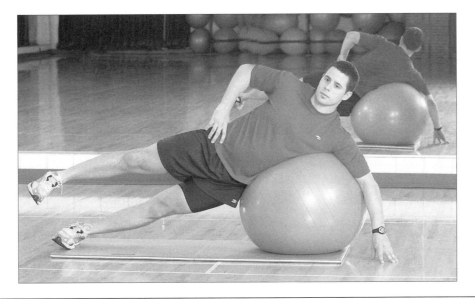

Figure 6.52 Side-lying hip abduction.

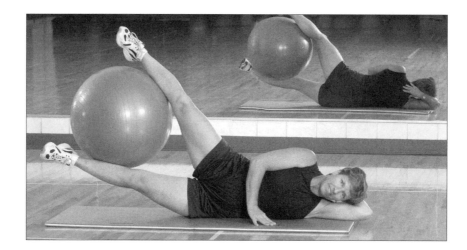

Figure 6.53 Side-lying hip adduction.

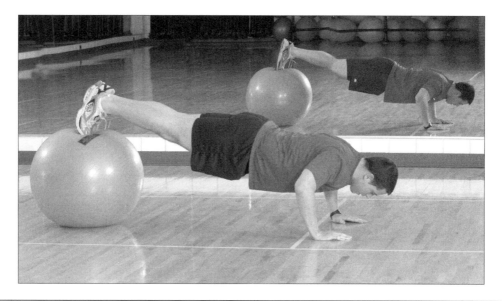

Figure 6.54 Prone push-up.

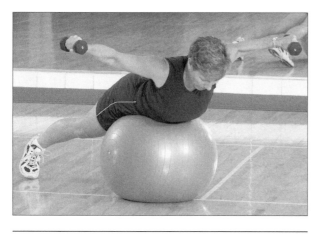

Figure 6.55 Prone reverse fly.

ball under lower ribs and arms at sides, elbows straight, wrists neutral, and neck in line with spine. Lift straight arms up toward ceiling. For additional challenge, lift one leg.

10. Prone back extensions: erector spinae (see figure 6.57). Lie prone with hands behind ears and smoothly extend spine.

11. Supine abdominal crunches: rectus abdominis (see figure 6.58). Lie supine on ball and perform abdominal curl-ups. Difficulty may be decreased by moving into inclined position or increased by moving into declined position or by lifting one leg. Obliques also may be challenged by performing crunches with rotation.

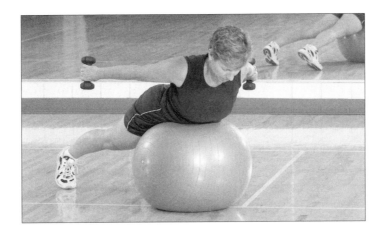

Figure 6.56 Prone shoulder extensions.

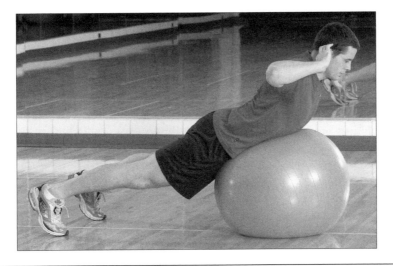

Figure 6.57 Prone back extensions.

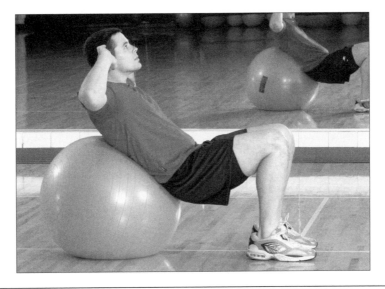

Figure 6.58 Supine abdominal crunches.

CUEING METHODS

The type of cueing required for muscle conditioning is different from that required for leading cardio exercise to music. When you are leading step or high/low, for example, good anticipatory cueing is essential; this type of cue lets your class know about upcoming moves before they actually happen, helping to ensure that your class moves safely together as a unit. During muscle conditioning, however, anticipatory cues are much less important than delivering many alignment, safety, and motivational cues.

Some instructors fall into the monotonous trap of counting every repetition throughout all the muscle exercises. There are so many other valuable things to say. We recommend that you save counting for the last set or the last few repetitions. For example, tell your class that they have eight more biceps curls and that you want them to go to the point of fatigue, squeezing their biceps as hard as possible for the last eight repetitions. Then, counting backward from 8, increase the intensity in your voice and add a motivational cue or two to encourage participants to achieve muscle overload by the last repetition. Remember, motivational cues are used liberally by experienced instructors. You can do it!

Additionally, the muscle-conditioning portion of class is an ideal time to face your class, because complex choreography is not an issue. Facing your class is more personal and more direct than facing the mirror and generally provides you with better visibility of your students' alignment. After demonstrating proper form and alignment yourself in the first few repetitions of an exercise, walk around your class to check everyone's form and give personal modifications for individuals if necessary. This is an excellent time to address participants by name and give encouragement! Following are some of the basic types of cues.

Alignment Cues

Here are some examples of alignment cues that are useful during squats: "Be sure your knees are behind your toes and your weight is directed back toward your heels. Point your tailbone toward the back wall. Tighten up those abdominals and lift your chest." Visual and tactile cues are very useful here as well.

When describing knee alignment, point to your knees; you might also demonstrate incorrect knee alignment, drawing an imaginary line from the hyperflexed knee to the floor and then repositioning your knees correctly. Place your fingers over your tailbone, showing how the tailbone should point toward the back wall. Touch your abdominals to indicate abdominal support. Alignment can be thought of as "joint" alignment. If you are at a loss as to what to say, verbally describe the alignment of all the joints. Even in a simple biceps curl, students need to be mindful of their lower body alignment. How should their knees be positioned? Their pelvis? Spine, shoulders, neck, wrists?

Safety Cues

A safety cue educates your participants about how to make the exercise safer and prevent injury. For example, during squats you could say, "Keeping both hands on the thighs, or alternating front raises with one hand on the thigh while squatting, helps protect your lower back. Maintaining an abdominal contraction while squatting also supports the lower back and guards against injury."

Motivational Cues

Motivational cues can make the difference for some participants: "Great job!" "I really like how all of you are keeping your knees in good alignment!" "You people are terrific!" "All right!" Many instructors cue on every (or almost every) repetition of muscle conditioning exercise. Additional cues that offer encouragement include these: "Squeeze!" "Contract!" "Press." "Breathe!" "Oh yeah!" "Release." "Make it look like work!" "Consciously tighten that muscle!" "Go!" "You can do it!"

The following list includes some examples of cueing that we use during strengthening segments to optimize educational opportunities:

- Perform this exercise slowly, smoothly, and with control.
- Breathe in, and as you begin the movement, perform the work, lift the weight, or pull against the resistance—exhale!

- The number of repetitions is not as important as tuning in to the area you are working.

- When you feel increased warmth, tingling, or tightness, stop!

- Correct form is more important than the number of repetitions or amount of weight.

- You can do one side until fatigued; then switch to the other side or alternate sides each time.

- If you are a beginner, stop when you get tired, or change sides even though the rest of the class keeps going.

- Even though we are doing many repetitions, this type of exercise will not remove fat from this area. To remove fat, you need aerobic exercise. This exercise will help you tone and shape muscles and allow you to tuck in, pull up, and contour your body.

Looking closer at verbal and physical cues will help you understand that there is more than one way to communicate and direct movement. Verbal cues include cueing movement with appropriate terminology and instruction as previously discussed. When you are teaching a standing outer thigh leg lift to strengthen the gluteus medius, include the following verbal cues:

- Ask participants to contract the stabilizers (abdominals, gluteus maximus).

- Give appropriate alignment cues joint by joint.

- Remind participants that the range of motion of the movement is around 45°, so lift with the side of the heel. If the toe comes up, that's hip flexion, which works the quads and hip flexors.

- Keep the movements slow and controlled and alternate sides to promote better participant comfort and muscle balance.

Physical, "hands on" cues are another way to give participants feedback on their form. When you give physical cues, walk around the room and observe participants from different angles. Gently placing your hands on a participant's shoulders to remind them to relax their shoulder blades is an example of a physical cue. Before touching, be sure to ask the participant's permission. Always be encouraging and positive when giving any cue.

PRACTICE DRILL

Pick an exercise that is easy to cue (e.g., biceps curls) and see how many alignment, safety, and motivational cues you can find. Practice teaching this exercise with visual cueing, plus the cues you found.

Chapter Wrap-Up

Outlined in this chapter are the variables that are common to most muscle strength and conditioning segments of group exercise. Knowing muscle anatomy and joint actions, selecting exercises and equipment, and demonstrating and cueing specific exercises are all important for leading an effective muscle-conditioning segment. Many group exercise classes include this component either before or after the cardiorespiratory component. The application of the principles we have discussed in this chapter will be useful in building combination classes like step and strength, water interval, or high/low impact strength classes. The information, skills, and exercises discussed in this chapter are fundamental for a skilled group exercise leader. Muscle conditioning is a key component of fitness, and we highly recommend that all group instructors develop their abilities in this important area.

Written Assignment

Find two pictures of exercises out of fitness trade magazines and analyze these exercises for safety and effectiveness. List the muscle name, action, and range of motion. Hand in the picture with your analysis.

Practical Assignment

Pick three exercises from three of the previously mentioned muscle groups and teach them to a small group. Use appropriate music, and give plenty of alignment, safety, visual, and motivational cues for each exercise. Walk around your group and modify the exercises as necessary.

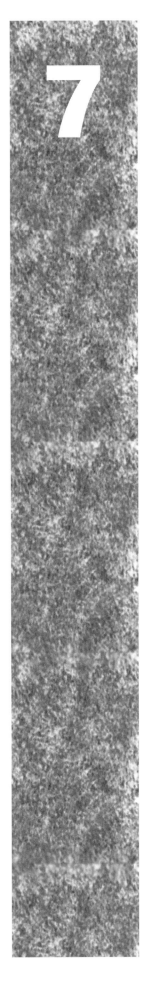

Flexibility Training

Chapter Objectives

By the end of this chapter, you will

- ■ be familiar with basic safety issues in flexibility training,

- ■ know a variety of flexibility exercises appropriate for the group setting,

- ■ be able to demonstrate and cue these exercises with proper form and alignment and use music appropriately, and

- ■ understand relaxation, visualization, and deep breathing techniques.

Flexibility training is an integral part of any exercise session; it helps release tight muscles and can help reduce the risk of injury by correcting muscle imbalances (see "Benefits of Flexibility Training"). There are several points during a group exercise class where stretching is appropriate. These include warm-up, postcardio cool-down, after resistance training a specific muscle or muscle group, and at the end of class. Alternatively, learning to teach an entire class specifically for the development of flexibility and relaxation can expand your opportunities as a group leader. Teach your class how to release and relax each muscle as well as how to breathe deeply and slowly, releasing excess tension, and you'll have many grateful students!

The main points on the group exercise class evaluation form (appendix A) under the flexibility training and cool-down segments are found in figure 7.1 and discussed here.

1. Chooses appropriate music ❑
2. Includes static stretching ❑
3. Appropriately emphasizes relaxation and visualization ❑

Figure 7.1 Flexibility training and cool-down.

BENEFITS OF FLEXIBILITY TRAINING

- Enhanced performance of daily activities
- Decreased low back pain
- Increased motor performance
- Injury prevention
- Reduced muscle tension
- Increased relaxation
- Increased range of motion
- Decreased muscle soreness
- Decreased stress and tension
- Improved posture

Exercises should stretch the muscle groups that have been used in the group exercise activity. For instance, after an indoor cycling class, stretching the quads, calves, and hamstrings makes sense because they are the major muscles used for cycling. In a kickboxing class, participants should stretch the muscles that surround the hip because they are used in kicking movements; it is also important to stretch the anterior chest muscles, which are used in punching.

How long should the stretches be held? Shrier and Gossal (2000) suggested performing one static stretch per major muscle group and holding the stretch for 15 to 30 s. The ACSM position statement (2006) suggests holding static stretches for 15 to 30 s and performing two to four repetitions per muscle group. It is not always possible to perform four repetitions; however, if you are leading a stretching-only class, this number of stretches is ideal.

SAFETY ISSUES

Participants must take precautions when stretching. Ballistic (bouncing) stretching and passive overstretching can be dangerous. Researchers have shown that ballistic stretches are significantly less effective than other stretching methods (Wallin et al. 1985). Passive overstretching and ballistic stretching can initiate the stretch reflex. Special receptors (Golgi tendon organs and muscle spindles) within the muscle fiber detect sudden stretches and excessive tension of the muscle (ACSM 2001). There is a complicated continual interplay between opposing muscle groups that leads to precise controlled and coordinated movement. During this interplay, if a muscle is activated by a sudden stretch or if it is continually overlengthened, then the system stimulates the muscle to contract rather than lengthen and maintains the contraction to oppose the force of excessive lengthening. Simply put, if you overstretch or bounce and stretch, then the muscle shortens to protect itself. Keep pulling on a shortened muscle and it will either cramp up or rip and tear—but it will not lengthen. This process is often referred to as the myotatic stretch reflex (figure 7.2). This is an involuntary reflex that happens at the spinal cord level; we cannot mentally override it no matter how hard we try.

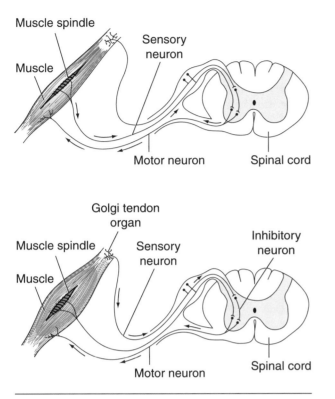

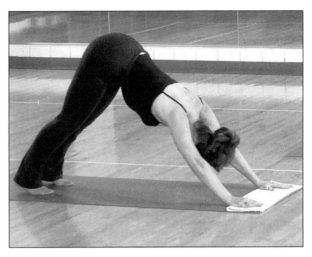

Figure 7.3 Take precaution when introducing high-risk yoga moves in traditional group exercise classes.

Figure 7.2 Special receptors are active during strong contraction or stretch. They inhibit or facilitate contraction in order to protect the muscle.

Stretching should be comfortable. Encourage proper form by giving cues like this: "Move to the position where you can feel the muscle stretch slightly, then hold. Your muscles should not feel like a rubber band ready to snap. If you are shaking, then reduce the intensity of the stretch." A student-centered teacher will give exercise options. An instructor should model average flexibility so participants do not imitate form they cannot safely match. As with any other activity it is important to move participants ahead appropriately. Yoga is a good example of an activity that has many high-risk stretches. They are taught progressively, however, so the body adapts to them over time. Putting some of the more difficult and controversial yoga moves into a traditional group exercise setting can be dangerous (figure 7.3).

Reminding participants of proper alignment while stretching helps to promote overall body stability and balance and enhances the effectiveness of the stretching experience. At least two to three verbal cues are needed on every stretch to make sure body positioning is effective. For example, for a standing hamstring stretch (figure 7.4), cue participants to tilt the pelvis anteriorly to lengthen the hamstring muscle. Sullivan and colleagues (1992) studied anterior and posterior pelvic tilt positioning using two types of stretching techniques and found that the anterior pelvic position was the most important variable for enhancing hamstring flexibility.

To help keep joints safe from injury, avoid these activities:

- Hyperextended knees or elbows
- Excessive use of momentum
- Inappropriate torque (a rotational, twisting force applied to a joint; e.g. the knee in the hurdler's stretch)
- Hyperflexing (bending past 90°) the knee in a weight-bearing position (e.g., a runner's lunge stretch performed with the knee past the toes)
- Unsupported forward flexion of the spine (no toe touches without low back support: place hands on thighs, shins, or floor)
- Unsupported forward spinal flexion with rotation (e.g., windmills)
- Unsupported spinal lateral flexion

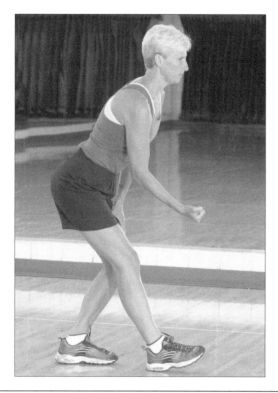

Figure 7.4 Standing hamstring stretch with anterior pelvic tilt. Instructors must always keep in mind the tenets of good alignment and use injury prevention strategies for the major joints.

- Ballistic stretching
- Deep squats (hips below knees)
- Extreme lumbar hyperextension (e.g., cobra position)

- Cervical spinal hyperextension
- Loaded cervical spinal flexion (e.g., plow)

In all of the preceding examples, the risk outweighs the benefit for most individuals. Consider the issue of appropriateness when providing stretches for your class. For example, the only groups for whom the hurdler's stretch is appropriate are track teams that are training to run hurdles in competition! For all other groups, the benefits of the hurdler's stretch are outweighed by the risk to the medial collateral ligaments of the knee (when overstretched, these lax ligaments lead to knee instability, which can lead to serious knee injuries). Instead of using the hurdler's stretch, teach your classes the modified version (much safer for the knees) or provide participants with a completely different hamstring stretch (see figure 7.5).

Other stretching recommendations include these:

- Stretch only to the point of mild tension, never pain. Stretching should feel good!
- Encourage your participants to tune in and listen to their bodies.
- Encourage muscle balance (this was discussed in chapter 3).
- If a participant has extremely flexible muscles around a joint, encourage her or him to focus on developing strong muscles around the joint instead of more and more mobility. Flexibility without balanced strength can lead to injury.

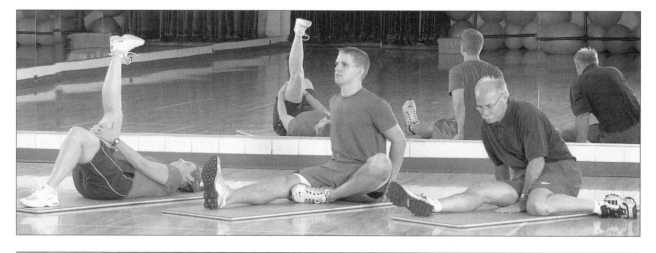

Figure 7.5 *(left)* Basic hamstring stretch, *(center)* modified stretch for hamstrings, *(right)* hurdlers stretch for hamstrings.

■ Ensure that the body is sufficiently warm before deep, sustained stretching.

■ Stretching does not need to be held as long in the warm-up segment.

The final flexibility portion of class is the point when stretching for long-term improvement is optimal. Students are warm and are more psychologcally ready to relax and hold a given stretch. Here the focus is on providing a variety of stretches held for long durations (15-60 s each). Studies show

See the DVD for a flexibility and cool-down segment example. Major muscle groups covered include inner/outer thigh, low back, hamstrings, abdominals, quadriceps, hip flexor, upper back, neck, deltoids, triceps, and pectorals; breathing, relaxation, and visualization are covered as well.

that flexibility improvement is related to both the frequency of stretching and the duration of each stretch (Bandy and Irion 1994, Feland 2000). We have found that one of the best techniques for comfortable stretching that helps to reduce stress is to have your students count their breaths while holding a position, usually three to five deep, slow breaths per stretch. Suggest that they imagine all their

stress and tension (both muscular and otherwise) draining out of and away from their bodies with each prolonged exhalation, leaving them more and more relaxed and refreshed.

FLEXIBILITY TRAINING EXERCISES

Refer to appendix F and tables 6.1 through 6.7 in chapter 6 for the joint actions of each muscle. When designing flexibility exercises, take the muscle being stretched into the opposite position of the concentric joint action listed in the joint action charts. For example, if you have just given your class lateral raises and overhead presses for the deltoids (shoulder abduction exercises), then an appropriate stretch would involve shoulder adduction, which is the opposite position from the concentric muscle-shortening action of the exercises. If you understand this principle, then you can come up with your own stretches for any muscle group (just make certain that you also abide by the safety guidelines given previously). Most of the following examples include a standing stretch (appropriate for both warm-up and the final portion of class) and a floor stretch (generally not used during most warm-ups) for each major muscle group.

DELTOID STRETCHES

These stretches are for the anterior, medial, and posterior deltoids (see figure 7.6).

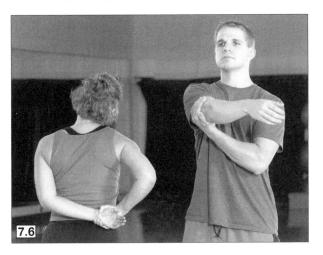
7.6

Cues: *(left)* For medial and anterior deltoids: Stand in the same ideal alignment and bend one elbow behind. Gently press the arm across and toward the back of the body. Try adding a tilt of your head to the opposite side for a great side of the neck (upper trapezius) stretch! *(right)* For medial and posterior deltoids: Stand with feet shoulder-width apart, knees slightly flexed, and pelvis, spine, and neck in neutral. Keep shoulder blades down and maintain a large space between shoulders and ears. Gently press your arm across and in toward the torso.

FYI: These stretches also may be performed seated.

LATISSIMUS DORSI STRETCHES

Figure 7.7 illustrates latissimus dorsi stretches.

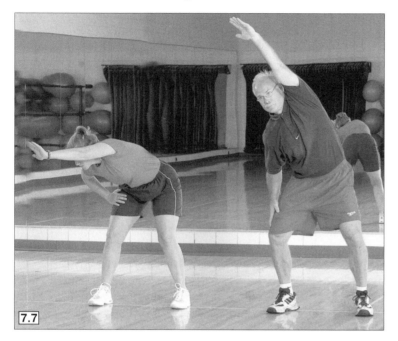

7.7

Cues: *(left)* Stand with feet shoulder-width apart, knees bent, and pelvis tucked under (posterior pelvic tilt). Curve (flex) your spine, pull abdominals in, and reach one arm up and out in front, allowing the upper back to round and curve slightly to one side to increase the lengthened feeling through the lats. Keep the opposite hand on the thigh to support the low back. *(right)* Stand with feet shoulder-width apart, knees slightly bent, and pelvis, spine, and neck in neutral. Place one hand on outer thigh and reach your other hand overhead. Lengthen your right side as you lift up, separating ribs away from hips; perform a comfortable, gradual side bend, allowing neck to continue the line of the spine. Leave hand on thigh to help support the low back.

FYI: These stretches also may be performed seated.

PECTORALIS MAJOR STRETCHES

See figure 7.8 for pectoralis major stretches.

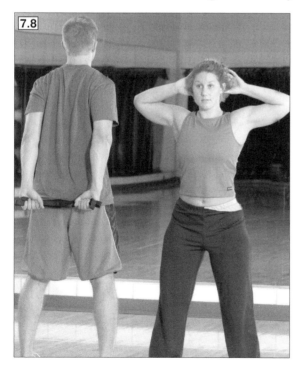

7.8

Cues: *(left)* Stand with feet hip- or shoulder-width apart, knees soft, and pelvis, spine, and neck in neutral. Bring arms behind your body, clasping hands together if possible (although this is not essential). Keep shoulders down and abdominals contracted, to avoid arching the lower back. Hold a towel or strap if desired to help increase the stretch. *(right)* Stand with feet shoulder-width apart, knees soft, and pelvis, spine, and neck in neutral alignment. Place hands behind ears with elbows high and shoulders down, and gently open the elbows toward the back, while lifting and opening the chest. Feel your shoulder blades scrunching together in the back as the chest muscles stretch.

FYI: These stretches may be performed in the seated position.

TRAPEZIUS STRETCHES

Figure 7.9 demonstrates trapezius stretches,

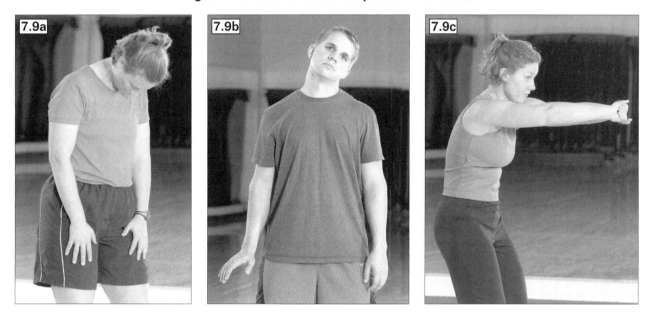

Cues: *(a)* For the upper trapezius, stand in the same good alignment as previous exercise and gently tip your head forward (cervical spinal flexion), chin toward chest. Do not allow your upper back to round forward; this is only for the neck. If desired, hands can be lightly placed on the top of the head without pulling. Experiment with slightly and carefully tipping your head diagonally (in the direction of your left little toe and then your right little toe) to release neck and shoulder tension. *(b)* For the upper trapezius, stand with feet shoulder-width apart, knees soft, and pelvis and spine in neutral. Consciously press your shoulder blades down. Tilt your head sideways (lateral flexion) to the left and feel a comfortable stretch on the right side of your neck. If you like, gently rest your left hand on your head to increase the stretch sensation (do not pull). Repeat on the other side. *(c)* For the middle trapezius and rhomboids, stand with knees flexed, pelvis slightly tucked under (posterior pelvic tilt), back rounded and flexed, and hands clasped together directly in front of your chest. Allow your shoulder blades to come apart as far as possible. Contract the abdominals, navel to spine, and allow your head to gently continue the line of the spine. Maintain your upper body over your hips (avoiding unsupported forward spinal flexion).

BICEPS STRETCHES

See figure 7.10 for biceps stretches.

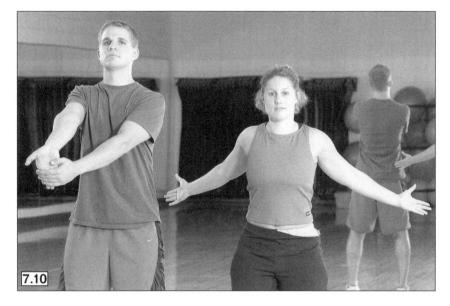

Cues: *(left)* Stand with feet shoulder-width apart, knees soft, and pelvis, spine, neck, and scapulae in neutral. Hold one arm out in front of your body (shoulder flexion) with the elbow straight and use your other hand to gently support the wrist, extending your wrist if desired. *(right)* Stand in the same alignment; reach your arms behind you with your elbows extended and shoulders externally rotated, palms facing forward and up (thumbs up). Allow the biceps muscles to lengthen.

TRICEPS STRETCHES

Triceps stretches are illustrated in figure 7.11.

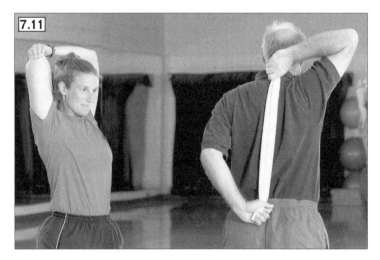

Cues: *(left)* Stand with feet shoulder-width apart, knees flexed, tailbone pointing straight down, abdominals in, and spine in neutral. Point one elbow toward the ceiling and reach your hand down your back. Gently support the stretch by placing your other hand on either your upper arm or elbow. Keep the head and neck in alignment; avoid hunching the shoulders with head forward. Keep shoulders down and away from the ears. *(right)* This is a more intense triceps stretch that also stretches the anterior deltoids and external rotators on the opposite side: Stand in the same ideal alignment described previously, pointing one elbow toward the ceiling. Bending your other elbow and pointing it toward the floor, position that same shoulder in extension and internal rotation, reaching your hand upward along your spine toward your opposite hand. Try using a towel or strap to help move the hands toward each other and deepen the stretch.

FYI: This stretch can dramatically identify muscle imbalances in right to left sides. Many people will have one side that is noticeably tighter than the other—keep stretching! Try not to force this stretch, particularly on the side with the elbow pointing down; the weaker external rotator cuff muscles are in a strong stretch on this side, and injuries may easily occur with intense stretching. Gradually release from the stretch.

RECTUS ABDOMINIS STRETCHES

Figure 7.12 shows rectus abdominis stretches.

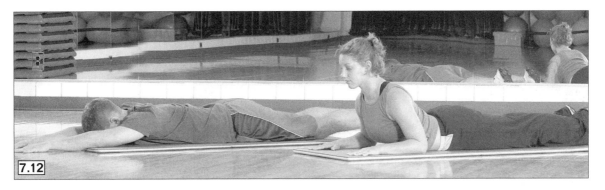

Cues: Lie prone and prop yourself up onto your elbows, stretching the spine up and away from your hips. Lengthen the neck and allow it to continue as a natural extension of the spine (avoid cervical spinal hyperextension). Press down against the floor with your forearms to lower shoulders away from the ears; slide shoulder blades down your back. If this position is uncomfortable, modify it by reaching your arms out in front and lifting your upper torso just slightly off the floor, lengthening the abdominals. Keep neck in alignment.

FYI: The full cobra pose, used in yoga, is an advanced version of these stretches. Since the cobra pose has a greater tendency to overstretch the long ligaments of the spine, we do not recommend including it in a group exercise class.

OBLIQUE STRETCHES

See figure 7.13 for oblique stretches.

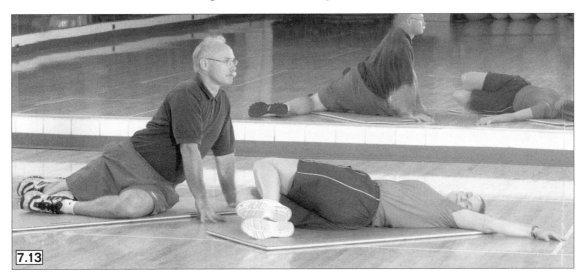

Cues: *(left)* Sit with your knees bent, one hip externally rotated (open) and the other hip internally rotated. Walk your hands around to the externally rotated side as far as is comfortable, stretching the obliques as well as the latissimus dorsi. Allow your arm to reach up and over in this position if desired. *(right)* Lie supine with both knees bent in toward torso. Allow knees to slowly drop off toward the floor. Reach your opposite arm off and away to the other side, turning your head in that direction. Breathe deeply, relax, and enjoy this multiple-muscle stretch (the pectorals, hip abductors, erector spinae, and rectus abdominis are all being stretched, as well as the obliques).

ERECTOR SPINAE STRETCHES

Figure 7.14 illustrates three types of erector spinae stretches.

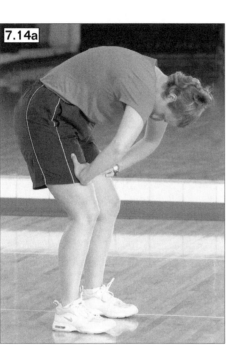

Cues: (a) Stand with feet shoulder-width apart, knees bent. Placing hands on thighs, tuck your pelvis (posterior pelvic tilt) and round (flex) your spine, pulling your navel in. Allow your head and neck to be a natural extension of the spine and your hands to support your back, as you press your waist backward, lengthening the lower back muscles. (b) Kneel on all fours and perform the angry cat stretch, flexing your spine upward and contracting your abdominals up and in. Keep your pelvis tucked under, tailbone pointing down, and allow your head and neck to flex gently as well, fol-lowing the line of the spine. Press your waist back and up to increase the low back stretch. (c) Lie supine and hug both knees in to your chest, hands behind knees. Allow your spine to flex and your tail-bone to curve upward. If comfortable, gently rock side to side, back and forth, or in a circular pattern, massaging the low back muscles. Head and neck rest in neutral alignment on the floor.

FYI: Encourage your participants to find torso (low back and abdominal) stretches that make their backs feel good. Provide them with several options and let them find their preference.

ILIOPSOAS (HIP FLEXOR) STRETCHES

See figure 7.15 for hip flexor stretches.

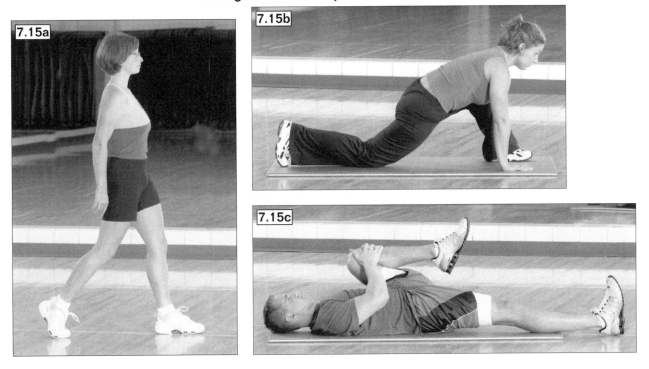

Cues: *(a)* Stand with feet staggered, as pictured. Have your feet far enough apart so that your front knee is not overbent (the front knee should be directly over the heel, with the lower leg perpendicular to floor). Turn all joints in the same direction: Toes, knees, hips, and shoulders all face the same way. Firmly squeeze the buttocks muscles and press your pelvis into a posterior pelvic tilt (tailbone tips slightly forward and under), with abdominals securely in and torso upright with neutral spine, scapulae, and neck. Feel the hip flexor muscles lengthen and stretch across the front of the right hip. If necessary, stand by a wall for balance. For a more intense version, move this position into a runner's lunge, bringing the back foot even farther back. The front knee will now make a right angle with the shin perpendicular and the thigh will be parallel to the floor. Keep the torso as upright as possible, hands on floor or balanced on thighs. Optionally, the back knee may be placed on the floor (although avoid placing it directly on a wood floor—use a mat for cushioning). *(b)* If you choose to show the runner's lunge variation first, always also show the easier version, as many participants will be uncomfortable in the runner's lunge. Pay special attention to the front (bent) knee, as overbending is a common mistake and can lead to knee problems. The rectus femoris is also stretched in these examples. *(c)* Lie supine on floor with one knee pulled into chest (hands behind thigh) and the other leg stretched out straight on the floor. Lie with spine and neck in neutral and abdominals contracted. Gently attempt to press the back of the straight knee toward the floor while maintaining the bent knee pressed into the chest. Feel the hip flexor stretch on the top of the extended hip.

QUADRICEPS STRETCHES

Standing and side-lying quadriceps stretches are illustrated in figure 7.16.

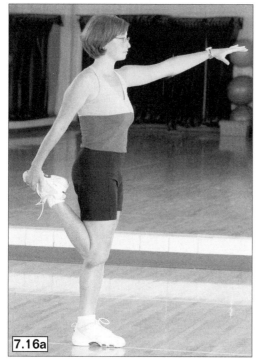

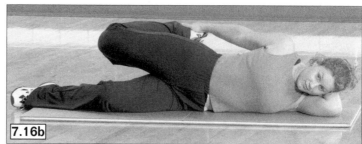

Cues: (a) Stand on one foot with knee soft, abdominals contracted, and pelvis, spine, neck, and scapulae in neutral. Grasp other foot with hand (usually the same side, although either hand is acceptable as long as it feels comfortable) and gently pull heel into buttocks, making certain that hip, knee, and ankle joints are all in a line (no torque) with the knee pointing toward the floor. Check to see that your hips and shoulders are level and even. If balance is a problem, stand near the wall for support. If you cannot comfortably reach your foot or ankle, try holding your pants or socks, or place your foot on a bench or chair and then squeeze your buttocks, tucking your pelvis posteriorly. (b) Lie on your side and grasp your top foot with your top hand, flexing the knee and gently pulling it toward your buttocks. Keep your hips stacked, abdominals in, and spine and neck in neutral, with your bottom arm bent under your head (do not place your head up on your hand, because this takes your neck out of alignment).

FYI: Another excellent position for quadriceps stretching is prone. The participant simply places one hand under his or her forehead (avoid cervical hyperextension) and reaches back with the other, grasping the same side ankle and gently pulling it in toward the buttocks.

BUTTOCKS AND HAMSTRING STRETCHES

See figure 7.17 for three types of hamstring stretches.

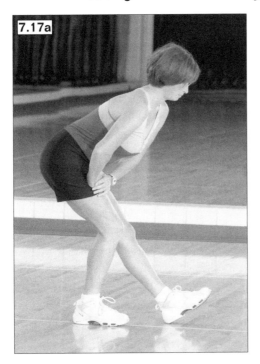

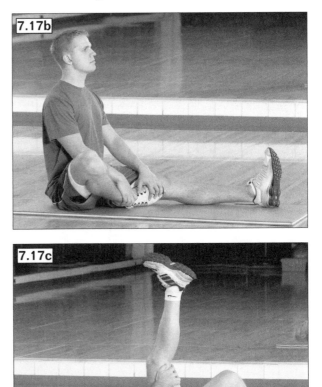

Cues: (a) Stand with feet hip-width apart, with the heel of one foot in line with the toes of the other foot. Press the tailbone backward, as if preparing to sit or squat, keeping hips and shoulders square. Hinging at the hips (no spinal flexion), fold the torso forward with a long, neutral spine, abdominals contracted and both hands on the thigh of the bent knee (this helps protect the low back). Your leg with the bent knee is the support leg, whereas the other leg is the stretching leg (knee is straight but not hyperextended). Your foot may be dorsiflexed or plantar flexed. Keep hips square and hip-hinge your torso in the direction of the straight leg so you are stretching along the longitudinal line of the hamstring muscle. (b) Lie supine with one knee bent and foot on the floor, with the spine, neck, and scapulae in neutral. With the other knee straight (but not hyperextended), gently pull your leg in toward your torso (foot may be pointed or flexed). (c) Sit perfectly upright on sitting bones (ischial tuberosities); this helps your pelvis, spine, and neck to be in neutral alignment. If you find it difficult to sit upright without slumping, wedge a towel slightly under the tailbone or use a stretch strap (or towel) around the feet, enabling you to pull yourself upright. (It is harmful to your spine to slouch in this position.) Keeping hips square and one knee bent out to side, hip-hinge as much as possible in the direction of your extended leg, keeping your spine long and straight, chest lifted, and head and neck a natural extension of the spine.

FYI: Be familiar with the modifications for seated hamstring stretches: Many participants won't be able to perform them with acceptable alignment, which will risk hurting their backs. Use props (a wedge or towel under the edge of the buttocks, with the strap around the feet), have participants place their hands behind the body for support (instead of reaching forward), or simply choose an alternative hamstring stretch (such as figure 7.17b) that is easier to do with good alignment. The seated stretch can be performed either unilaterally or bilaterally (both legs in front), although the bilateral position is potentially more stressful to the low back.

HIP ABDUCTOR (GLUTEUS MEDIUS) STRETCHES

Two types of hip abductor stretches are illustrated in figure 7.18.

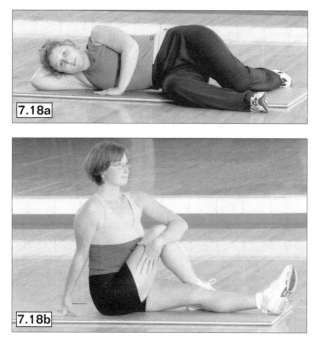

Cues: (a) Lie on your side with your arm comfortably under your head, hips stacked, and spine in neutral. Flex the bottom hip so that your bottom leg is in front of your body (knee can be bent). Place your top leg in a straight line with your torso and bend the knee. Gently lower the bent top knee toward the floor, maintaining level, stacked hips and avoiding any lateral spinal flexion. Do not let your top leg move in front of or in back of the torso; it needs to be in exactly the same plane for the most effective outer thigh stretch. (b) Sit in good alignment, up on the sitting bones, with spine, neck, and scapulae in neutral and one leg extended out in front. Bring your other knee diagonally across your torso, attempting to press the knee into the opposite shoulder. Feel the stretch in the right outer thigh and buttock muscles.

HIP ADDUCTOR STRETCHES

See figure 7.19 for hip adductor stretches.

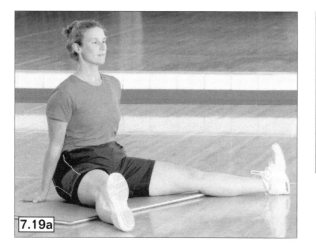

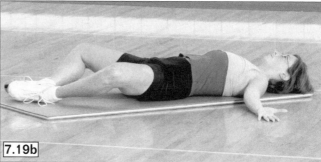

Cues: (a) Sit on the floor in straddle position, legs wide apart, weight securely on sitting bones (ischial tuberosities). Place hands on floor behind body, if necessary, to help place your pelvis, spine, scapulae, and neck in neutral, directly in line with the sitting bones. Rotate hips open so kneecaps face the ceiling; feet may be pointed or flexed.

Hinging at hips, not waist (no spinal flexion), point tailbone backward and bring torso forward, maintaining neutral alignment. The farther you are able to hinge the hips and bring the torso forward, the more you'll need to place your hands in front for support. (b) Lie supine with knees bent, feet on floor, and pelvis, spine, scapulae, and neck in neutral. Allow the legs to open (abduct) until you feel a comfortable inner thigh stretch; feet stay together on the floor, with knees bent.

CALF STRETCHES

Calf stretches are shown in figure 7.20.

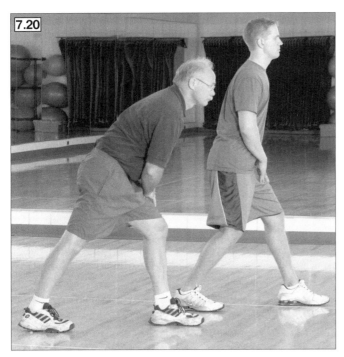

Cues: *(left)* Stand with feet staggered, one foot behind. Adjust the distance between your feet so that your back heel comfortably reaches the floor, yet your front knee is not overbending (the front knee should be directly over the heel, with lower leg perpendicular to floor). Turn all joints in the same direction: Toes, knees, hips, and shoulders all face the same way. Place both hands on your front thigh and check to see that you have one long line from heel to head, spine in neutral. Contract your abdominals and keep the chest slightly lifted, shoulders back and down. This stretch also may be performed with hands on a wall. *(right)* Stand in the same position described previously; however, let your back knee bend as far as is comfortable, maintaining your back heel down and all your joints in alignment—pointing in the same direction. Performing this stretch with a bent knee provides a deeper stretch for the soleus muscle and helps lengthen the Achilles tendon (which is often too tight).

SHIN STRETCHES

See figure 7.21 for shin stretches.

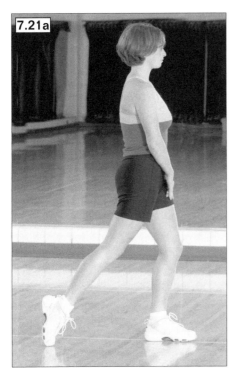

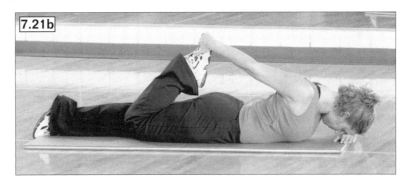

Cues: *(a)* Stand in the calf stretch position described previously, feet staggered with one foot behind. Maintaining one long line from back foot to head, abdominals contracted, balance on the front leg while pointing the back foot (ankle plantar flexion). Keep all joints in line and avoid letting the ankle collapse to the right or left side. Feel the stretch through the shin and down through the top (front) of the foot. *(b)* Lie prone in the prone quadriceps stretch position, one hand under your forehead and the other hand holding your foot. Point your foot as you gently bring the heel toward the buttocks, feeling the stretch not only in the quadriceps but also in the shin (anterior tibialis) and the top (front) surface of the foot.

▨ **PRACTICE DRILL** ▨

Get with a partner and practice each one of the preceding stretches. Study the pictures, cues, and information given. Perform each stretch with excellent form and alignment. Write down two cues for every major muscle group reviewed in this chapter.

CUEING METHODS

Proper alignment and safety cues are critical for leading beneficial flexibility exercises, as are visual cues. Motivational cues, although still important, are generally not used as liberally and enthusiastically as in the muscle conditioning and cardio portions of class, where students often need continual encouragement to reach muscle overload and work at the proper intensity. Instead, you'll want to give more descriptive cues that promote enhanced body awareness. Following are some examples:

Alignment Cues

"When performing a seated hamstring stretch, sit up high on your sitting bones and hinge at the hips, not the waist. Place your hands slightly behind your body to assist you in lengthening the spine and placing it in neutral. Shoulder blades are down, shoulders are square, and neck continues the line of the spine. Make certain your kneecap is facing up." Notice that most of these cues tell the participants where to position their specific joints and how to hold their bodies in space. In most stretches, no matter what muscle is being stretched, you need to detail each joint's correct alignment. Pointing to specific parts of your own body and demonstrating correct versus incorrect alignment is also helpful, especially for those participants who are visual learners.

Safety Cues

"It's important to sit up straight and maintain a neutral spine. Rounding and hunching your back (bending at the waist) and then reaching forward with your arms out in front are actually harmful to your spine and may lead to back pain. It's always safest to support your spine with your hands either behind or next to your hips on the floor, or, if you're very flexible, with your hands on your legs or on the floor in front of you." This type of cue alerts your student to potential risks and educates them about proper biomechanics. Here is another good place to offer modifications so that all participants in your class perform the stretch that is appropriate for them.

Motivational Cues

"That's right, you've got it!" "I really like how you modified that stretch!" "Excellent job, everyone!" These types of cues help participants feel successful, build their confidence, and create a positive environment for exercise. Remember, part of your role is to be a supportive encourager and motivator of people!

Descriptive Cues

This type of cue uses imagery and visualization and can help your students achieve better alignment, relax, integrate body and mind, and reach a state of inner peace. Descriptive cues are particularly effective during the final stretch segment of class. Here are some examples: "Feel as if the crown of your head were attached to a silken cord, connecting you to the ceiling, lengthening your entire spine and neck." "Breathing deeply, filling your entire body with fresh, clean oxygen; very slowly exhale, allowing each muscle to release and let go as you deepen your stretch." "Sinking and melting deeper into the stretch, imagine that all tension is being exhaled, from the backs of your thighs, your hips and buttocks, your lower back, your shoulders, and your head and neck." Notice that many words are used ending in -ing. This is a very different way of cueing than the telling or directive style that is often needed during the cardio or muscle conditioning segments of class. Additionally, to help encourage relaxation and mind–body integration, you'll probably need to change your voice. The final stretching and relaxation portion of class is the time to use a softer, slower, more soothing voice.

Here are some ideas for general cueing when stretching:

- Stretching should be comfortable. It should not hurt or cause pain.
- During this stretch you may not feel anything but comfort—that's OK! You are maintaining flexibility and preventing injury.

- Avoid bouncing or overstretching, because either of these will shorten or contract the muscles. Shortened muscles cannot be stretched, so you are defeating the purpose and risking injury.

- Stretch to the point of tension; then hold the stretch and relax.

- Listen to your body. Pay attention to comfort, relaxation, and easy stretching.

- Your goal is not to touch your foot but rather to keep your knee straight and your back in good alignment to stretch optimally and safely.

- Check your position—are your toes straight ahead? Is your knee straight? Is your leg straight out in front of you?

- Hold each stretch for 5 to 15 s during the warm-up and 20 to 30 s for increasing flexibility; if you do not like counting, take three to four deep breaths while holding each stretch.

- Position yourself so that you can achieve maximum muscle relaxation and minimize the effects of gravity during the stretch.

- At any time during the exercise period or during any activity, if a muscle is tight, stop and stretch!

- Close your eyes and feel your muscle tension dissolve with each exhale.

RELAXATION AND VISUALIZATION

The hardest part for most participants is getting to an exercise class. When the class is finished they usually feel good about coming, and this feeling keeps them coming back. They have taken time to care for themselves and thus have taken another step toward healthier living. The relaxation and visualization segment is where you can help participants complete their journey (see "Music for Flexibility Training").

In this portion of class, one of your goals is to facilitate the relaxation response. The relaxation response is a physiological response where the blood pressure, heart rate, and breathing rate decrease, muscle tension dissipates, and alpha brain wave patterns are altered. It has been suggested that a quiet environment, a peaceful mental focus (such as focusing on each muscle "letting go"), a passive attitude (accomplished by reducing distractions), and a comfortable position are necessary to elicit the relaxation response (Benson 1980). Yoga practitioners for thousands of years have recommended deep, abdominal breathing to help bring about a relaxed state. In an abdominal or diaphragmatic breath, the diaphragm (a horizontal muscle that divides the chest cavity from the abdominal cavity) drops down toward the abdomen on a deep inhale, causing the abdominal organs and abdominal wall to move outward. When exhaling, the diaphragm rises back up into the chest cavity, pressing air out of the lungs, and the abdominal wall and internal organs pull back in toward the spine (see figure 7.22). A helpful image for many people is that of a balloon inside the abdomen. When you put air into a balloon, it enlarges, just like the abdomen during inhalation. When you take air out of a balloon, it becomes smaller, as does the abdominal area during a deep exhalation as the navel pulls toward the spine. You will find that many participants are confused about deep breathing and may habitually reverse the process. However, correct abdominal breathing is how everyone breathes when sleeping peacefully and is our most natural state. It is very worthwhile to patiently work with your class to teach them about this valuable and healthful practice.

MUSIC FOR FLEXIBILITY TRAINING

To help facilitate deep, slow, safe, and effective stretching, use calming and relaxing music. Choose music that doesn't have a strong or driving beat, and turn down the volume so you can easily be heard. Music without a distinct beat is often labeled *amorphous* and is usually instrumental only. New Age music, easy listening mellow rock, soft jazz, and classical adagios (the slow, peaceful part of a symphony or concerto) are all good choices.

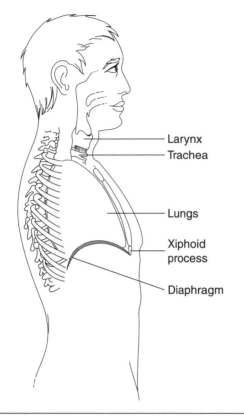

Figure 7.22 The diaphragm lowers when inhaling and rises when exhaling. In deep breathing, this causes the abdominal wall to move.

During a group exercise class, participants have worked hard, increasing the blood flow of nutrients and oxygen to the exercising muscles. As each minute of the class passes, it is easier for anxieties, worries, and stressors of the day to be released. Participants may have switched from logical and calculating functions to operating more spontaneously, with fluid thought. Take the last few minutes of every class to let participants relax or reenergize before returning to their duties and commitments. These relaxation moments can be structured or free-flowing, philosophical or quiet.

Silence or quiet, slow soothing music might be enough. Storytelling, guided imagery, or creative visualization might help deepen the sensation as you describe quiet forests, gentle breezes, a warm fire, or a cozy room. Starbursts, bright, intense sunlight, or the power of a wave or waterfall might suggest the energy necessary to continue with the day's activities. Partner massage, group stories, deep breathing, or progressively tightening and releasing muscle groups may help participants find any remaining tensions, areas of pain, or resistance to change. While the participants are receptive, use the time to compliment them on their hard work and reinforce their positive lifestyles or help them perform a mental exercise to increase their self-esteem and personal power. Consider reading inspirational quotes or poetry. Include social announcements about birthdays and upcoming events or compliment a regular participant about his or her attendance. Tell the class about your life to create a cohesive, family-like atmosphere. Instructors need to find a comfort zone and use these last few minutes to end the exercise experience on a positive note, allowing participants to take their encounter past the allotted time.

Chapter Wrap-Up

Flexibility is an essential component of fitness. In this chapter we covered safety issues and recommendations related to stretching, specific stretches for each major muscle group, cueing for flexibility, and breathing and relaxation techniques. We hope you will integrate this information so that you and your students can enjoy the benefits of stretching.

Written Assignment

Prepare in writing a stretch for each major muscle group listed in this chapter. List at least one safety, alignment, motivational, and descriptive cue for each stretch.

Practical Assignment

Be prepared to teach a stretch for any of the major muscle groups listed in this chapter to a small group using appropriate cues.

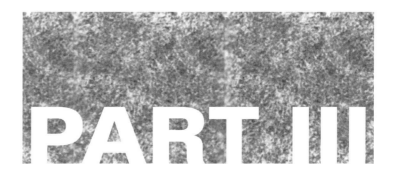

PART III

Practical Teaching Skills

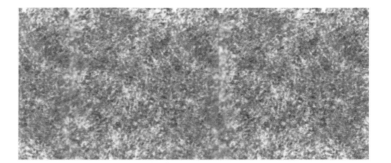

High/Low Impact

Chapter Objectives

By the end of this chapter, you will

- be able to teach basic moves for high/low impact classes,

- understand safety issues and use good alignment and technique in high/low impact classes,

- understand the elements of variation,

- know how to create smooth transitions,

- be able to build basic high/low impact combinations,

- know how to use different choreographic techniques,

- be familiar with different training systems for high/low impact classes,

- be able to cue basic moves in a high/low impact class, and

- be able to teach a 2-min high/low impact routine with at least two 32-count blocks and proper cueing.

In a high/low impact class, large muscle movements are performed to promote the benefits of cardiorespiratory fitness. These movements are typically dancelike in nature and can be executed while jumping (high impact) or by keeping one foot on the floor at all times (low impact). High/low impact classes may be labeled in a variety of ways such as cardio conditioning, aerobic dance, or simply high/low impact aerobics. Learning the skills necessary to teach high/low impact classes provides the foundation of group exercise instruction for many group leaders. The basic skills described in this chapter such as anticipatory cueing, smooth transitioning, and choreography building techniques can apply to most other forms of group exercise, including step, kickboxing, muscle conditioning, water exercise, slide, and NIA. The main points on the group exercise class evaluation form (appendix A) for high/low impact programs are found in figure 8.1.

Key Points for Warm-Up Segment

1. Gradually increases intensity ❏

2. Uses a variety of muscle groups and minimizes repetitive movements ❏

3. Promotes participant interaction and encourages fun ❏

4. Demonstrates movement options and gives clear verbal cues and directions ❏

5. Gradually decreases intensity during postcardio cool-down ❏

6. Uses an appropriate music tempo of 134-158 beats/min ❏

Figure 8.1 Group exercise class evaluation form for high/low impact programs.

TECHNIQUE AND SAFETY

To minimize repetitive stress on the joints and to prevent boredom (for both the instructor and the participants!), the best instructors constantly vary their moves and patterns. Too much of any one move can create excessive wear on the joints. A

☑ **BACKGROUND CHECK**

Before working your way through this chapter, you should do the following:

READ
❏ chapter 4: Warm-Up,
❏ the music section in chapter 3 (pp. 31-37).

PRACTICE
❏ the music drills in chapter 3 (pp. 34-35).

fundamental consideration for varying moves and patterns is to ensure that they are balanced; balance forward moves with backward moves, balance right and left sides, and balance right and left leads. To protect the joints, avoid too much high impact, too many jumps on one leg in a row (no more than eight), and too many repetitive moves that stress the musculoskeletal system. Moves such as jumping jacks, ski jumps, and scissors deliver large impact forces to the joints. Combine these types of moves with a totally different move (such as a march) for the safest class.

Demonstrate proper technique at all times to avoid injuries. When performing high-impact moves, roll through the entire foot with each jump, bringing the heels to the floor. This toe–ball–heel landing pattern helps to distribute the impact forces more evenly over the whole foot. Be careful with lateral foot movements such as grapevines and shuffles, especially on a carpeted surface. These types of moves can increase the risk of a lateral ankle sprain, especially if participants are fatigued. When performing lunges, keep the back heel up to prevent excessive eccentric loading of the calf muscles (potentially leading to Achilles tendinitis). It is also wise to avoid ankle weights during high/low impact classes due to the increased risk of injury. If light hand weights are used, chose a reduced music speed (such as 138 beats/min) to minimize the risk of upper body injuries. Hand weights less than 3 lb have not been shown to significantly affect caloric expenditure in high/low impact activities (Yoke et al. 1988). Hand weights greater than 3 lb are not recommended during high/low impact activities because of the increased potential for upper body injury. Avoid keeping arms overhead for prolonged periods of time; in addition to increasing the risk of shoulder joint injuries, this can elicit the pressor response—elevating the heart rate without a corresponding increase in oxygen consumption. Avoid knee and elbow hyperextension, both of which can result from excessive momentum (e.g., during kicks or rapid press-outs).

In addition to considering joints and injury prevention, good instructors are aware of potential safety issues caused by the difficulty of the move or the participant's ability. Keep all moves fluid and under control. Be careful with sudden directional changes; always provide clear, advance cueing to prevent falls and collisions. Finally, always provide an option for turning steps, such as pivot turns. Some participants become dizzy and disoriented with this type of move.

☑ TECHNIQUE AND SAFETY CHECK

To help keep your classes safe, observe the following recommendations.

REMEMBER TO

- ❏ provide a variety of moves (front to back, side to side, and right to left),
- ❏ roll through the entire foot with each jump,
- ❏ be careful with lateral foot movements,
- ❏ keep the back heel up when performing lunges,
- ❏ be careful with sudden directional changes, and
- ❏ always give an option for turning steps.

AVOID

- ❏ too much high impact,
- ❏ too many jumps on one leg in a row (no more than eight),
- ❏ too many repetitive moves that stress the musculoskeletal system,
- ❏ excessive momentum,
- ❏ knee and elbow hyperextension,
- ❏ keeping arms overhead for prolonged periods of time, and
- ❏ using ankle weights.

BASIC MOVES

A skilled high/low impact instructor has a large repertoire of high/low impact moves that allow for endless variety and creativity. Most of these moves can be performed at low to moderate impact (one foot is always on the floor during the move) or high impact (both feet leave the floor during the move). For example, a grapevine can be performed with one foot always on the ground (low impact) or jumping from foot to foot, which would be high impact. In so-called moderate impact, one foot remains in contact with the floor, but a springy, bouncing motion is performed, rolling toe–ball–heel and back again with the feet during each repetition. Research has shown that low- to moderate-impact cardio routines, when performed with full range of motion and appropriate choreography, can provide a cardiorespiratory stimulus similar to high-impact routines (Clapp and Little 1994; Otto et al. 1986, 1988; Parker et al. 1989; Williford et al. 1989a, 1998b; Yoke et al. 1988, 1989). Instructors may choose to lead routines or classes that are entirely high impact, entirely low impact, or a combination of both styles. Following is an introduction to basic lower and upper body moves for high/low impact classes.

Lower Body

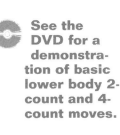 **See the DVD for a demonstration of basic lower body 2-count and 4-count moves.**

Lower body moves and patterns can be roughly divided into 2-count moves and 4-count moves, as in table 8.1 and on the DVD. These moves have many variations, as we see in the next section.

An aerobic or cardiorespiratory exercise is one in which large, major muscle groups move repetitively through full range of motion for a prolonged period of time. Therefore, keep the lower body moving at all times during a high/low impact class, because lower body muscles contain more muscle mass than upper body muscles and will consume more oxygen, providing a stronger cardiorespiratory stimulus. Studies have shown that simply staying in one place with minimal lower body involvement while vigorously pumping the arms brings up the heart rate but does not significantly increase oxygen consumption or caloric expenditure (Parker et al. 1989).

Table 8.1 Lower Body 2- and 4-Count Moves

2-count moves	4-count moves
Walk, march, or jog	Grapevine
Step-touch	Walk front for 3, tap on 4 (also known as a hustle)
Hamstring curl	V-step (also known as "out, out, in, in")
Knee lift (front or side)	Mambo
Kick (front, side, or back)	Box step (also known as jazz square)
Heel dig (front or side)	
Toe tap (front or side)	Charleston
Jumping jack	Shuffle
Heel jack	Power squats
Twist	Cha-cha
Pony	Rocking horse
Kickball change	Jig
Lunge	
Pendulum (ticktock)	
Scissors	
Ski jumps	
Plié	

Upper Body

In high/low impact activities, arms can move bilaterally (right and left sides perform the same movement simultaneously, as in biceps curls with both arms) or unilaterally (right and left sides either move individually or perform different movements simultaneously, as in alternating biceps curls).

In addition to bilateral or unilateral arm movement, the upper body moves can complement or move in opposition to the lower body movements. For example, when one is performing knee lifts, the right arm could reach up at the same time the right knee lifts up (complementary arms), or the right arm could reach up while the left knee is lifting (opposition arms). Upper body moves

> See the DVD for a demonstration of high/low arm patterns. These patterns can be used in other modalities as well.

also can be categorized as low-range, midrange, and high-range movements, as in biceps curls (arms at sides), front raises to shoulder height, and overhead presses, respectively.

⚜ PRACTICE DRILL ⚜

Practice the lower body moves listed previously in both their low- and high-impact variations. Then practice adding different arm movements: low, middle, and high range, unilateral and bilateral, opposition and complementary. See DVD for a demonstration of this drill.

ELEMENTS OF VARIATION

Understanding the elements of variation can help you get more mileage out of your basic moves. Almost every basic move can be altered in numerous ways for variety, interest, additional challenge, and fun! Variations give the illusion of brand-new moves and choreography, when in fact you are only tweaking moves that are already familiar to your participants. The primary elements of variation are lever variations, plane variations, directional variations, rhythm variations, intensity variations, and style variations.

Lever Variation

Performing a lever variation simply means moving from a short lever move to a long lever move, or vice versa. For example, progressing from a knee lift to a kick is a lower body lever change; similarly, moving from a bilateral front raise to a bilateral biceps curl illustrates an upper body lever change variation. This element of variation does not work for all moves.

Plane Variation

Changing the plane of movement while performing essentially the same move is a plane variation. When you change a front kick to a side kick or change a front raise to a lateral raise, you are executing a plane variation. The basic planes are frontal (abduction and adduction movements), sagittal (flexion and extension movements), horizontal (horizontal shoulder adduction and abduction or twisting movements), and diagonal movements. This variation does not work for all moves (see figure 8.2).

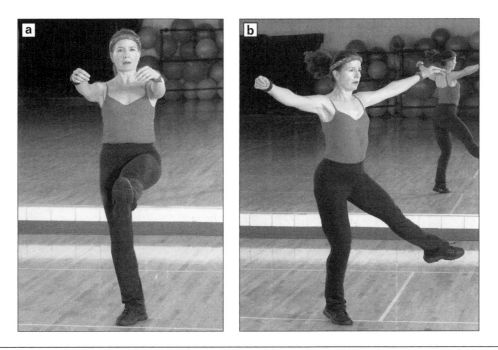

Figure 8.2 Moving from the sagittal to the frontal plane.

Directional Variation

A directional variation can mean changing the direction of the movement: If you are facing front, perform the same move facing the side or back, or if you are traveling forward (e.g., as in a hustle), travel diagonally instead. A directional variation can also mean traveling with the move instead of performing it in one place: for example, moving while performing alternating knee lifts instead of remaining in one place. This is an excellent strategy for increasing intensity and energy expenditure. It's amazing how common and familiar moves (e.g., knee lifts) can feel completely different by varying the direction! Some moves will naturally feel better when you are moving in a certain direction; jumping jacks, for instance, feel much more uncomfortable when moving forward than backward. A simple traveling combination might go like this: four jumping jacks backward (8 counts), then march or jog forward (8 counts). Repeat for a complete 32-count phrase.

Rhythm Variation

Rhythm variations involve either changing the rhythm of the move or adding sound. An example of a rhythmic move change would be to switch from alternating single-knee lifts (a 2-count move) to alternating double-knee lifts (a move that takes 4 counts). Other moves that can easily go from

single to double and back again include hamstring curls, step-touches, and lunges. Experiment with rhythmic sound variations: Try adding single and then double or triple claps to some moves. Snaps and stomps are also fun. Or, ask participants to yell, whoop, or grunt at various points in the song; this technique has the potential to totally energize your class! (Always keep your group's demographics and individual characteristics in mind; some people may be uncomfortable with making sounds, whereas others will enjoy it.)

Intensity Variation

You can increase physiological intensity in a number of ways, by

- increasing the lever length,
- increasing the range of motion,
- increasing the speed of the move (or of the music itself),
- taking bigger steps when traveling as well as taking wider steps in "stationary" moves such as step-touches, or
- changing the literal "level" of the move, also known as vertical displacement.

For example, in a low-impact move such as a step-touch, the center of gravity remains on the same level as one steps side to side. However, if the participant changes the move to high impact

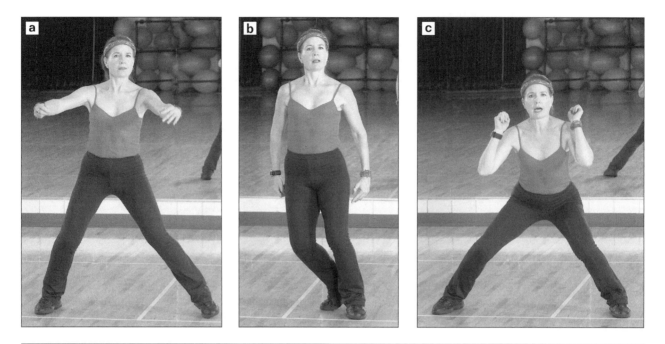

Figure 8.3 (a) Basic step-touch, (b) high-impact step-touch, which actually becomes a "pony" or triple step, (c) low-impact step-touch with knees flexed.

(as in a side-to-side pony or triple step), the center of gravity moves up and down and more muscle mass is involved, thus increasing the intensity. Vertical displacement can also occur in a downward direction, exemplified by bending the knees more during a low-impact step-touch so that the emphasis is down–up (instead of up–down), shifting the center of gravity downward and requiring more muscle mass activation without jumping. Many low-impact moves lend themselves to this type of intensity variation: hamstring curls, knee lifts, kicks, and lunges. Conversely, of course, moves can become lower intensity by decreasing any of these variables (see figure 8.3).

Physiological intensity is not necessarily the same as complexity or psychological intensity. A combination can be quite intense in terms of heart rate, oxygen consumption, and caloric expenditure without having complex choreography. Ironically, a very technical or complex combo with many intricate foot and arm patterns can actually lower the intensity, because participants must focus intently on memorizing what comes next and on not appearing clumsy. Later in this chapter

See the DVD for a practice drill showing elements of variation (lever, plane, directional, rhythmic, intensity, and style variations).

we discuss sequencing and choreographic issues in greater depth.

Style Variation

Potentially, one of the most enjoyable ways to vary your moves is by playing with the style. A grapevine, for instance, can look and feel completely different when performed with a funky style versus an athletic or sporty style, even though it's essentially the same move! Other styles include Latin (salsa), hip-hop, dance, martial arts, country, jazz, Irish, or African. Expand your repertoire of styles and increase your fun potential!

■ PRACTICE DRILL ■

Play your favorite music (with a strong beat) and begin with a basic move such as a march, step-touch, or grapevine. Add upper body movements. On every 8th or 16th beat, change your move slightly by varying the lever, plane, direction, rhythm, intensity, or style. For example, go from a basic step-touch with lateral raise arms to a plane change: Arms perform front raises. Then try a direction change: Move the step-touch (with front raises) diagonally to the front of the room and back again. Hold the basic move. Vary this by changing the rhythm: Take two step-touches to the right and then two to the left. Add an additional rhythm change by clapping on the 4th count each time. Return to the basic move. Have fun with a style change: Emphasize the upbeat by stomping the inside foot on the step-touch while loosening the arms (allowing the elbows to flex slightly on the upbeat) and popping the torso slightly with an upbeat hip-hop style! When you feel you've exhausted the possibilities, go to another move and try more elements of variation.

SMOOTH TRANSITIONS

Skilled instructors teach so that their moves flow seamlessly from one to the other, making it easier to cue and easier for participants to follow, thus enhancing participant success. Spend time on the drills in this section to build your skill at connecting moves. For the smoothest transitions, keep it simple! It's best if you change only one thing at a time (e.g., change only the arms, or only the legs, or only the lead foot).

Connecting End Points

Some moves just naturally transition into other moves. Most of the elements of variation, described earlier, provide for smooth transitions: Executing a plane change from a front kick to a side kick is an example of a smooth lower body transition. The subtle change from a front kick with a front raise to a side kick with a lateral raise is easy for almost every participant to grasp and requires a minimum of cueing. Notice that each move has a starting point and an end point. The smoothest transitions connect moves that have one of these points in common.

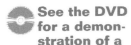 **See the DVD for a demonstration of a smooth transitions drill.** For example, a bilateral front raise starts with the arms down and ends with the arms up at shoulder height in the sagittal plane (2-count move). A lateral raise also starts with the arms down but ends with the arms up at shoulder height in the frontal plane (2-count move). These two moves flow together well because they share a common starting point and end point—arms down. It's easy and natural to go back and forth between these two moves; in fact, you could even create a combination 4-count upper body move by putting these two moves together and repeating the 4 counts over and over.

> ### ✖ PRACTICE DRILL ✖
>
> With the feet stationary, practice transitioning from one upper body 2-count move to another, making sure that each move has a common denominator (starting point or ending point) with the previous move. Perform each 2-count move at least four to eight times (which would be 8-16 counts), and challenge yourself by connecting at least eight different upper body moves sequentially. If necessary, pause briefly between moves to find a move with a common end point, but keep practicing to eventually eliminate the pause. See DVD for an example of this drill.

> ### ✖ PRACTICE DRILL ✖
>
> Start with a simple lower body move (e.g., a march) and add a simple upper body move such as bilateral biceps curls. After 8 or 16 counts, change the upper body while you maintain the lower body move, experimenting until you find an upper body movement that shares a common connecting point and flows smoothly and naturally (as in the previous drill). Notice if it feels right to your body. Continue 8 or 16 more counts, and then, maintaining your new upper body move, smoothly transition to a new lower body move. In this drill, only half the body changes at a time. Remember, you are working for smoothness; think of it as finding moves that flow so naturally that cueing is completely unnecessary. As you improve your skill, increase the speed of your transitions and switch to a new upper body move or a new lower body move every 4 counts.

Leading Foot

Another factor in creating smooth transitions and easy-to-follow choreography is to maintain an awareness of which foot is leading at all times. In other words, you'll enhance your participants' success if you always lead with the same foot in each move throughout a combination. So, if you start with a step-touch to the right (right foot leads off on the 1st count, or downbeat), then you'll also need to start your grapevine to the right, if that's your next move. Trying to start with a grapevine to the left after leading right in a step-touch will confuse your participants and make the combination harder to follow. In addition to constantly hearing the downbeat in the back of your mind, stay aware of your lead foot and make sure it's contacting the floor on the downbeats of the music. After performing your combination all the way through with the right foot leading, balance your body's neuromuscular and biomechanical systems by performing the entire combo with the left foot leading.

Connector Moves

You may have noticed that in some lower body moves, the feet do the same thing at the same time; examples include pliés, jumping jacks, and double-time bouncy heel lifts (see figure 8.4). These symmetrical moves are valuable as filler moves and can help you switch your leading foot if you haven't built a lead change into your combination. Because both feet are doing the same thing at the same time, it's easy to start the next move on either the right foot or the left foot.

Other types of moves are so basic that they can be used over and over as fillers to ease transitions

between moves and to create participant security. A walk, march, or jog is a good filler. A good beginner combo might be walk 8 counts, four knee lifts (8 counts), walk 8 counts, step-touch four times (8 counts), walk 8 counts, four hamstring curls (8 counts), walk 8 counts, four kicks (8 counts). This adds up to two 32-count phrases, or 64 counts. An 8-count walk is interspersed between all the other moves, which can enhance participant confidence and provide a psychological break from complex choreography. (Incidentally, these 8-count walks could be made more interesting by traveling, adding impact, changing the style, or adding arm variations.) Once participants become comfortable with the combination, try removing all the filler moves (the walks). What you'll have left is a 32-count combination that is more complex: four knee lifts, four step-touches, four hamstring curls, and four kicks.

Every instructor needs filler moves as reliable standbys for those times when the brain seems to stop working; you simply can't remember what's supposed to come next! If this happens, you can always return to the safety of a walk, march, or jog.

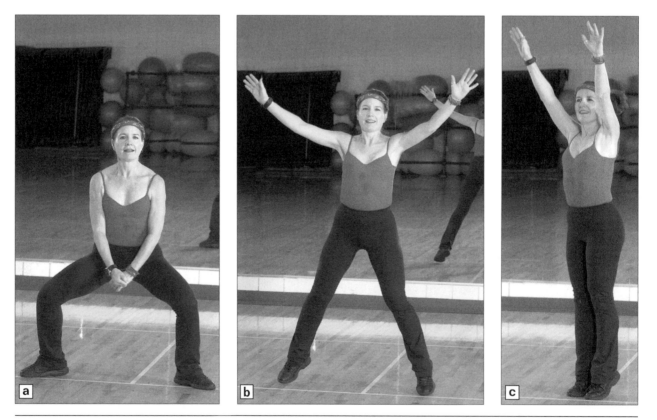

Figure 8.4 (a) Plié (flex knees, down, up, down, up), (b) jumping jack, (c) bouncy heel raises (flex knees down, up, down, up—may add a "jump shot" action with upper body).

Moves That Don't Fit Easily

Some moves simply don't fit well together. When designing a combination, you may have to incorporate one or two transition moves for the easiest to follow and smoothest choreography. For example, moving from a plié to a front kick is awkward; transitional moves are needed for a more natural flow between these two moves. A possible solution could be plié (8 counts), step toe touch side (8 counts), step toe touch front (8 counts), and then step kick front (8 counts).

BUILDING BASIC COMBINATIONS

Many instructors prefer to teach high/low impact classes with combinations of moves; usually these combinations have been designed and practiced before class using the structure of the 32-count phrase. Here are the typical steps used in designing a high/low impact combination:

1. Start with four lower body moves that flow together smoothly. Make sure each move fills 8 counts for a total of 32 counts. Practice to find the smoothest arrangement of the four moves, adding transitional moves and eliminating moves that don't fit as necessary, but staying within the 32-count framework.

2. Find upper body movements that go with the lower body combination.

3. Check to see that your combination
   - provides a balance of complex and simple moves,
   - can be modified to provide appropriate intensity and complexity variations,
   - flows smoothly,
   - is easy to cue (see cueing section on pages 133-138), and
   - can be "broken down" easily (more about this later).

4. Repeat this process with another 32-count combination, sometimes referred to as a *block*. If you plan to eventually link several blocks of 32-count combos together, you will need to see that they have common end points and

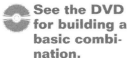 **See the DVD for building a basic combination.**

starting points for smooth transitions between blocks.

Showing Modifications

Skilled instructors are adept at providing intensity and complexity modifications to accommodate different participant skill and fitness levels. Generally, it is recommended that instructors teach at an intermediate level and demonstrate intensity variations for both more and less fit exercisers. See the section on intensity variation on page 125 and "Intensity Drill."

INTENSITY DRILL

A group instructor should occasionally incorporate an intensity drill into the class routine; this way participants will be more likely to take responsibility for themselves and modify moves to fit their own needs.

Show a basic move such as a hamstring curl and cue, "Show me this move at low intensity." Watch participants do the move for a moment and then say, "Now show me the same move at medium intensity." And later, "Can you show me this move performed at high intensity?" (It helps build participant confidence if you call out suggestions for increasing and decreasing intensity during the drill.) Then have participants show medium intensity again and finally low-intensity modifications, so they know how to both increase and decrease the intensity of the hamstring curl. Repeat with other simple moves such as knee lifts, grapevines, or even a basic march.

In addition, the more complex your choreography, the more important your ability to show modifications and break down your routines (see the next section). This is particularly true with moves that pivot or turn, as some participants tend to get dizzy or disoriented. (A 4-count pivot turn can always be modified to a 4-count mambo, or even a march, for instance.)

Breaking Down and Building Combinations

A combination is said to be "broken down" when an instructor takes the finished choreography and essentially works backward. In other words, many participants generally can't grasp the final, most complex, most intense version of your routine the first time you show it. Instead, you start the combo with the most basic, simplest moves and gradually build in intensity and complexity until participants are performing the final product. This may take quite a while, depending on the choreography and your participants' skill levels. Design all your routines so that they can be easily broken down into their basic components. Some practitioners call this the "part to whole" method. Practice teaching your routines as if you were leading novice participants through your combinations for the first time. Here's an example of how to break down a 32-count combination that contains a rather complex move: The final version of the combination is as follows:

1. Facing the left corner, perform two kick-ball-changes (right leg performs full range of motion [ROM] kick while right foot is leading) followed by one box step (jazz square). (This is the complex move). Upper body performs alternating punches on kick-ball-change; arms sweep backward on box step—8 counts all together. See the DVD under basic moves for a demonstration.

2. Repeat for another 8 counts.

3. Facing front, step-touch right and left, repeat. Upper body performs full ROM lateral raise—8 counts.

4. Perform four jumping jacks, turning so last jack faces right corner. Upper body performs overhead presses—8 counts. You have now completed 32 counts all together.

5. Repeat the entire combination on the other side, leading with left foot.

Here's how to break down this combination:

1. Start by repeating the kick-ball-change move over and over again, right foot leading. Drill this move without arms until the majority of your class can perform it correctly. (You could even break this move down further by teaching it half time.)

2. Now drill the box step, continuing to repeat the move until it appears that most of your participants are comfortable with it.

3. Next, combine the two moves: two kick-ball-changes followed by one box step.

Again, repeat this two-move pattern over and over until participants have it.

4. Adding on, perform four sets of right and left step-touches for a count of 16.

5. Then perform eight jumping jacks for a count of 16.

6. Now that your participants know the four movement patterns you'll be using, start the beginning of the combo at the top of the next 32-count phrase (still leading right), and lead your group in an expanded version of the final combination: four sets of the two kick-ball-changes followed by a box step combo (32 counts), four sets of right and left step-touches (16 counts), and eight jumping jacks (16 counts).

7. Repeat this expanded version; add upper body movements.

8. Repeat the combination again; asking for more energy and greater ROM on the kick part of the kick-ball-change.

9. Finally, reduce the combo to its intended version: two sets of the two kick-ball-changes followed by a box step combo (16 counts), two sets of right and left step-touches (8 counts), and four jumping jacks (8 counts).

Participants now should be familiar enough with the routine that they are ready to try it with the left foot leading. Because of the initial complexity of this routine and to balance left with right, it's probably wise to go through all the preceding nine steps on the left side.

The preceding combination illustrates the concept of balancing complex with simple moves. Because the kick-ball-change requires agility and feels so complex to most participants, the simple step-touches and jumping jacks provide a nice physiological and psychological balance. In addition, any decrease in intensity required by the complex footwork in the first moves can be balanced with the jacks at the end of the combination.

Teaching techniques used in this example include *adding on* and *repetition reduction*. After the class has learned a move, pattern, or short sequence, the instructor adds a new move or pattern to the existing sequence, gradually putting together the final product. Because most participants need repetition of a move in order to learn it (particularly if it is complex), skilled instructors teach combinations in expanded versions with many repetitions of each move. In other words, a combo that is intended to be 32 counts might be drilled in a 64-count or 128-count version. In beginner classes, the combo might remain expanded; it is not even always necessary to reduce it to its most complex form. The process of reducing the number of repetitions to the most complex, 32-count version is called *repetition reduction*. This process also goes under the name of *pyramid building:* You start the sequence with large numbers of repetitions and gradually reduce the number of repetitions until the desired combination is achieved.

See the DVD for a choreography overview for high-low impact moves.

ADDITIONAL CHOREOGRAPHY TECHNIQUES

Although combination building is the most common way to teach high/low impact classes, it is not the only method. Other choreographic teaching techniques (in addition to adding on, repetition reduction, and breaking down a combo, as discussed earlier) include layering, using building blocks, and playing flip-flop. All of these techniques are usually planned and practiced in advance of your actual class. Another choreographic technique, called freestyle or linear choreography, is extemporaneous.

Freestyle Choreography

The freestyle method, also known as using linear progressions, is a valid and effective technique. Whereas combination-style choreography is usually planned and organized into patterns, freestyle choreography is spontaneous and delivered "on the spot," without an emphasis on pattern development. In freestyle, one move flows smoothly into the next move, which flows into the next move, and on and on without much repetition.

See the DVD for a practice drill on freestyle choreography.

Although this technique demands skill on the part of the instructor, it is psychologically easier for participants, who don't have to remember complex moves and patterns. In well-led freestyle, exercisers don't have to worry so much about appearing clumsy or inept, because they are always at least half right! This is because, ideally, the instructor only changes one thing at a time: either changing the upper body movement while the lower body movements remains the same, or changing the lower body while the upper body is maintained. This kind of linear progression allows participants to commit more fully to the moves with greater intensity, potentially resulting in an even better training effect and higher caloric expenditure than might be possible with combination choreography.

The best way to improve your skill at freestyle is, of course, to practice. The drills described in the section on elements of variation and in the section on combining endpoints in smooth transitions are particularly useful. Here's an example of freestyle choreography:

1. Start with a basic march.
2. Add arms pressing front.
3. Keeping the arm movement, change the lower body to a heel dig front.
4. Keeping the lower body, change the arms to an overhead press.
5. Maintaining the upper body, change the legs to toe touch side.
6. Staying with the leg movement, change the arms to side press-outs.
7. Keeping the arms, change the lower body to heel digs to the side.
8. Keeping the lower body, change the arms to long lever lateral raises.
9. Maintaining the upper body, change the legs to a high-impact heel jack.
10. Maintaining the upper body, change to a jumping jack.
11. Change the legs once more to a step-touch (same upper body).
12. Keeping the step-touch, change the arms to unilateral overhead presses.

This example generally alternates upper and lower body changes, but you may sequence your changes however you like as long as you provide variety and muscle balance, avoiding excessive repetitions of moves that are stressful to the musculoskeletal system. Each move or change (be sure to initiate on the 1st count of an 8-count phrase) can be performed for 4, 8, 16, or even 32 counts, depending on your class. As always, an appropriate intensity level must be maintained: Too many low-intensity moves in a row results in a low-intensity progression.

Notice that each move in the example transitions smoothly into the next. Not only is this easier for participants to successfully follow, but it's much easier for you to cue! In fact, good freestyle requires a minimum of cueing; participants simply have to keep moving and watching and they will naturally move with you. This provides an ideal format for those times when you want to promote group interaction and sociability while working out or when you want to make class announcements or educational points. Because it's not as necessary to give anticipatory cues (cues that let exercisers know what the next move is), you can talk about other subjects with your class. Freestyle is especially useful during the warm-up as well as at any point when you sense that participants are experiencing "brain strain" from too much concentration and memorization of complex choreography. Many instructors intentionally intersperse freestyle between choreographed routines to give their class psychological breaks and to help boost intensity levels. The freestyle technique is also great for less experienced or coordinated participants because they don't have to remember specific sequences.

Layering

The layering technique is used when you add more and more complexity to a move or combination. Each layer is repeated until participants appear confident, and then complexity is increased. See the following example of layering:

1. Perform 3 counts of walking-in-place with a knee lift on the 4th count. Repeat other side.
2. Layer with a directional variation: Travel forward repeating the move twice for a total of 8 counts and then travel backward repeating the move twice for 8 counts.
3. Increase the complexity by keeping the pattern only on the 8 counts forward; walk for 8 counts backward without any knee lifts.

4. Layer by adding a hop on the 4th and 8th counts forward (on the knee lifts) while abducting the arms to shoulder height.
5. Layer by adding jazz style to the forward movements. While hopping and lifting the left knee, twist the spine and adduct the knee across the body, showing the left hip; while hopping and lifting the right knee, twist the spine and adduct the knee across the body, showing the right hip.
6. Layer the backward 8-count walk by performing a pivot turn on counts 5, 6, 7, and 8 (finish facing frontward).

As you can see, the same 16 counts are performed over and over, but gradually the patterns become more interesting, stylistic, and complex.

Building Blocks and Linking

A block can be defined as a 32-count combination of moves. Instructors can create several blocks and then link them together for one long combination (e.g., A + B + C + D). When using many blocks and linking them together, name your combos or associate them with key words or numbers to help your students with recall. For example, you could cue your class, "Now let's do Carol's combo" (named after Carol); then, "Next the shuffle routine" (this routine has a shuffle in it); and then, "It's time for the traveler" (combo with large traveling moves).

Flip-Flop

This technique works well for combinations that have clearly defined elements such as high- and low-impact or stationary and traveling moves. After participants have become very familiar with the initial combination, flip-flop the key elements; for example, change all the low-impact moves to high impact and all the high-impact moves to low impact, thus gaining more mileage from existing combos.

TRAINING SYSTEMS

The major training systems used in the design of a high/low impact class are continuous or steady-state training; interval intensity training, which may be either timed or sporadic; interval cardio modality training (usually timed); and interval cardio and strength training.

Continuous or Steady-State Training

In this format, different choreographic techniques may be used to produce one long, continuous endurance workout with few intensity variations. Even though low- and high-impact moves may be used throughout, the overall effect is steady; participants are usually encouraged to work in their target heart rate zone at a moderate to high level without major fluctuations (see figure 8.5).

Interval Intensity Training

In this system, intensity levels can fluctuate between high, low, and moderate. The instructor provides high-intensity patterns or short intense combos for an anaerobic (power) interval. This interval may last for 15, 30, or 60 s, during which participants are encouraged to challenge themselves, perhaps pushing into the top range of their target heart rate zone (or even beyond, for advanced participants). Patterns used during the intervals may include plyometric, bounding, or power-type moves. The cardio conditioning segment can be organized into regular timed intervals (e.g., a 4-min song with a typical high\low combination, followed by a 1-min power interval, with this sequence repeated five times), or the intervals can be interspersed randomly throughout the high/low impact portion of the class.

Interval Training With Differing Cardio Modalities

This system is a great way to incorporate cross-training and alleviate boredom. A typical format might be 4 min of high/low impact followed by 4 min of step, repeated for 32 mins. Other modalities to consider include kickboxing, slide, and jump rope.

Intervals of Cardio and Strength Training

Another popular system for overall class organization is to alternate timed intervals of cardio training with strength training stations: for example, 4 min of high/low impact, 4 min of squats and lunges, 4 min of high/low impact, and then 4 min of biceps and deltoids.

CUEING METHODS

Proper cueing is essential for a successful high/low impact class. Class members will have different learning styles; most will learn best by watching you, others will learn by hearing your verbal instruction, and others will learn by doing (visual, auditory, and kinesthetic styles, respectively). Use as many styles as possible, and enlarge your teaching vocabulary so that you can say the same thing in multiple ways. Several types of cues are necessary, including anticipatory, movement, motivational, educational, alignment, and safety verbal cues, plus visual cues. In this section we also discuss the advantages and disadvantages of mirroring your class.

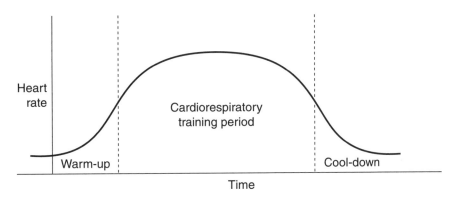

Figure 8.5 Steady-state training.

Anticipatory Cueing

An anticipatory cue tells your participants when to do the next movement and what that next movement will be. Learning to deliver timely and appropriate anticipatory cues often takes considerable practice, so be patient and practice the drills given in this book, and you will eventually become an instructor who is easy to follow. To give good anticipatory cues, you must understand music structure and be able to hear the beat, the downbeat, and the 4-, 8-, and 32-count phrases. (Refer to chapter 3 for a discussion of this information.)

It's easiest for your class if you count backward when cueing an upcoming new move or transition. If you count, "4, 3, 2, and _____," your participants know that after "_____" (where the 1 would be) there will be a new move. This helps them to pay attention and be ready to change and move with the rest of the class. If your anticipatory cue is short (e.g., step-touch), only one beat might be needed, as in, "4, 3, 2, step-touch." Longer cues (e.g., grapevine right, arms up) take more time to say and therefore will need more beats: "4, 3, grapevine right, arms up."

Practice Anticipatory Cueing

Additionally, instructors don't usually speak on every single beat for anticipatory cueing; not only is this usually too wordy and confusing, it is hard on your voice! Instead, count backward on every other beat of your 8-count phrase as shown in figure 8.6. Practice this example by clapping your hands on every beat while you speak in rhythm at the suggested times. This method of counting on every other beat works very well when you are performing 2-count moves.

Practice Cueing 2-Count Moves

Starting without music, march, feeling your lead foot (e.g., right) coming down on every other beat (a march is a 2-count move). Begin to practice the cue given in figure 8.6 ("4, 3, 2, step-touch"), saying "4" when your lead foot strikes the floor (this is a downbeat and the first beat of an 8-count phrase). If all goes well, you will be ready to step-touch to the right at the end of the 8 counts, leading off on the new move (step-touch) with your right, or lead, foot on the downbeat. Notice the paradox: You are saying one thing while your body does something else. This probably won't

feel natural at first, but keep practicing—it's a skill worth acquiring if you want your participants to all do the same thing at the same time and feel satisfied with your class!

After mastering the march to step-touch while cueing, see if you can continue the step-touch and, when ready, cue back to a march. Note that you may continue step-touching for as many counts as you like, starting the anticipatory cue, "4, 3, 2, _____" when you are ready to change (see figure 8.6). Be sure to say "4" when your lead foot (e.g., right) is striking the floor and stepping right (always be mindful of your lead foot).

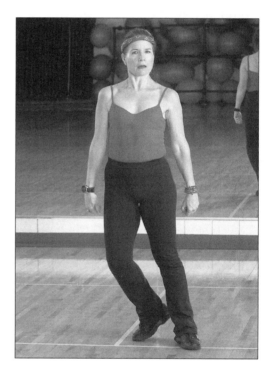

Counts	8	7	6	5	4	3	2	1	8
Footstrike	(March) R	L	R	L	R	L	R	L	(Step-touch) R
Cue	"4,		3,		2,	step	touch"		

Figure 8.6 Practice march to step-touch while cueing.

Now when you start to march, the right foot is still leading with the footstrike on the downbeat or the actual first count of the 8-count phrase (which, as explained, is counted backward in 4s to make it easier for your participants). Be aware that to finish the 8 counts, your right foot performs a tap or touch immediately before leading right in the march (the end of your last step-touch). This is called *finishing the movement phrase* and is a key component in keeping you on the downbeat. If you forget to perform this tap or touch, you will no longer be moving with the music and your participants will eventually become confused. It's actually much simpler than it sounds; performing these moves to music will feel quite natural. You don't even need to mention this extra tap or touch to your students; they'll just unconsciously do it as long as you're moving with the downbeats.

Before trying this drill with music, go back and forth between these two moves (marching and step-touching), continuing each move as long as necessary for you to collect your thoughts and cue properly. Practice leading with your other foot, as well. Another basic pattern for initial practice is march to wide march and back again to march, cueing, "4, 3, march it wide," and then, "4, 3, march it back in." Experiment with speaking in rhythm. You want to start to hear the ticktock of the constant rhythmic beat at all times in your head while teaching. Eventually this drill can be expanded to a wide variety of 2-count moves (see the sample list in table 8.1).

Practice these drills with a friend who will pretend to be your student. This person's responses can give you instant feedback about the timeliness and effectiveness of your cues. Then, repeat the entire drill with music. Pick popular music (preferably a commercially mixed group exercise tape) with a strong, easy-to-hear beat to help you integrate this basic cueing exercise. These drills and speaking in rhythm may have a slightly robotic feel. This is appropriate in the early stages of learning to cue, when hearing and moving on the downbeat may not yet be habitual and spontaneous for you.

✓ TECHNIQUE CHECK

When cueing, be sure to

- ❏ hear the downbeat and the 8-count phrase,
- ❏ initiate new moves at the top of the 8-count phrase on the downbeat,
- ❏ initiate these new moves with your lead foot,

- ❏ finish all moves (e.g., the last tap or touch),
- ❏ cue backward starting with 4,
- ❏ speak in rhythm (at least initially), and
- ❏ cue the next move while you're still performing the current move.

Practice Cueing 4-Count Moves

The process of learning to cue 4-count moves is similar to the drills described previously; however, instead of counting on every other beat, you count on every 4th beat. For example, perform grapevines, right and left continuously, leading with the right foot. When ready to change to the next move, such as a march, begin counting backward, starting with 4 when the right (lead) foot initiates a grapevine to the right. This time, however, count each individual grapevine, or every 4th count, as shown in figure 8.7.

Finish by marching right, which should be your lead foot. Notice again the final tap of the right foot just before the march; this tap finishes the last grapevine and is essential to keep you moving with the music. When marching, return to the 2-count cueing you have already learned, saying, "4, 3, 2, grapevine" to cue the grapevine, at which point you'll again switch to the 4-count cueing (see figure 8.7). Practice moving back and forth between 2- and 4-count moves until the anticipatory cueing feels comfortable. A grapevine is a perfect move to simultaneously practice visual cueing, which we'll discuss shortly. Participants will be grateful if you point in the direction of the initial grapevine (to help them get started) and if you hold up fingers (4, 3, 2, 1) to let them know when the next change will occur.

Another cueing drill that entails switching from 2-count to 4-count anticipatory cueing involves moving from singles to doubles and back to singles again. Several movement patterns work here, including knee lifts, hamstring curls, lunges, and step-touches. Start with single hamstring curls, for instance, and cue every 2 counts: "4, 3, 2, now doubles." Each double hamstring curl requires 4 counts. When ready to return to singles, cue as directed previously on every 4 counts: "4, 3, 2, 1, now single."

See the DVD for a practice drill on cueing 2-count and 4-count moves.

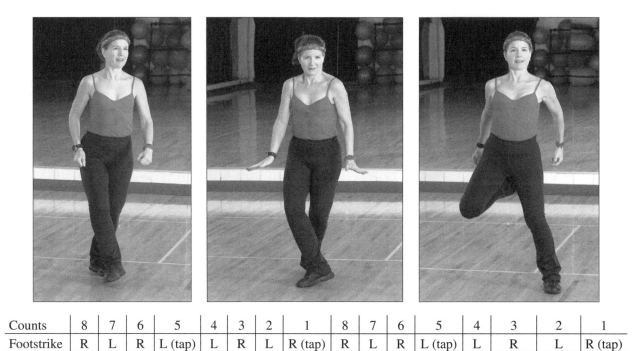

Counts	8	7	6	5	4	3	2	1	8	7	6	5	4	3	2	1
Footstrike	R	L	R	L (tap)	L	R	L	R (tap)	R	L	R	L (tap)	L	R	L	R (tap)
Cue	"4,				3,				2,				1,	march	right"	

Figure 8.7 Practice grapevine to march while cueing.

Movement Cues

A movement cue verbalizes what is seemingly obvious. Many participants need this verbal reinforcement to enhance their confidence and success. A movement cue can point out the footwork, either with rhythmic counts (as in a cha-cha: "the feet go 1, 2, 1, 2, 3—1, 2, 1, 2, 3") or rights and lefts (e.g., when lunging: "right foot back, left foot back, right foot back, left foot back"), or a movement cue can provide basic directions (as in a double lunge: "feet go down, up, down, switch—down, up, down, switch"). Such cues may be repeated over and over with appropriate rhythmic emphasis until participants perform the pattern correctly. Movement cues also include naming the move or step (e.g., "pivot turn" or "twist") and stating an actual direction, as in "grapevine right," although in such cases we recommend always accompanying the words *right* and *left* with the visual cue of pointing. (Some participants experience confusion and anxiety when suddenly asked to move right or left. This can be eased or eliminated entirely by pointing, which is a visual cue.)

Motivational Cues

The sole purpose of a motivational cue is to increase your participants' self-confidence and enjoyment and to encourage a sense of play! Your speech should be liberally sprinkled with encouraging words and phrases: "Great," "Super," "Well done," "Fantastic job," "You people look terrific," "Outstanding." Some instructors give as many motivational cues as one every 8 to 16 counts! No wonder their classes are so popular! Additionally, many instructors cut loose with whoops, trills, yahoos, hup-hup, and other noises just for fun. If you have a good time in class, the chances are good that your students will too!

Educational Cues

An educational cue delivers relevant information about the workout itself or about other topics related to fitness or wellness. Reviewing the benefits of aerobic training while leading your class in simple freestyle moves is an excellent way to incorporate education into your teaching. And, of course, it's essential to give intensity guidelines and recommendations throughout your class. Muscle identification ("these are your hamstrings") and hydration information are other examples of educational cueing.

Alignment and Safety Cues

Skilled instructors constantly deliver alignment and safety pointers. Common misalignments during cardio training include forward head (chin jut), rounded and hunched shoulders, shoulders that elevate when reaching overhead, hyperextended elbows and knees, and lack of spinal and pelvic stability (particularly during knee lifts and kicks). When participants perform lunges or repeaters, the hips, knees, and toes all need to point in the same direction. Safety cues include reminding participants to bring their heels down when jumping, avoid excessive momentum, stay in control, keep their fists relaxed, listen to their bodies, work at their own pace, and stay hydrated. It's nearly impossible to give too many of these types of cues! See the technique and safety section earlier in this chapter for more ideas.

Visual Cues

Do everything possible to ensure your participants' success. If the majority of class members consistently have trouble following or grasping new moves, the difficulty is probably not with the individuals in the class but with the instructor. Such problems can be traced to the instructor's moves, transitions, sequencing, ability to understand and work with the music, and especially ability to cue correctly. Thus, you will want to work hard to make your cueing crystal clear. One major way to help participants move with you at all times is to use visual cueing in conjunction with verbal cueing. This is essential when you work with large groups or without a microphone, and in addition it can save your voice. A number of visual cues have been developed and are used commonly by high/low impact instructors (Webb 1989). These include using hand signals for counting, showing direction, turning, holding a move, tapping the thigh of the lead leg, calling for everyone's attention ("watch me"), and pointing to various parts of your own body to indicate proper alignment (see figure 8.8).

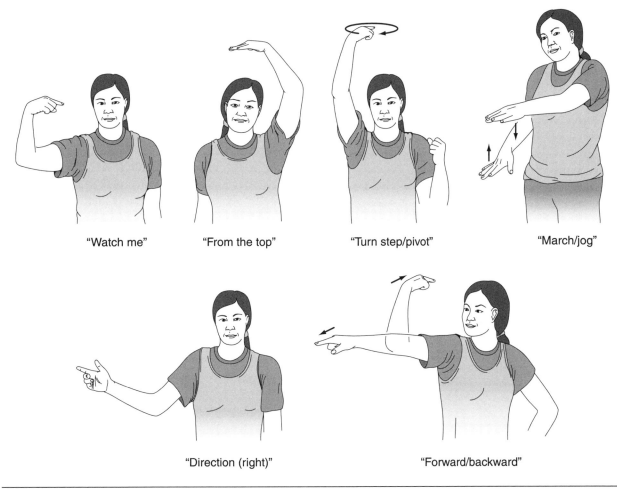

"Watch me"   "From the top"   "Turn step/pivot"   "March/jog"

"Direction (right)"   "Forward/backward"

Figure 8.8 Visual cues.

Most people are visual learners. This means that they tend to unconsciously copy your body language, including your alignment, physical energy, and movement style. This is good if you have excellent alignment and physical energy; however, it can be problematic if you use incorrect alignment or technique.

PRACTICE DRILL

Play your favorite music with a strong beat. Facing a partner, choose a familiar move (such as a walk or step-touch), continue the move for 4 to 16 counts, and then transition through several new moves (this works best if your transitions are smooth and natural and you use the elements of variation). Try not to speak at all, using only visual cueing to communicate. This includes having an animated face and a high level of enthusiasm!

When you face your partner or a class, you are using the technique of *mirror imaging*. Mirror imaging is another valuable group leadership skill that takes practice. Advantages of mirror imaging include more personal and direct eye contact with your students, better vocal projection, and less temptation to become mesmerized by your own image in the mirror. Facing your class shows that you are a student-centered instructor and makes your job seem less like a performance. We recommend facing your class as much as possible, especially during the warm-up, when you are leading freestyle choreography, and during the muscle conditioning and flexibility portions of your class. The major disadvantage of facing your class is that if your high/low impact combinations are relatively complex, it's often more difficult for your class to follow. In other words, their success is more likely if you face away from them during intricate choreography.

Mirroring takes practice. When you want your class to move right, you'll need to point left with your left hand, even as you are saying "right." If you want them to march forward, you'll need to move backward as you motion them to come toward you. Your directional cues will be reversed for you but not for your class. For practice, repeat all the drills described in this chapter while facing a partner.

Movement Previews

When you are teaching more complex choreography, sometimes a movement preview is useful. As participants continue with a familiar move, you demonstrate (preview) the new move or the more complex variation for them. In other words, they see it before they do it. For example, while participants perform grapevines, you preview the more complex layer by demonstrating grapevines with a turn.

COMPREHENSION CHECK

Here are the key points for cueing:
- As much as possible, cue both verbally and visually.
- Use a microphone whenever possible.
- After you become proficient at cueing, avoid endless counting. Instead, use your time whenever possible to deliver other types of cues (e.g., alignment, motivational).
- Always count down instead of up.
- Keep cues relatively short and to the point.
- Initiate cues on the downbeat and time them so the new move is also on the downbeat.

Chapter Wrap-Up

This chapter has covered the most important practical techniques for leading a high/low impact cardio group exercise class. Most of the topics and techniques described are applicable to other types of group exercise such as step, slide, NIA, and kickboxing.

When developing your high/low impact class segment, check yourself against the group exercise class evaluation form to be sure you've met the basic criteria for leading cardio segments. To become proficient at leading group exercise, you must practice, experiment, and keep challenging yourself. The rewards are worth it; you will soon lead a class that your participants will want to take over and over again!

Key Points for Leading High/Low Impact Classes Based on the Group Exercise Evaluation Form.

- Gradually increase intensity from the warm-up into the main portion of the cardio segment. Avoid giving high-intensity moves such as jumping jacks and lunges right away.
- Use a variety of muscle groups and minimize repetitive movements. Use muscles on the front, back, and sides of the body to avoid overuse injuries. For example, if you've given a combination with a large number of knee lifts, make certain the next combination includes a large number of hamstring curls!
- Demonstrate good form, alignment, and technique. Remember that your class will be subconsciously copying your body! Be impeccable with your alignment.
- Give movement options and modifications. Jumping in place on both feet, for example, can easily become a march. A pony can become a step-touch and vice versa.
- Use music appropriately. The tempo range for high/low impact is approximately 134 to 158 beats/min. The faster the music, the less your participants will be able to go through their full ranges of motion, and the sloppier their form may become. Always keep safety in mind. Using music appropriately also means moving on the beat, downbeat, and the 32-count phrase so the class feels natural and has a comfortable flow.
- Give clear cues and verbal directions, including visual, anticipatory, movement, motivational, safety, and alignment cues.
- Promote participant interaction and encourage fun. Use circles, hand slaps, and name calls; ask for each person's favorite move! Use freestyle choreography to ask how your class is doing and to talk about upcoming events. Design routines with noises (e.g., uh-huh uh-huh, hey, trills) built in!
- Gradually decrease intensity during postcardio cool-down. Taper off from vigorous high-intensity and peak moves. Return to low-impact, low-intensity moves such as walking, step-touches, and heel digs, keeping arms low. Include standing static stretches for the calves, hamstrings, hip flexors, low back, and chest muscles in the postcardio cool-down.

Written Assignment

Prepare a high/low impact group exercise lesson plan using the group exercise class evaluation form cardio segment. Write specific moves (at least four 32-count blocks) to a favorite piece of high/low impact music.

Practical Assignment

Prepare a 2-min high/low routine to present. Use at least two 32-count blocks of simple choreography. Incorporate anticipatory cueing (on the downbeat), visual cueing, and at least one other cueing technique.

Step Training

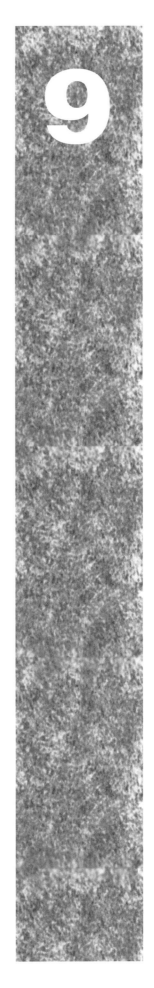

9

Chapter Objectives

By the end of this chapter, you will

- ■ understand how to warm up for step training,

- ■ be able to teach basic moves and patterns for step,

- ■ be able to build basic combinations and choreography for a step class,

- ■ be able to teach a 2-min step routine with appropriate content, alignment, technique, and cueing using appropriate music, and

- ■ be able to identify proper alignment, technique, and safety recommendations for step training.

Cardio step classes are an increasingly popular training modality since their inception in 1990; approximately 66% of fitness facilities offer step aerobic programming (IDEA 2002). Step classes promote cardiorespiratory fitness, muscle endurance, coordination, balance, and several health benefits (see "Step Training Research Findings"). Many participants enjoy the rhythmic sound, exact patterning, and high energy of a step class. Your marketability as a group exercise leader may increase if you learn how to teach motivating step class. The main points on the group exercise class evaluation form for step are found in figure 9.1.

Key Points for Warm-Up Segment

1. Includes appropriate amount of dynamic movement ❑
2. Provides rehearsal moves ❑
3. Stretches major muscle groups in a biomechanically sound manner with appropriate instructions ❑
4. Gives clear cues and verbal directions ❑
5. Uses an appropriate music tempo of 118-128 beats/min ❑

Key Points for Cardio Segment

1. Gradually increases intensity ❑
2. Uses a variety of muscle groups and minimizes repetitive movements ❑
3. Promotes participant interaction and encourages fun ❑
4. Demonstrates movement options and gives clear verbal cues and directions ❑
5. Gradually decreases intensity during postcardio cool-down ❑
6. Uses an appropriate music tempo of 118-128 beats/min ❑

Figure 9.1 Main points for step from the group exercise class evaluation form.

Before working your way through this chapter, you should do the following:

READ

❑ chapter 4: Warm-Up,

❑ the music section in chapter 3 (pp. 31-35), and

❑ the choreographic technique sections in chapter 8 (pp. 124-133).

PRACTICE

❑ the music drills in chapter 3 (pp. 34-35) and

❑ the cueing drills in chapter 8 (pp. 134-138).

WARM-UP

Warm-ups for step training follow the same recommendations outlined in chapter 4: preparing the heart, lungs, and all major muscles for vigorous activity using a combination of dynamic movements and stretches. However, an optimal step warm-up also incorporates the bench, thus specifically readying the body for the step workout to follow. This is achieved by using a *floor mix*, that is, a mixture of step and low-impact moves. A simple floor mix pattern is shown in table 9.1.

Dynamic Movement and Rehearsal Moves

The grapevine is performed on the floor, whereas the tap-up, tap-down is a rehearsal move that uses the step. This type of sequencing specifically and gradually prepares the mind and body for more intense step moves. Because the warm-up is to be performed at a lower intensity than the cardio-conditioning portion of class, the number of step moves used and the sequencing of the floor mix are important factors. Avoid continuous stepping in the warm-up because it is stressful to unprepared joints and can increase the heart rate too quickly. Instead, intersperse low-impact moves with step moves.

STEP TRAINING RESEARCH FINDINGS

Many research studies have shown that step (or bench) training can provide an excellent and predictable cardiorespiratory stimulus with important health benefits (Kin Isler et al. 2001, Kraemer et al. 2001). A number of these studies have specifically measured energy expenditure at various step heights and have found that step training meets the ACSM criteria for the achievement of cardiorespiratory fitness (Olson et al. 1991, Stanforth et al. 1991, Woodby-Brown et al. 1993). Research shows that intensity and caloric expenditure increase with increased step height (Stanforth, Stanforth, and Velasquez 1993, Wang et al. 1993, Woodby-Brown et al. 1993). Specific moves and patterns as well as the inclusion of arm movements influence the energy cost (Calarco et al. 1991, Francis et al. 1994, Olson et al. 1991), as does the addition of propulsion to common step moves (Greenlaw et al. 1995). Some researchers have found that increased music tempo results in increased energy consumption (Scharff-Olson, Williford, Duey, et al. 1997, Stanforth et al. 1991), whereas others have measured the cost of stepping while holding hand weights (Kravitz et al. 1995, Olson et al. 1991, Workman et al. 1993), finding that 2-lb hand weights do not significantly influence the energy cost of stepping.

Yet other studies have measured the impact forces on the feet when a participant is performing step. Francis et al. (1994) found that the feet undergo approximately the same peak vertical forces when stepping on a 10-in. step as when walking at a 3 mph pace, which is roughly 1.25 times body weight. However, the lead foot (first foot down off the step) absorbs a greater impact force—1.75 times body weight. This is one reason why it's so important to frequently change the lead foot. Other researchers have found that vertical ground reaction forces increase with increasing step height and with the addition of propulsion (Johnson et al. 1993, Moses et al. 1993, Scharff-Olson, Williford, Duey, et al. 1997). The forces on the knees when stepping also have been examined (Francis et al. 1994), and researchers have found that increasing forces are incurred with increasing angle of knee flexion.

At least one researcher has collected data on step instructors (Kravitz 1994), finding a relatively low percent body fat and favorable upper and lower body strength. Other researchers have examined the effect of step intensity on mood, finding less fatigue and anger in participants who exercised at higher intensities and reduced state anxiety after step training (Hale and Raglin 2002).

◼ PRACTICE DRILL ◼

Design and practice a simple floor mix 32-count combination suitable for a step warm-up, using no more than four moves, for example, one floor move, one step move, one floor move, and one step move.

Stretching Major Muscle Groups

Ideally, some of your warm-up stretches should use the step; common stretches on the bench include those for the hamstrings, hip flexor, and calf muscles (see figure 9.2). The ideal time to increase flexibility is in the final cool-down

Table 9.1 Floor Mix Pattern for a Step Warm-Up

Move	Foot pattern	No. of counts
Grapevine R (on floor)	R, L, R, tap	4
Tap up, tap down (on step)	Up, tap, down, tap	4
Grapevine L (on floor)	L, R, L, tap	4
Tap up, tap down (on step)	Up, tap, down, tap	4

Note. R = right; L = left.

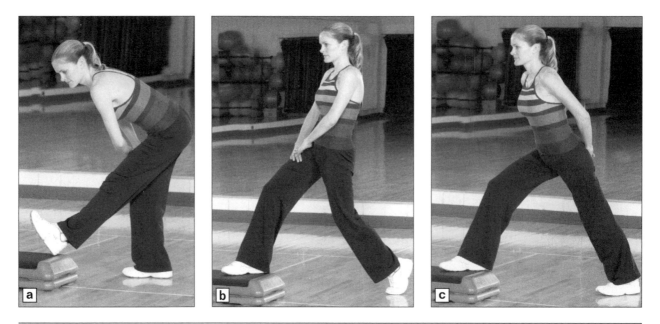

Figure 9.2   (a) Hamstring stretch, (b) hip flexor (iliopsoas) stretch, (c) calf (gastrocnemius) stretch.

portion of class. Stretching during the warm-up is performed simply to take all the joints and muscles through their full range of motion before vigorous exercise. A warm-up stretch is more about extensibility than flexibility and therefore doesn't need to be held as long (8 counts are usually sufficient). Include stretches for the areas that are commonly tight and most heavily used in a step class: calves (both gastrocnemius and soleus), shins, hamstrings, quadriceps, hip flexors, low back, and anterior chest muscles.

▓ PRACTICE DRILL ▓

Design a warm-up segment that incorporates stretches for the calf and hip flexor muscles using the step. Precede the calf stretch by limbering the ankle (lifting and lowering the heel) and precede the hip flexor stretch by limbering the pelvis and hip.

Verbal Cues and Tempo

Cueing during the warm-up is critical. You will be setting the tone for the workout, motivating your class to get going, and educating them about safety and proper alignment. Your voice should be audible, upbeat, encouraging, and energetic. See chapter 8 for a thorough discussion of the various types of cues. Music tempo in a step warm-up is approximately the same as in the step cardio segment: 118 to 128 beats/min.

✓ TECHNIQUE AND SAFETY CHECK

Here are some step warm-up recommendations:

❑ Use the step for at least one low- to moderate-intensity floor mix.

❑ Avoid continuous stepping until the body is thoroughly warm.

❑ Use the step for some of your static stretches.

❑ Stretch the areas that are commonly tight or are heavily used in step: calves, hip flexors, hamstrings, low back, and chest.

TECHNIQUE AND SAFETY

Good step alignment and technique include maintaining neutral spine and neck, with the head and eyes up, and keeping abdominals

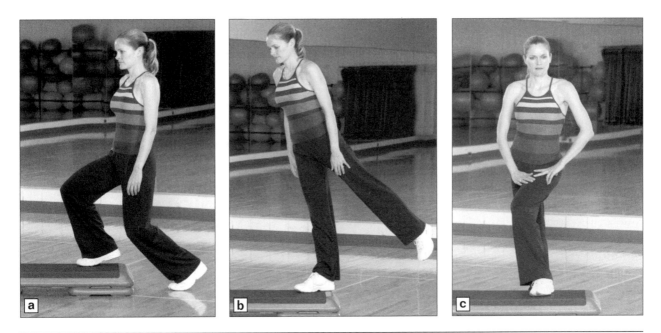

Figure 9.3 Avoid the following: knee (a) hyperflexed, (b) hyperextended, and (c) twisted.

lifted and contracted. As always, avoid hyperextending, hyperflexing, or twisting the knees (see figure 9.3). Keep all joints facing the same direction with shoulders down, even, and relaxed. Use a full body lean when stepping up; visualize one long line from heel to head (see figure 9.4).

You can greatly enhance the safety of your class by avoiding stepping forward off the step; research has shown that much higher impact forces are generated when one is stepping forward off the bench than when stepping backward while facing the step (Francis et al. 1992). Always step lightly on the platform and avoid pounding the feet hard. In addition, step to the center of the platform, and make sure the heel doesn't hang off the back of the step; this helps protect the Achilles tendon. When stepping up, go to full extension of the knees (without hyperextending them). And to minimize the risk of patellar tendinitis, always keep the angle of knee flexion greater than 90°. Stay close enough to the step so that heels can be comfortably brought all the way to the floor on the step-down (landing and rolling through toe, ball, and heel). Your feet should land approximately one shoe length away from the step. Step down without bouncing. Bouncing when you land on the floor increases the eccentric muscle loading and forceful stretching of the Achilles

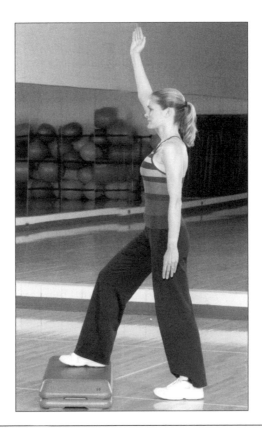

Figure 9.4 Good alignment on a step.

tendon and may lead to Achilles tendinitis. Encourage your participants to jump up on the step instead! Avoid forcing your heels down to the floor during lunges and repeaters. In this case, the ball of the foot contacts the floor while the heel remains lifted. Forcing the heels down may increase the risk of Achilles tendinitis due to the forceful stretching and eccentric loading of the tendon. When performing pivot turns on the step, unload the lower leg by simultaneously hopping so the foot is not in contact with the step during the actual turn.

Help participants choose the proper step height. Step heights greater than 8 in. should be reserved for those with long legs or advanced levels of fitness (see table 9.2). It's also a good idea to change the lead leg frequently to minimize repetitive stress to the leg stepping down off the bench. Finally, keep the tempo of your step music slow enough so that all participants are able to step safely with good technique and alignment. Several organizations recommend step speeds no greater than 126 beats/min. This can be a challenging issue in clubs where participants are used to stepping at much faster speeds. However, research clearly shows that effective workouts are possible at speeds under 126 beats/min, with the added benefit of decreased impact forces and enhanced safety for partici-

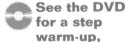 **See the DVD for a step warm-up, which is also outlined in appendix G.**

pants. Look where you are stepping by glancing down occasionally with your eyes while keeping your head up. Avoid high numbers of moves that stress the musculoskeletal system, such as repeaters with more than five repetitions. Limit lunges and other stressful propulsive moves to 1 min or less, depending on your participants. Avoid using hand weights while stepping; while caloric expenditure increases are minimal, the risk of injury is significantly greater with hand weights (Olson et al. 1991, Step Reebok 1997, Workman et al. 1993).

TECHNIQUE AND SAFETY CHECK

To help keep your classes safe, observe the following recommendations.

REMEMBER TO

- ☐ maintain neutral spine and neck, with head and eyes up,
- ☐ keep abdominals lifted and contracted,
- ☐ keep all joints facing the same direction,
- ☐ keep shoulders down, even, and relaxed,
- ☐ use a full body lean when stepping up,
- ☐ step to the center of the platform,
- ☐ keep the angle of knee flexion greater than 90°,
- ☐ help participants choose the proper step height, and
- ☐ change the lead leg frequently.

AVOID

- ☐ hyperextending, hyperflexing, or twisting the knees,
- ☐ stepping forward off the step,
- ☐ pounding the feet hard, and
- ☐ step speeds greater than 126 beats/min.

BASIC MOVES

There are six basic locations around the step from which to perform step moves. The six basic approaches to the step are front, end, side, corner, top, and astride (see figure 9.5).

Lower Body

The use of a step in group exercise presents many options for basic moves of the lower body. The

Table 9.2 Guidelines for Step Height and Step Speed

Participant level	Step height (in.)	Step speed (beats/min)
Novice (new to exercise)	4	118-122
Beginner (regular exerciser who has never done step)	<6	<124
Intermediate (regular stepper)	<8	<126
Advanced (regular, skilled stepper)	<10	<128

Note. Adapted from the 1997 Revised Guidelines for Step Reebok.

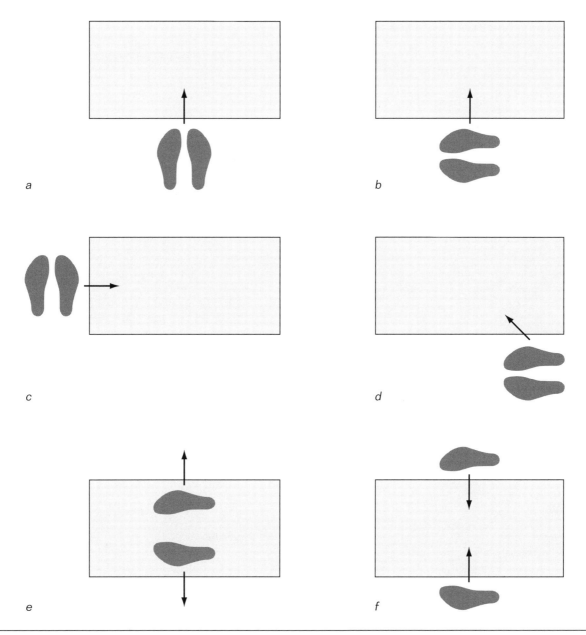

Figure 9.5 Step locations: *(a)* front, *(b)* side, *(c)* end, *(d)* corner, *(e)* top, and *(f)* astride.

DVD presents the basic lower body moves in step training. Lower body moves on the step are all 4-count moves unless otherwise noted. Lower body moves are listed in table 9.3. These moves near the bottom of the list may be more difficult to teach, may be more complex, or may require different approaches and are better suited for a more experienced instructor.

See the DVD for basic lower body step moves.

Most of these moves and patterns can be performed with either a *single* or *alternating lead*. Single lead means that the move is executed in such a way that the same foot continues to lead, for example,

Table 9.3 Moves for Instructors

Moves	Typical approaches
Basic step	Front, end, corner
V-step	Front
Tap up, tap down	Side, end, corner, front
Lift step (knee lift to the front, side, or back; a kick to the front, side, or back)	Front, side, end, corner, astride, top
Turn step	Side
Over the top	Side
Repeater	Front, side, corner, end, astride (8 counts)
Lunge	Top (2 counts) can face front or side
Straddle down	Top
Straddle up	Astride
Across the top	End
Corner to corner	Corner
L-step	Front, end, side
A-step	Corner, side
Charleston	Front, corner, side
Over the top pivot	Side

V-step with no tap-down, up with right foot, up left, down right, down left, up again with the right foot, and so on. In an alternating lead, however, a tap-down is performed on the 4th count so that the lead foot changes, as in this V-step: up right, up left, down right, down tap left, up left, up right, down left, down tap right, and so on.

Additionally, *propulsion* or *power moves* can be added to many patterns to increase the intensity if desired. This simply means to jump up on the step, which requires significantly more energy (never jump off the step because this increases joint stress—see the key points section on safety recommendations for step training). Good moves for adding propulsion include basic step, lift steps, over the top, across the top, L-steps, tap-ups, lunges, and pivot turns.

Upper Body

As with high/low impact moves, there are endless variations of upper body moves in step. Review chapter 8 for a discussion of unilateral and bilateral moves, complementary and opposition arms, and low-, mid-, and high-range arm movements. Common arm moves and step patterns include these:

- Bilateral biceps curls with basic step
- Externally and internally rotated shoulders (out, out, in, in) with V-step
- Overhead press (clap on 4th count) with turn step
- Bilateral shoulder circumduction with over the top
- Chest presses with lunges facing front

It's generally easiest for participants if you teach the lower body movements first, only adding the arms when everyone is comfortable with the lower body patterns.

PRACTICE DRILL

Using the short combination you designed in the previous drill (see p. 147) add simple upper body moves.

BASIC COMBINATIONS AND CHOREOGRAPHY TECHNIQUES

The elements of variation discussed in chapter 8 provide an unlimited number of variations for step moves and patterns. You can vary your moves by changing

- the lever,
- the plane,
- the direction (and, in step, the approach),
- the rhythm,
- the intensity (add propulsion), and
- the style (see pp. 124-126 in chapter 8).

For example, see how a hamstring curl (knee lift to the back) on the step, front approach, can be varied: (1) increase the lever, resulting in hip extension, (2) change the plane for a "side-out" (long lever leg lift to the side), (3) add the element of direction by angling the body diagonally to alternating corners, (4) change the rhythm by performing a hesitation move before each alternating side-out, (5) increase the intensity by adding propulsion (jump up) on each side-out, and (6) play with the style by performing a funky "shimmy" movement with the shoulders on the hesitation, then dorsiflexing the foot and pressing the heels of the hands down on the side-out.

Drilling the elements of variation can result in entirely new moves and patterns and even new combinations! It's easiest to provide smooth transitions when one move begins where the previous move finished (i.e., end points and starting points connect). Moves that share the same approach usually connect well to each other; for example,

over the top and tap-up, tap-down can both be performed from the side approach and thus flow well together.

PRACTICE DRILL

Take one basic move and add (or subtract) an element of variation. Perform each move at least four times (16 counts) before adding or subtracting another element of variation. Make your transitions smooth and natural with end points and starting points connecting (see the section on pp. 127-129 in chapter 8 on smooth transitions). Challenge yourself by changing first an element of variation for the upper body, then one for the lower body, and then one for the upper body, building a *linear progression*.

Teaching With the Music

It is essential to teach with the music in step class. Because almost all step moves are 4 or 8 counts, participants will naturally want to initiate moves on the 1st downbeat of 8-, 16-, and 32-count phrases. Using step music with an easy-to-hear, strong beat, practice often until hearing this downbeat and the musical divisions into counts of 4 becomes second nature for you. Teaching on the beat and with the music keeps you and your students from becoming frustrated and discouraged; your patterns will be easier to follow and more enjoyable. Many students instinctively feel that something is wrong when an instructor is not on the downbeat, although they may not be able to articulate why. Refer to chapter 3 for a thorough discussion of beats, downbeats, measures, and 8-, 16-, and 32-count phrases.

32-Count Blocks

As in high/low impact choreography, step choreography usually consists of blocks of 32-count combinations. These blocks can be repeated over and over, expanded or reduced, or linked together for long, complex combinations. Movements within the blocks can be layered for increasing complexity or changed using the elements of variation. Different choreographic techniques and class structures were discussed in chapter 8. Here's an example of a 32-count block:

1. Facing front: three basic steps, leading right (12 counts; to increase complexity, add a different arm move for each basic step)

2. One half time squat with right foot on bench (facing left side for squat, then facing front on return; 4 counts)

3. Repeat other side, leading left (total 16 counts)

This could be linked to another 32-count block:

1. Facing front: two alternating knee lifts (8 counts)

2. One three-knee repeater (8 counts)

3. Two alternating knee lifts (8 counts)

4. One three-knee repeater other side (8 counts)

See the DVD for a sample 32-count step practice drill. These two blocks could alternate with each other, or you could link them to more blocks for a longer combination.

PRACTICE DRILL

Using a favorite premixed step tape with a strong beat (see the sidebar in chapter 3 for a list of companies that produce step tapes), put together two 32-count blocks of simple choreography. Be sure to start your routine at the "top of the phrase," the 1st downbeat of the 32-count phrase.

Repetition Reduction

Another important technique in skillful step teaching is *repetition reduction*. As discussed in chapter 8, each move is repeated several times until participants are comfortable, and then the number of repetitions is gradually reduced. This can result in a complex combination that requires everyone to concentrate! Here's a relatively simple example:

1. Start with four alternating V-steps and four alternating knee lifts.

2. Reduce to two alternating V-steps and two alternating knee lifts.

3. Reduce further to one V-step and one knee lift.

Holding Patterns

A holding pattern is simply a move (such as a basic step or an over the top) repeated over and over for a brief period of time, allowing both the instructor and the participants to collect their thoughts and return to the desired intensity level. Using a holding pattern provides an ideal time for you to communicate with your students, giving alignment, technique, educational, or motivational cues as necessary.

Intensity Issues

Compared with traditional high/low impact programs, step has workloads that are easier to measure because of the known variable of the step height. As you might suspect, the higher the step, the greater the intensity and the higher the vertical ground reaction forces (Johnson et al. 1993). Students need to use a step that provides a sufficient cardiorespiratory challenge while also allowing them to move with good form and alignment and minimize the risk of injury. Higher platform heights have been associated with knee discomfort attributable to the increased angle of knee flexion (Francis et al. 1994). It is recommended that beginner steppers start with the platform only (4 in.) and gradually progress to a higher step as they become more conditioned and familiar with proper step biomechanics (AFAA 2002).

Intensity is also affected by the specific moves and sequences used in *step choreography*, as well as by changes in lever length, elevated arm movements, increased traveling, and propulsion or power-type moves. Moves that involve more traveling over and around the step and those with more vertical displacement, such as lunges, have been found to have a greater energy cost than moves that involve less knee flexion and extension, such as basic steps. (Note the energy cost of the moves listed in table 9.4.)

Music speed, or tempo, can affect intensity, although most experts do not recommend using a music tempo greater than 126 beats/min because of the increased risk of injury. Participants have a more difficult time completing their movements with full range of motion and can compromise their alignment and stepping technique, increas-

Table 9.4 Energy Costs of Step Training Moves

	Basic step	Traveling with alternating lead	Over the top	Knee lift	Lunges	Repeaters
$\dot{V}O_2$ (ml/kg/min)	26.2	35.5	26.6	28.7	32.7	32.0
METS	7.5	10.1	7.6	8.2	9.3	9.1
HR	141	167	143	147	162	157
RPE	9.5	12.1	11.0	10.8	11.9	11.9

Note. METS = metabolic equivalents; HR = heart rate; RPE = rating of perceived exertion.

Adapted, with permission, from Calarco et al., 1991.

ing the likelihood of injuries such as Achilles tendinitis (see section on technique and safety).

TRAINING SYSTEMS

There are several ways a step class can be formatted, including step super-circuit, step intervals, step alternated with high/low impact intervals, and double step (participants use more than one step). Following are descriptions of step circuit and step interval formats.

Step Circuit

In a step circuit or super-circuit class, several minutes of step may be alternated with several minutes of muscle conditioning work for a complete workout (Kraemer et al. 2001). Here's a sample step circuit class: warm-up (10 min); step (4 min); squats, pliés, and lunges on the floor with weights (4 min); step (4 min); latissimus dorsi and deltoid exercises with weights (4 min); step (4 min); standing chest exercises such as wall push-ups, plus upper back exercises with tubing (4 min); step (4 min); biceps and triceps exercises with weights or tubing (4 min); step (4 min); postcardio cool-down (4 min); abdominals and low back on the floor (5 min); and stretch on the floor (5 min). Total time is 60 min.

Step Intervals

In this type of class, "power" intervals are randomly or regularly interspersed throughout the step portion. The power interval typically lasts 30 to 60 s and consists of a simple move or pattern repeated over and over. Participants are given intensity options that allow them to work at very high levels during the interval if desired. A good example of a power interval combination is as follows: Facing front, perform two lift steps (knee lift with a tap-down) with the right foot leading for 8 counts, follow with four jumping jacks on the floor for 8 counts, repeat the two lift steps with the left foot leading for 8 counts, and then do four more jumping jacks for 8 counts. This simple combination can then be demonstrated with at least three intensity options: (1) perform without jumping—the jacks become low-impact toe touches to the side, (2) perform lift steps with a jump-up on the step (arms low) and perform regular jacks on the floor, and (3) perform lift steps with a jump-up on the step (arms high) and perform "fly" or cheerleader jacks on the floor with arms circumducting. Allow your students to select the intensity option that requires more work than during the regular step portion of class but is still appropriate for them.

Chapter Wrap-Up

The basic teaching strategies for step include providing a warm-up that incorporates rehearsal moves (generally in the form of a floor mix) and teaching small parts of your combination first, usually in 8- or 16-count blocks. Drill these parts, using the principle of repetition, until participants have learned the movements. Teach the lower body first and then add the upper body moves. Then teach the 32-count block, using repetition reduction until participants have learned the movements. Layer your combination with the elements of variation, changing the lever, plane, direction or approach, rhythm, style, or intensity. Repeat this process with the next 32-count block, adding on as desired (A + B + C + D). Use holding patterns between blocks to enhance your communication with your class and to help avoid "brain strain." Practicing these teaching techniques will help you to become a creative and effective step instructor.

Key Points for Leading Step Classes From the Group Exercise Class Evaluation Form

- Gradually increase intensity. After the warm-up and as you begin the cardio segment, gradually increase intensity until you reach the peak part of the cardio stimulus. In other words, plyometric intervals, lunges, and other high-intensity moves do not belong near the beginning of the cardio portion.

- Use a variety of muscle groups and minimize repetitive movements. Avoid high numbers of any move in a row; this can lead to overuse injuries and muscle imbalances. Follow four knee lifts on the step with four hip extensions on the step, for example.

- Demonstrate good form, alignment, and technique on the step. You must be a good role model for your students, because they will unconsciously copy your form and alignment. Stand tall, move with precision, and avoid bouncing down off the step.

- Use step music appropriately. Use a recommended tempo (118-128 beats/min) that allows all participants to complete full range of motion safely and with control. In addition, keep practicing to get better at moving on the beat, initiating new moves at the beginning of phrases, and using the 32-count phrase.

- Give clear cues and verbal directions, including anticipatory cues, safety and alignment information, directional cues, and motivational cues. Remember that for big anticipatory cues you usually count backward starting with 4, as in, "4, 3, 2, knee lift." That way, your class will perform the knee lift together on the downbeat of the next phrase.

- Promote participant interaction and encourage fun. Have students call out their names, say "hi" to their neighbors, and occasionally count with you. Ask them questions, as in, "Everybody feeling fine?"

- Gradually decrease intensity during postcardio cool-down. This can be done by avoiding high-intensity moves and eventually moving off the step. A simple example is to march 4 counts on the step and then march 4 counts on the floor, repeating several times, finishing with marching only on the floor. Incorporate some static stretches while standing, especially stretches for the calves, hip flexors, hamstrings, and low back.

Written Assignment

Prepare a step group exercise lesson plan using the group exercise class evaluation form cardio segment. Write out specific moves for at least four 32-count phrases to a favorite piece of step music.

Practical Assignment

Prepare a 2-min step routine. Use at least one 32-count block and teach it using the techniques of repetition, repetition reduction, holding patterns, and layering.

Kickboxing

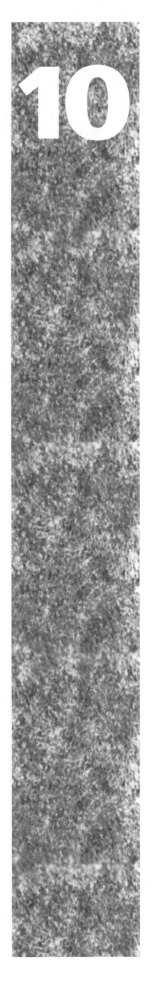

Chapter Objectives

By the end of this chapter, you will

- ■ understand how to warm up for kickboxing,

- ■ be able to teach basic moves for kickboxing,

- ■ know how to build basic choreographic patterns and recognize other class formats for a kickboxing class,

- ■ be able to identify proper alignment, technique, and safety concerns for kickboxing, and

- ■ be able to teach a 2-min kickboxing routine with appropriate content, alignment, technique, and cueing using appropriate music.

Kickboxing is a group exercise modality that has grown in popularity through the late 1990s and into the 21st century. The term *kickboxing* can encompass a wide variety of martial arts fitness workouts, and some of the popular forms include aeroboxing, cardio karate, box step, and Tae-Bo. The goal of most students in a kickboxing class is to promote health and fitness. Most participants aren't taking class with the intention of actually fighting. Therefore, the basic moves in a group kickboxing class are slightly modified from classical martial arts styles to enhance safety and reduce the risk of injury. We recommend going beyond basic group exercise training and certification and pursuing additional training in specific kickboxing techniques if you plan to teach this format. A well-taught kickboxing class can be a great workout and can be fun and highly stimulating for you and your students (see "Kick-

boxing Research Findings"). The main points on the group exercise class evaluation form for kickboxing are found in figure 10.1.

✓ **BACKGROUND CHECK**

Before working your way through this chapter, you should do the following:

READ

❏ chapter 4: Warm-Up,

❏ the music section in chapter 3 (pp. 31-35).

PRACTICE

❏ the music drills in chapter 3 (pp. 34-35) and

❏ the cueing drills in chapter 8 (pp. 134-138).

Key Points for Warm-Up Segment

1. Includes appropriate amount of dynamic movement ❏
2. Provides rehearsal moves ❏
3. Stretches major muscle groups in a biomechanically sound manner with appropriate instructions ❏
4. Gives clear cues and verbal directions ❏
5. Uses an appropriate music tempo of 125-135 beats/min ❏

Key Points for Cardio Segment

1. Gradually increases intensity ❏
2. Uses a variety of muscle groups and minimizes repetitive movements ❏
3. Promotes participant interaction and encourages fun ❏
4. Demonstrates movement options and gives clear verbal cues and directions ❏
5. Gradually decreases intensity during postcardio cool-down ❏
6. Uses music appropriately 118-128 beats/min ❏

Figure 10.1 Group exercise class evaluation form for kickboxing.

KICKBOXING RESEARCH FINDINGS

A number of studies have examined the effectiveness of kickboxing for cardiorespiratory training (Adams et al. 1997, Albano and Terbizan 2001, Anning et al. 1999, Bellinger et al. 1997, Bissonnette et al. 1994, Franzese et al. 2000, Greene et al. 1999, Kravitz et al. 2000, O'Driscoll et al. 1999, Perez et al. 1999, Scharff-Olson et al. 2000). These studies have found that kickboxing can provide a workout that is sufficient to develop increased cardiorespiratory fitness. Significant findings from these studies include: (1) increasing the music speed from 60 to 120 beats/min while punching increased the cardiovascular responses, (2) combining punches with vigorous lower body moves such as shuffles, jacks, and squats resulted in a better cardiovascular stimulus than performing the punches alone, and (3) there was no significant difference in terms of energy cost between shadowboxing and boxing with a heavy bag.

Other researchers have examined injuries in kickboxing classes (Buschbacher and Shay 1999, Davis et al. 2002, McKinney-Vialpando 1999). A relatively high rate of injury (29.3% of participants and 31.3% of instructors) was found in the Davis et al. study, which included 572 participants. This study also found that risk of injury increased dramatically when the frequency of kickboxing was increased: 43% of participants reported injuries with four or more classes per week versus 25% of participants injured when the frequency was one to two classes per week. McKinney-Vialpando found that the faster the music speed, the greater the postexercise pain, and the higher the kicks, the greater the incidence of pain. Axe and crescent kicks were also found to cause pain in 22% of the study participants.

WARM-UP

Kickboxing warm-ups follow the same recommendations outlined in chapter 4 on warm-ups and thus include dynamic movements, rehearsal moves, and appropriate stretching. Alignment cues and a safe music speed are also very important in a kickboxing warm-up.

Dynamic Movement and Rehearsal Moves

The biggest difference between a kickboxing warm-up and other kinds of group exercise warm-ups is the inclusion of dynamic rehearsal moves specific to kickboxing. (A rehearsal move actually rehearses specific movement patterns at a low intensity that will be used later in the high-intensity portion of class.) These moves help prepare the body for the kickboxing workout to follow and include punches, jabs, hooks, and kicks, all performed at a slower speed than will be used during the actual workout. Focus on teaching proper form and technique while your class practices these basic movements. When teaching beginners, you may even consider teaching the basic punches and kicks without music to allow your students to learn proper form and alignment.

Following is a simple warm-up combination that uses rehearsal moves:

1. Using the ready position: four right arm punches performed with one punch every 4 counts; total counts = 16.

2. Repeat with left arm; total counts = 16.

3. Four step-touches; 16 counts.

4. Four hamstring curls; 16 counts.

5. Repeat.

PRACTICE DRILL

Create your own kickboxing warm-up. Pair a basic upper body move, such as a punch, jab, hook, or uppercut, with a basic lower body move, such as a march, step-touch, or grapevine.

Stretching Major Muscle Groups

Another important aspect of a kickboxing warm-up is the increased focus on limbering and stretching the muscles that are heavily used in most kickboxing drills; these muscles include the calves, hip flexors, inner thighs, hamstrings, low back, and anterior chest and shoulder complex. (For specific stretches see chapter 7.) It is particularly important to include dynamic, full range of motion movements and static stretches for these muscles because of the high number of repetitive drills found in a typical fitness-based kickboxing class. As always, the warm-up is an ideal time to stress proper alignment—in the punches and kicks as well as in the static stretches. Because the incidence of injury in kickboxing classes is relatively high (Davis et al. 2002), a proper warm-up and careful teaching of the basic moves are essential.

Verbal Cues and Tempo

Focus on delivering precise anatomical and educational cues when detailing alignment. A good tip is to briefly review several joints or areas of the body: For example, when holding a calf stretch you might say, "Hold the head high, with ears away from the shoulders, neck in line with the spine, shoulders down and back, abdominals in, one long line from head to heel, stretching heel down with the toes facing straight ahead, and hips square." Keep cues positive, telling your class what to do, not what *not* to do. Remember, also, that pointing to or touching parts of your body can be an effective way to cue alignment.

A music tempo of 125 to 135 beats/min is appropriate for most warm-ups. The tempo is fast enough to elevate heart rate, core temperature, and breathing rate but not so fast that participants will become winded or be unable to fully complete the moves.

TECHNIQUE AND SAFETY

Safety should always be a primary concern for instructors, especially in kickboxing, where the incidence of injury has been shown to be approximately 30% (Davis et al. 2002). Backs, knees, hips, and shoulders have all been reported as injury sites. Instructors should understand the common mechanisms of injury at these sites and take steps to avoid increasing their participants' risk of injury.

Eighty percent of Americans report low back pain at some point in their lives (Frymoyer and Cats-Baril 1991). Maintaining a stable, neutral spine while performing kicks and punches is key to preventing back problems in a kickboxing class. Abdominal and back muscles must be dynamically and statically trained to develop spinal stability, and participants must understand the concept of a neutral spine. Excessive hip flexor involvement from high numbers of kicks also can contribute to low back pain because the iliopsoas muscles attach on the lumbar spine. To prevent this problem, include hip flexor stretches in both the warm-up and cool-down portions of your class.

The incidence of knee pain can be reduced by teaching good kicking technique, emphasizing an active *retraction,* or knee flexion, phase immediately after the knee extends in a kick. Snapping or ballistically extending the knee with excessive momentum can overstretch the knee ligaments and create knee instability. Torque or sudden twisting moves where the foot is anchored but the knee

turns are also mechanisms of knee injury, overstretching the collateral knee ligaments. Always keep toes aligned in the direction of the knees.

Hip pain can result from a lack of muscle balance around the hip joint. Use the hip flexors and extensors as evenly as possible, as well as the hip adductors and abductors and the hip internal and external rotators. Provide plenty of appropriate stretches for these muscles, avoid excessive repetitions of kicks, and always teach a thorough warm-up.

Reduce the incidence of shoulder pain by teaching good punching technique (retracting the arm immediately after each punch) and by training the external rotator cuff and posterior deltoid muscles with specific exercises to counterbalance all the forward motion involved in punching. Additionally, shoulder pain is more likely when the shoulder girdle isn't properly stabilized. Instruct participants to punch with the scapulae down, and give isolation exercises for the middle trapezius and rhomboids (scapular retractors) as well as plenty of stretching for the anterior chest muscles. Too many kickboxing classes without proper stretching, muscle conditioning, and body awareness can definitely result in a hunchbacked, rounded shoulder appearance (excessive kyphosis). With proper instruction, however, you can avoid promoting this type of poor posture and help your students avoid injuries.

□ provide plenty of stretches for hip flexor, hamstring, calf, low back, upper trapezius, and chest,

□ provide strengthening exercises for the middle trapezius, rhomboid, posterior deltoid, abdominal, and low back muscles,

□ give equal numbers of punches and kicks on both sides and kick in both front and back directions, and

□ start with only one kickboxing class per week and gradually increase the number, if desired, up to three classes per week.

AVOID

□ a "snapping" motion when kicking and punching,

□ advanced and high kicks for all but the most skilled participants, and

□ music speeds greater than 138 beats/min.

BASIC MOVES

Although the standard kickboxing moves can be performed in a variety of different martial arts styles (see figure 10.2), we recommend modifying some of these traditional moves to allow for proper joint alignment and decrease the risk of injury.

■ American boxing	■ Taekwondo
■ Thai kickboxing	■ Aikido
■ Karate	■ Kung fu
■ Judo	■ Jujitsu

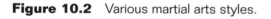

Figure 10.2 Various martial arts styles.

Initial Positioning

All kickboxing moves start from one of two basic positions: the *ready position* (body faces forward with feet parallel) or the *staggered position* (body is slightly angled to the side with one foot back). In both positions, the elbows are flexed with the fists close together protecting the face and neck (the forearms should make a V shape). The core muscles (abdominals and lower back) are engaged at all times, and the shoulder blades are slightly protracted (causing a slight rounding of the upper back and shoulders). Knees are slightly flexed (see figure 10.3).

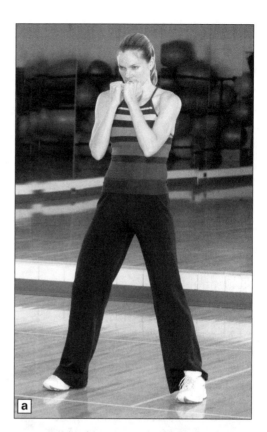

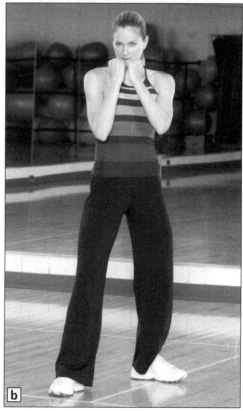

Figure 10.3 (a) Ready position and (b) staggered position.

Four Basic Punches

There are four basic punches in kickboxing: the jab, the cross-jab or cross-punch, the hook, and the uppercut. To protect the upper body joints in fitness settings, these punches are performed with a concentric contraction in both directions. In other words, there are two phases to a punch:

1. The punch itself, where the elbow extends (triceps contracts) and the fist moves away from the body
2. The retraction phase, where the elbow flexes (biceps contracts) and the fist is pulled quickly back into the body

This technique prevents the elbow from hyperextending when one is shadowboxing (punching air) and helps protect the elbow and shoulder joints. Additionally, it is safer to modify the full palm-down, pronated position of a classic punch to a slightly angled three-quarter turn of the wrist, with the thumb slightly higher than the littlest finger, according to Buschbacher and Shay (1999). Be especially careful when incorporating equipment into your classes such as weighted gloves, focus mitts, or punching bags. Weighted punches and contact punches greatly increase the risk of injuries such as muscle strains, ligament sprains, surface abrasions, and jamming and dislocations of the wrist and finger joints. We recommend that weighted and contact punching be reserved for advanced classes only.

The *jab* is a straight punch to the front. If you are in the ready position, the torso rotates; if you are in the staggered position, the torso doesn't need to rotate (see figure 10.4).

The *cross-jab* is typically performed from the staggered position, with the heel of the back foot up, allowing the whole body to pivot as the punch is thrown. As the spine and hip rotate forward, the cross-jab crosses the midline of the body with the shoulder following through (see figure 10.5).

In the *hook,* the elbow is lifted with the shoulder joint abducted at approximately 90°. The fist and arm curve around, following a horizontal line in front of the shoulders or face. Keep the fist either pronated (palm facing down) or in the recommended midpronated (palm facing the body) position with the elbow remaining flexed. The torso and hip rotate in the direction of the punch (see figure 10.6).

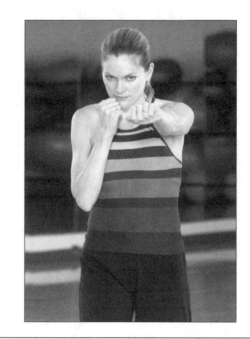

Figure 10.4 Jab punch.

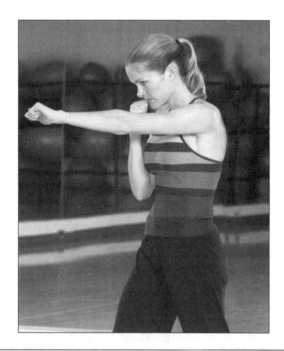

Figure 10.5 Cross-jab punch.

In the *uppercut,* the elbow also stays flexed but is kept down near the ribcage. The fist is supinated with the palm facing the body. Initiate this punch by allowing the shoulder to extend and the arm to move behind the torso (elbow is still flexed) before the actual punch. Tilting the pelvis, lifting the heel, and slightly rotating the torso will increase power (see figure 10.7).

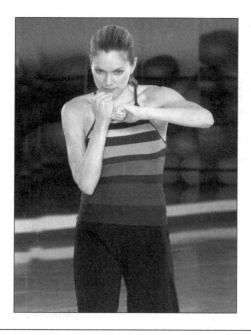

Figure 10.6 Hook punch.

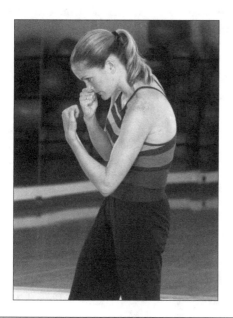

Figure 10.7 Uppercut punch.

Four Basic Kicks

The four basic kicks used in a typical kickboxing class are the front kick, back kick, side kick, and roundhouse kick. To decrease the risk of injury to the knee joint, it is recommended that the knee extension phase of the kick be immediately followed by a quick retraction of the leg. In other words, performing an almost reflexive and conscious knee flexion movement can help prevent ballistic knee hyperextension while the participant is kicking air. To perform proper kicks, the participant must have strong supporting leg and core (torso) muscles as well as adequate flexibility and the ability to balance on one leg. Remember, most martial artists take years to perfect their kicking technique and begin performing advanced kicks such as crescent, axe, hitch, and spin hook kicks only after extended study. Discourage beginners and less fit participants from attempting repetitive and advanced kicks too soon. We also recommend that head-high kicks be reserved for advanced participants, because these kicks require great flexibility, strength, balance, and coordination, and they increase the risk of hamstring pulls and back pain. You will probably need to demonstrate kicks at waist height or lower to reduce the risk of competitive students exceeding their own range of motion. It's also a good idea to slowly break down the kick movement for your students, as follows:

1. Flex the hip.
2. Extend the knee (avoiding hyperextension).
3. Quickly flex the knee.
4. Extend the hip and return the leg to neutral standing position (see figure 10.8).

In the *front kick*, the kicking leg moves directly to the front, while the body remains squared, with hips and shoulders facing forward. The kicking hip flexes but the spine remains in neutral alignment (no rounding). For advanced participants with the flexibility and strength to kick head high, a backward lean is permitted; however, participants must maintain neutral spinal alignment throughout. The ankle should be dorsiflexed with the point of contact at the ball of the foot, and the leg should be retracted quickly.

The *back kick* involves externally rotating the hip of the kicking leg while flexing forward on the standing hip; immediately retract the leg after

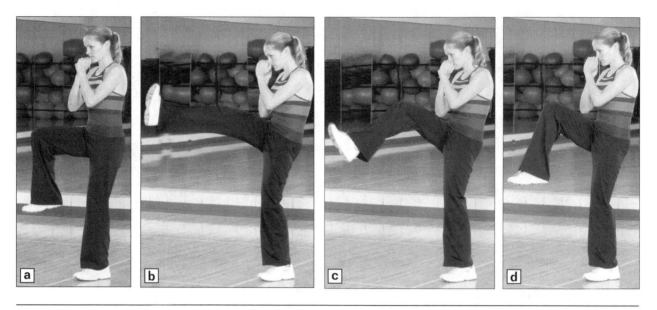

Figure 10.8 Phases of the front kick: (a) flex hip, (b) extend knee, (c) flex knee, (d) extend hip and return leg to neutral standing position.

kicking. Maintain neutral spinal alignment (no spinal flexion) while leaning forward. The point of contact is the heel of the back foot with the ankle dorsiflexed (see figure 10.9).

When a participant is performing a *side kick,* the point of contact is the ball of the foot (ankle is dorsiflexed). Depending on the height of the kick, a side (lateral) lean is acceptable; however, keep the spine in neutral without rounding. The kick-

ing hip internally rotates so that the knee faces forward; extend the knee after abducting the hip to the desired height (see figure 10.10).

The *roundhouse kick* involves working from a "turned out" (externally rotated) position of both hips. Make certain that knees are aligned in the same direction as the toes to avoid unnecessary torque or twisting of the knee and ankle joints. Externally rotate and flex the hip of the kicking

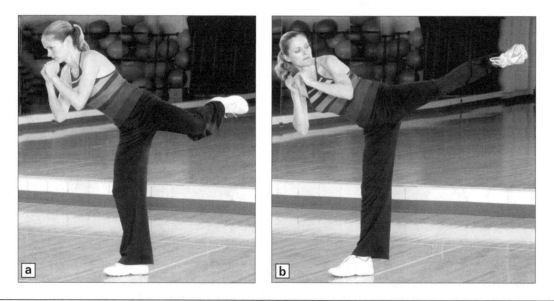

Figure 10.9 Phases of back kick: (a) standing in hip extension and knee flexion and (b) knee extended at waist height.

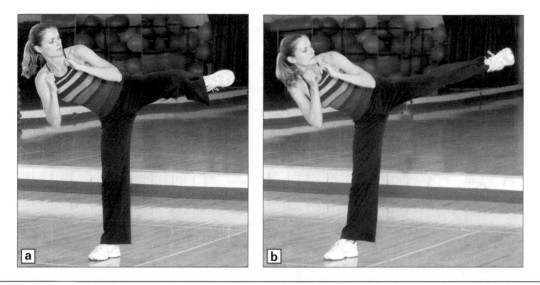

Figure 10.10 Phases of side kick: (a) standing in hip and knee flexion and (b) knee extended at waist height.

leg while performing lateral spinal flexion; imagine contact with the top of the foot (the forefoot) and keep the ankle plantar-flexed. Quickly retract the leg to finish (see figure 10.11).

PRACTICE DRILL

Using your favorite music at approximately 130 beats/min, practice the four kicks on every 4th beat as follows:

- Four right kicks front (16 counts), four left kicks front (16 counts), step-touch for 16 counts, march for 16 counts
- Four right kicks back (16 counts), four left kicks back (16 counts), step-touch for 16 counts, march for 16 counts
- Four right kicks side, four left kicks side, step-touch for 16 counts, march for 16 counts
- Four right roundhouse kicks, four left roundhouse kicks, step-touch for 16 counts, march for 16 counts

---

Other Basic Moves

Other moves and activities common to kickboxing include boxer's shuffle, jumping rope, bob and weave, and lateral slip.

The *boxer's shuffle* is a foot pattern intended to help maintain an increased heart rate and develop speed and agility; you can use it when developing kickboxing combinations. With feet hip-width apart and parallel, quickly move sideways without crossing the feet.

Jumping rope is often used to increase heart rate, power, stamina, and agility. In most kickboxing classes, the jump rope segments are in timed intervals (e.g., 3-5 min). During this interval, you can show different jump rope moves such as jogging, hopping twice on one foot and then the other, a hop kick with alternating feet, bilateral jumping, bilateral jumping while twisting, and jumping jacks, all while jumping over the rope! Even traveling moves such as grapevines, and power moves such as jumping high while circling the rope twice around the body (called salt and pepper), can be performed while jumping rope. For those participants who haven't yet coordinated the rope movement with jumping (it takes practice!), the jump rope motion can be simulated with twirling wrists and arms held close to the rib cage. Remind students to land properly with a toe–ball–heel descent, bringing heels all the way down and landing softly. Alternatively, beginners and those who don't want to perform high impact can jog in place or simply march. Jump rope intervals can be quite intense, so ease your participants into jumping rope with shorter intervals and be sure to spread the intervals throughout the class.

The *bob and weave* is simply a movement performed by the upper body and torso while

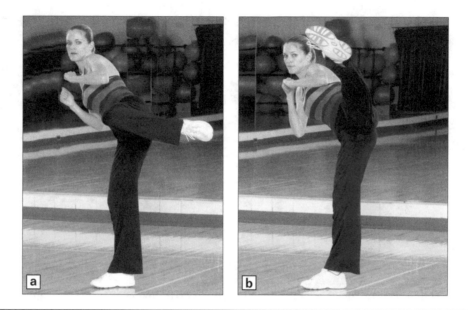

Figure 10.11 Phases of the roundhouse kick: *(a)* standing hip and knee flexion and *(b)* standing with knee extended.

 See the DVD for a demonstration of basic punches, kicks, and movements (jab, cross-jab, hook, uppercut, front kick, back kick, side kick, boxer's shuffle, bob and weave, lateral slip, and jump rope).

the feet are parallel or staggered; the upper body "ducks" under an imaginary punch, bobbing from one side to the other.

The *lateral slip* is performed by laterally flexing the spine side to side without bobbing down and up. The feet remain anchored, usually in a parallel position.

BASIC COMBINATIONS AND CHOREOGRAPHY TECHNIQUES

Building basic combinations in kickboxing is simply a matter of combining the basic moves. Many instructors also enjoy interspersing standard high/low moves such as grapevines, hustles, step-touches, hamstring curls, V-steps, and jumping jacks (see chapter 8 for a description of these moves) with the punching and kicking segments. When designing your choreography, use a variety of moves

 See the DVD for a demonstration of a kickboxing combination sample.

and avoid high numbers of repetitions. Because most kickboxing classes are intended to provide a cardiorespiratory stimulus, the intensity should be gradually increased before you include peak moves and should be gradually decreased at the end of class or before participants perform floor work. Peak moves include kicks, jumping jacks, and jump rope intervals. A basic sample kickboxing combination is shown in table 10.1.

OTHER KICKBOXING FORMATS

Some instructors prefer not to teach preplanned choreography on a 32-count block like the routine outlined in table 10.1. Instead, they may teach a more military or "combat" style, which includes repetitive drills that may or may not use music or follow the musical beat. For example, the class might include 10 min of punching practice (with or without a bag), 3 min of jump rope, 10 min of

Table 10.1 Sample Kickboxing Combination

Move	Foot pattern	Upper body	No. of counts
Shuffle right	R, L, R, L, R, L, R, pause	Cross jab L on 7	8
Shuffle left	L, R, L, R, L, R, L, pause	Cross jab R on 7	8
Repeat			16
Front kick	R, L kick, L, R, L, R kick, R, L	Ready position	8
Repeat			8
Repeat			8
Repeat			8
Bob and weave	Staggered position	Ready position	8
Lateral slip	Staggered position	Ready position	8
Repeat bob and weave			8
Repeat lateral slip			8
Jab	Ready position	Jab R, L, R, L (every 4 counts)	16
Hook	Ready position	Hook R, L, R, L (every 4 counts)	16
Repeat entire combination			

Note. R = right; L = left.

kicking, 3 min of jump rope, 10 min of punching, 3 min of jump rope, and 10 min of kicking. When using this style, include movements in a variety of directions and limit the number of repetitions to avoid overuse injuries.

Other formats include step kickboxing classes (intervals of step alternated with intervals of kickboxing), equipment-based classes (intervals of punching with bags or focus mitts and intervals of kicking shields or bags), and classes with partner drills, circles, and other group formations. Many kickboxing classes incorporate push-ups, abdominal work, or other muscle conditioning after the kickboxing portion of class.

Chapter Wrap-Up

A kickboxing class can be a fun, energizing, and challenging way to exercise in a group. However, instructors must keep safety concerns a priority to ensure an enjoyable experience for all participants. Learn to throw proper punches and kicks and teach them carefully to your classes, emphasizing correct alignment and technique at all times.

Key Points From the Group Exercise Class Evaluation Form

- Gradually increase intensity. In kickboxing, this means avoiding high-intensity drills, high kicks, and jump rope intervals for the first several minutes of the cardio stimulus. Review the first Practice Drill in this chapter and see if you can gradually increase the intensity of this combo by increasing the range of motion, traveling, or impact of the floor pattern.

- Use a variety of muscle groups and minimize repetitive movements. Review your combination from the last Practice Drill in this chapter (see p. 163) to be sure you considered muscle balance, variety, and safety.

- Demonstrate good form, alignment, and technique for kickboxing. Keep practicing so that excellent alignment and technique become second nature to you.

- Use music appropriately. Keep your music speed less than 138 beats/min for the cardio segment. Music that is too fast makes it difficult for participants to move safely with good alignment. If you choose to teach to the music, move on the downbeat and use 32-count phrases to enhance participant success.

- Give clear cues and verbal directions. Anticipatory cues, discussed in chapter 8, are particularly important when teaching combinations. An example, spoken in rhythm is, "4, 3, 2, right hook." (The word *hook* is spoken on the last beat.)

- Promote participant interaction and encourage fun. Try different room arrangements such as having two groups of participants face each other while practicing punches, or have the class stand in one large circle for kicking drills.

- Gradually decrease intensity during the postcardio cool-down with lower intensity moves and patterns similar to those used in the warm-up. Decrease music speed, range of motion, traveling, impact, and overhead arm moves as you return to resting conditions. Walking in place, step-touches, and heel digs all can be performed at a low intensity while keeping the arms low.

Written Assignment

Prepare a kickboxing group exercise lesson plan using the group exercise class evaluation form cardio segment. Write some specific moves (for at least 64 counts) that meet the criteria on the form.

Practical Assignment

Prepare a 2-min kickboxing routine with appropriate content, alignment, technique, and cueing using appropriate music. You will teach this routine to a group of four to five students.

Stationary Indoor Cycling

Chapter Objectives

By the end of this chapter, you will

- understand proper bike setup, riding alignment, and safety issues,

- understand how to warm up for stationary indoor cycling,

- be familiar with basic indoor cycling class techniques and music,

- be able to format different indoor cycling classes,

- understand cueing and coaching techniques on and off the bike, and

- be able to teach a 4-min indoor cycling segment with appropriate content, technique, and cueing using appropriate music.

Stationary indoor cycling (variously known by such trademarked names as Spinning, Cycle Reebok, and Power Pacing) is another modality for group exercise. Many clubs and facilities have a designated room just for indoor cycling, complete with specialized indoor bikes, sound systems, microphones, and even occasionally videotapes, disco or strobe lighting, and candles. Unlike more traditional forms of group exercise such as high/low impact or step, indoor cycling classes may be held in darkened rooms without mirrors. Here, the focus is less on how you look or how you compare with others in the room and more on your own personal workout experience. Or, as some instructors like to say, it's about the ride, or journey, itself and not the final result. Because there are no choreographed moves that all participants must do at the same time, it's much easier for indoor cyclists to personalize their workouts. Hence, several different fitness levels can be easily accommodated in the same class, with elite cyclists working out next to deconditioned novices. Stationary indoor cycling can provide an excellent cardiorespiratory workout, with up to 400 to 550 kcal burned per 45-min ride, not counting warm-up and cool-down. Many fitness facilities require a specific training and certification to teach a cycling class (see "Indoor Cycling Organizations and Certifications"). Teaching a stationary indoor cycling class can be fun and exhilarating for both you and your participants! The main points on the group exercise class evaluation form for stationary cycling are found in figure 11.1.

✓ BACKGROUND CHECK

Before working your way through this chapter, you should

☐ read chapter 4 on warm-up and
☐ read chapter 5 on cardiorespratory training.

WARM-UP

Building on the concepts and recommendations covered in chapter 4, a stationary indoor cycling warm-up consists primarily of dynamic movements, rehearsal moves, and some light prepara-

Key Points for Warm-Up Segment

- Uses an appropriate amount of dynamic movement.
- Gives rehearsal moves for indoor cycling.
- Stretches major muscle groups in a biomechanically sound manner.
- Gives clear cues and verbal directions.
- Uses an appropriate music tempo.

Key Points for Cardio Segment

- Gradually increases intensity.
- Uses a variety of cycling techniques and minimizes prolonged emphasis on any one technique.
- Demonstrates good form and alignment for indoor cycling.
- Uses music appropriately.
- Gives clear cues and verbal directions.
- Promotes participant interaction and encourages fun.
- Gradually decreases intensity during postcardio cool-down.

Figure 11.1 Group exercise class evaluation form for stationary cycling.

tory stretching, all taught with skillful cues at the appropriate tempo.

Dynamic Movement and Rehearsal Moves

The focus of a group cycling warm-up is on gradually increasing the intensity with a corresponding elevation in heart rate, ventilation, and oxygen consumption—all preparations for the cardiorespiratory workout to follow. This is initially accomplished by having participants sit upright on the bike with spine in neutral alignment while cycling to loosen up their legs. Bikes should be adjusted so there is light resistance and just enough tension on the flywheel for participants to stay in control. A typical indoor cycling

INDOOR CYCLING RESEARCH FINDINGS

Many studies have examined the cardiorespiratory and metabolic responses to group indoor cycling. Virtually all researchers have found that a stationary indoor cycling workout can provide a stimulus sufficient to meet ACSM guidelines for the development and maintenance of aerobic fitness, and most have reported high levels of caloric expenditure, up to 550 kcal per 45-min ride. Several investigations also measured responses to various positions and activities in a typical cycling class. Standing, climbing, high resistance settings, and jumping maneuvers elicited the highest heart rates, rating of perceived exertion (RPE), oxygen consumption, and caloric expenditures (Chinsky et al. 1998, Flanagan et al. 1998, Francis et al. 1999, Williford et al. 1999). Williford found that "speedplay and vigorous jumps/lifts may produce transient maximal effects." And in one study (Francis et al. 1999), energy cost was found not to be related to cadence; in other words, higher pedaling speeds did not appear to increase caloric expenditure. John and Schuler (1999) reported that the 6- to 20-point Borg RPE scale may be inaccurate when used by novices during group cycling; thus, either heart rate monitors or more detailed instruction regarding the RPE scale may be needed.

INDOOR CYCLING ORGANIZATIONS AND CERTIFICATIONS

Mad Dogg Athletics, Inc.
2111 Narcisus Court
Venice, CA 90291
800-847-SPIN
www.spinning.com

CycleReebok
800-REEBOK-1
www.reebokuniversity.com

The Nautilus Group
1400 NE 136 Ave.
Vancouver, WA 98684
360-694-7722
www.nautilusgroup.com

warm-up lasts approximately 4 to 8 min; intensity may be gradually increased toward the end of the warm-up by changing either the resistance or the pedaling speed.

Stretching Major Muscle Groups

We recommend performing some light preparatory stretching and dynamic movements for the upper body while cycling during the warm-up. These moves should include rolling the shoulders backward, stretching the pectoralis major (chest), and stretching the upper trapezius (neck) to counteract the rounded, hunched posture so often seen in cycling classes (see figure 11.2). Most instructors reserve lower body stretching for the end of a cycling class, when everyone is very warm and psychologically ready to relax and hold the static stretches. Stopping the rhythmic rehearsal movements of cycling to perform lower body static stretches would have the negative effect of decreasing the heart rate and oxygen consumption, exactly the opposite of the warm-up purpose. Therefore, we suggest waiting to stretch the lower body muscles until the end of class.

Verbal Cues and Tempo

The warm-up is an ideal time to teach proper alignment and riding technique as well as review intensity guidelines. Teach your class about neutral spine, neutral scapulae, and proper neck, elbow, and wrist alignment. Give technique pointers regarding pedaling, such as, "visualize your feet spinning in separate perfect circles" or "feel each foot moving front to back with each revolution" or "create a perfect balance between your right and left feet." Additionally, many participants need instruction regarding proper intensity. Now is the time to address heart rate

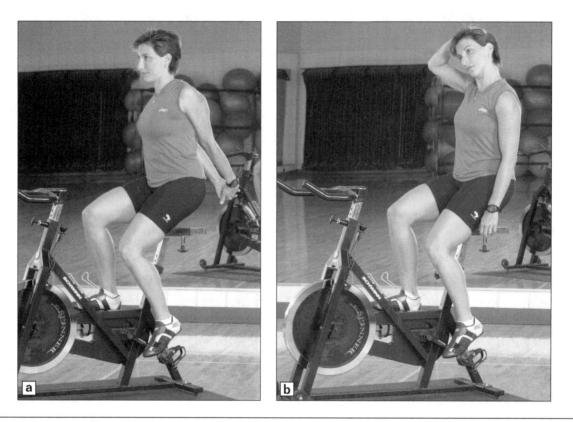

Figure 11.2 Upper body stretches: *(a)* pectoralis major stretch and *(b)* upper trapezius stretch with neck laterally flexed.

issues, perceived exertion, and the concept of listening to one's own body and working at the level that is right for each individual. Some instructors suggest that participants silently create an *intention,* or personal focus, for the workout ahead. Finally, make certain that all participants can hear you; be sure there's a proper balance between the music volume and the microphone volume.

An appropriate music tempo is one that allows participants to work comfortably at a low to medium intensity during the warm-up. There are no set guidelines for music speed, and participants can pedal off the beat or on the beat in three ways: (1) Each individual leg completes a downstroke on every other beat (slow), (2) each individual leg completes a downstroke on each beat (faster), and (3) double time, where both legs complete a downstroke on each beat (very fast). Because of the variability in how music is used, rigid tempo guidelines are somewhat meaningless. Instead, select warm-up music that is motivating, is fun to listen to, and encourages a comfortable pace at a low to moderate intensity.

☑ **TECHNIQUE AND SAFETY CHECK**

Stationary cycling warm-up recommendations are to

- ❏ gradually increase intensity,
- ❏ include some light preparatory stretching and dynamic movements for the upper body,
- ❏ teach proper alignment and cycling technique, and
- ❏ give intensity information and guidelines.

TECHNIQUE AND SAFETY

Before beginning a cycling class, make certain that each participant is properly aligned and adjusted on his or her bike. You should be available for at least 15 min before class to assist participants with bike setup, answer any questions, get to know new participants, and set up your own equipment (including music and microphones). The three main bike adjustments are the seat height, the fore and aft seat position, and the handlebar height. The *seat height* depends on the cyclist's leg length; the longer the leg, the higher the seat. In general, when the rider is seated on the bike with the balls of the feet on the center of the pedals, there should be a slight bend in the knee of the extended leg when pedaling. Experts suggest anywhere from 5° to 30° of flexion at the knee. If the seat height is too low, inadequate leg extension may cause knee problems, especially in the front of the knee. If the seat is too high, the rider's hips will rock back and forth; in addition, the risk of knee hyperextension is increased, which may cause pain at the back of the knee. Most participants err on the side of having the seat too low, to minimize saddle soreness. Encourage students to wear padded bike shorts or use gel-padded bike seats, and let them know that saddle soreness usually lasts for just the first few sessions. Proper seat height is key for healthy knees!

For *fore and aft* positioning, adjust the saddle so that the cyclist's front kneecap is aligned directly above the center of the pedal when the pedal is forward and the crank is horizontal (the nine o'clock position). Cycling with the saddle too far forward can also cause anterior knee problems. The correct fore and aft position also should allow the arms to comfortably reach the handlebars with the elbows slightly flexed.

Handlebar height is mostly a matter of personal preference, although beginners usually are more comfortable with the handlebars higher and the torso more upright. The upright, spinal neutral position is definitely recommended for those with back or neck problems. The lower the handlebars, the more the cyclist simulates a racing position, which creates favorable aerodynamics when the rider is outdoors but is obviously unnecessary when indoors. Teach your participants to ride with a relaxed grip and neutral wrists and to vary their hand positions. Additionally, encourage students to wear stiff-soled shoes that remain rigid over the pedal; students should position their feet so that the balls of the feet, not the arches, contact the pedals. Clipping onto the pedals or securely strapping the shoes into the foot cages can enhance pedaling efficiency. Because most

bikes are fixed gear and the pedals will continue to rotate if you take your feet off, remind your class to either keep their feet on the pedals until they stop or hold their feet away if they must detach from the pedal.

Always maintain neutral spinal alignment on the bike. The rider is in a neutral spine position (also known as ideal alignment) when the four natural curves of the back are in their proper relationship to each other. This is easiest, of course, when the rider is sitting upright with the torso perpendicular to the floor. When the rider is seated and riding with a forward lean, the spine should still be in neutral, albeit inclined at a 45° angle or so, depending on the activity. Avoid tucking the hips under (posterior pelvic tilt), which causes the back to round, or flex, and places much more strain on the structures of the back. Shoulders should be down and slightly retracted, also known as neutral scapular alignment. Avoid rounding, hunching, or allowing the shoulders to come up by the ears (see figure 11.3).

See the DVD for a cycle set-up demonstration.

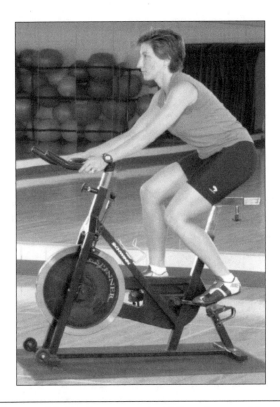

Figure 11.3 Proper seated bike alignment in the inclined position.

Remind participants to ride with a full water bottle and a towel. And, as with any new activity, recommend gradually increasing the frequency of their classes, starting with one or two per week and slowly increasing to three or four classes per week if desired.

✓ **TECHNIQUE AND SAFETY CHECK**

To help keep your classes safe, observe the following recommendations.

REMEMBER TO

☐ undertake a thorough, appropriate warm-up,

☐ maintain a neutral spine whether sitting upright, inclined forward, or standing,

☐ keep neck in line with the spine,

☐ adjust the bike properly,

☐ keep wrists in neutral and maintain a relaxed grip,

☐ wear proper footwear and contact pedals with balls of feet, and

☐ stay hydrated.

AVOID

☐ tucking hips under and

☐ neck hyperextension.

BASIC MOVES

The typical indoor cycling class is divided into several *segments,* which are usually designed to simulate aspects of an outdoor ride; these segments may be linked to specific songs, or "cuts" of music. Segments may include

- seated flat road,
- seated climb (hill),
- standing flat road run or jog,
- standing climb (hill),
- seated downhill or flush,
- rebounds, jumps, or lifts,
- seated and standing sprints (also known as spin-outs, fast hammers, or power drills),

Participants are often asked to visualize themselves performing these segments outdoors on a bike.

Many instructors create imaginary journeys and scenarios for cyclists to visualize: Images of tropical islands, mountain roads, green forests, sandy beaches, open fields and meadows can all be conducive to an improved workout and an enjoyable class experience. Visualization can also be used to improve breathing, alignment, muscle focus, mental awareness, and even self-empowerment! Have participants see in their mind's eye the goal they wish to accomplish and see themselves being successful. This can be a very powerful aspect of a group cycling class.

 See the DVD for basic cycling moves, instructions on seated flats, seated climb, cadence and resistance, standing climb, sprint, and rebounds.

The *seated flat* is the most basic technique in cycling. Participants can work at a variety of speeds, and the flat road can be used in the warm-up, cardio stimulus, and cool-down phases of class. The seated flat is perfect for cadence drills, alignment and pedaling work, endurance work, and "rhythm presses" (a pulsating, wave-like movement of the upper body). During the cardio stimulus, especially, the seated flat is usually performed in the basic riding position where the body is inclined at approximately 45°.

Seated and *standing hill climbs* are simulated by increasing the resistance on the bike. When performing seated climbs, the rider should shift the hips to the back of the saddle to avoid excessive pressure on the knees. When climbing and standing, the rider should move the hands forward on the handlebars and keep the hips in line over the seat (maintaining hip flexion). These segments are usually performed with a slow pedal revolution (50-70 rev/min) and can be quite strenuous, with the primary focus on strength.

In the *standing flat run* or *jog,* the resistance is light to medium with an endurance focus. Weight is balanced over the lower body while hands rest lightly on the handlebars. Instructors may require participants to remain vertical or slightly flexed at the hips (keep spine in neutral).

The *downhill* or *"flushing"* segment is usually short (1-3 min) and is used for recovery after a strenuous uphill climb. Flywheel tension is low, cyclists are seated, and the breathing rate and heart rate return to more moderate levels.

Rebounds, jumps, or *lifts* are used to increase intensity and are considered more advanced. Participants need to be completely familiar with seated and standing positions before attempting regular jumps. Jumps or lifts are most often taught on the beat at regular intervals: for example, stand up for 8 counts, sit down for 8 counts. The intervals can be short or long. An entire song or segment may be used for jumping, or you may use just part of a segment. Keep the lifting and lowering smooth, fluid, and even, working for smooth knee transitions between sitting and standing. Jumps are usually accomplished without changing the pedal cadence. Be aware that jumping can be hard on some participants' knees. We recommend limiting jumps in most cycling classes.

Sprints, spin-outs, fast hammers, and *power drills* may be performed either seated or standing. They may be used in intervals or randomly dispersed throughout a segment. When the rider is performing a sprint, the cadence changes to a very fast pace with light to moderate resistance—just enough to keep the hips from bouncing. Experienced participants may cross their anaerobic threshold and cycle with a near-maximal effort, focusing on speed and power.

PRACTICE DRILL

Using your favorite music, practice the seated flat road, seated and standing climbs, standing run, jumps, and sprints. Work on positioning your body in ideal alignment as you experiment with these positions and riding techniques (see figure 11.4).

FORMATTING INDOOR CYCLING CLASSES

Formatting a stationary cycling class is simply a matter of combining the basic moves with each other. These combinations become the ride profile, which is the structure, or organization, of the cycling workout. Always prepare your ride profile, with the accompanying music selections, in advance. However, be prepared to modify your class plan depending on the fitness and skill levels of the individuals in class; your profile is only a guideline and will be subject to change. Each class will be different and participants will have different needs. If you teach indoor cycling classes regularly, eventually you will have many different class profiles and a large selection of music from which to choose. You can be spontaneous and creative! Always gradually increase the intensity at the beginning and gradually decrease the intensity at the end of class. A sample 45-min ride profile is shown in table 11.1.

The music you choose for your cycling class is key to making your class a success. Unlike other types of group exercise where the music must be metered into even 32-count phrases for choreography purposes, in group cycling you may use virtually any style of music you choose. It may have an even number of beats or not. You can choose from pop, disco, rock 'n' roll, rhythm and blues, jazz, reggae, rap, Latin, country, folk,

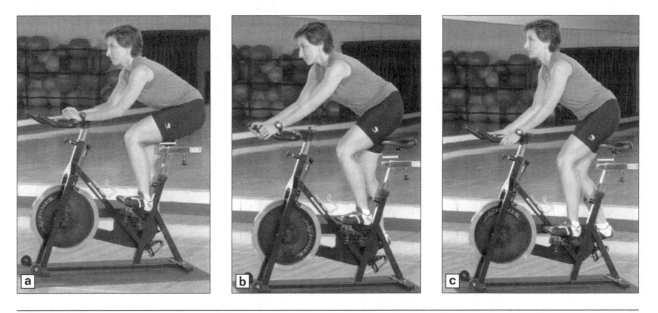

Figure 11.4 (*a*) Seated climb, (*b*) standing climb, and (*c*) standing run on the bike.

Table 11.1 Sample Ride Profile

Segment	Body position	Resistance	Music tempo	Music selection	Duration (min)
1. Warm-up	Seated	Light	Moderate	New Age	5
2. Climb	Standing	Moderate	Slow	Rock 'n' roll	4
3. Climb	Standing	Heavy	Slow	Rhythm and blues	4
4. Flat road	Seated	Moderate	Moderate to fast	Rock 'n' roll	6
5. Flat road	Standing	Moderate	Fast	Latin	4
6. Jumps	Seated or standing	Moderate	Moderate	Pop	4
7. Climb	Seated	Heavy	Slow	Funk	6
8. Downhill	Seated	Light	Slow	Classical	2
9. Sprints	Seated or standing	Moderate	Moderate	Rock 'n' roll	5
10. Cool-down	Seated	Light	Moderate	Pop	3
11. Stretch	Off bike		Slow	New Age	≥2

gospel, classical, New Age, world, and movie soundtracks. Find music that is motivating to you and to your students, music that makes everyone smile and want to work. It's usually best to include several different kinds of music in your workout to fit varying participant preferences and to go with the various class segments and moods you'll be creating. Connecting the music with the segments, moods, intensity, and journey can be the most fun yet challenging aspect of teaching an indoor cycling class.

Some instructors prefer to cross-train with their cycling classes. This can mean varying the focus on alternate days: for example, strength (hill) focus on Monday, endurance focus on Wednesday, and speed focus on Friday. Another approach is to combine indoor cycling with a different modality such as treading, rowing, muscle conditioning, Pilates, or yoga. In this type of format you might lead cycling for 30 min followed by yoga for another 30 min. The Keiser Power Pace cycling program recommends incorporating muscle-conditioning exercises into the bike workout itself, using free weights, rubber tubing, and bands.

INTENSITY

Another important training issue is *intensity*. One of the benefits of group indoor cycling is that each participant works at his or her own level, and there is much less pressure to conform to the group than in a traditional high/low impact class with mirrors, for example. Even so, you must give your students target heart rate zones and perceived exertion intensity guidelines and help them learn to assess themselves.

Many indoor cycling instructors strongly recommend the use of a heart rate monitor. Using heart rate monitors has a number of advantages as well as some disadvantages. Heart rate monitors can be very useful if students know their actual training zones. (A participant might know her actual training zone if she has had a graded exercise stress test—see the section on monitoring exercise intensity in chapter 5.) The monitors make it easy to keep track of heart rate at any time during the class without stopping, and they can provide an incentive to work harder when motivation falters. Unfortunately, most exercisers who use heart rate monitors assume that training zones given are accurate, when in fact standard heart rate formulas are suitable for only 75% of the population (McArdle et al. 2001). In the other 25% of the population, the target heart rate zones will be either overestimated or underestimated, sometimes significantly. Another limitation of the heart rate method involves the effects of medications (many either decrease or increase the heart rate). No one heart rate formula will fit every participant, so it's wise to use other methods as well. Help your students establish a workout intensity zone—a heart rate training zone, a perceived exertion zone, or both.

During the workout, you can suggest that your students work at a low level during the warm-up, cool-down, and downhills (this would be equivalent to the low end of their actual target heart rate zone, or an 8-12 on the 6-20 Borg RPE scale); a moderate level during flat roads and standing runs (middle of the zone or 12-14 RPE); and a high level during climbs, jumps, and power intervals (top of the zone or 15-18 RPE), for example. Some participants may choose to push past their anaerobic threshold during power surges; this should be reserved for advanced students only.

Remind your students that cycling intensity can always be modified by changing

1. their position (seated vs. standing),
2. their resistance, or
3. their pedaling cadence.

For example, when cadence goes up often resistance levels go down. Count cadence by tapping the thigh on each revolution. Slow cadence is 60-80 revolutions per minute (rpm), tempo is 80-100 rpm, and fast cadence is 100 or greater rpm. Let students know that even though you'll be giving intensity suggestions, it's important to exercise at their own pace. Many participants appreciate knowing how long each segment will last, so consider making an announcement such as, "We'll be working hard on the next hill for 5 minutes" before the more difficult sections.

Include a thorough *cool-down* period at the end of class. This is accomplished by gradually decreasing the intensity with little to no resistance while continuing to ride, allowing heart rates, breathing rates, oxygen consumption, and caloric expenditure to return toward normal values. We recommend statically stretching all major muscle groups at this time as well. Many instructors prefer to stretch the upper body muscles while slowly cycling on the bike and then dismount to stretch the lower body muscles. Include stretches for the hamstrings, quadriceps, hip flexors, calves, buttocks, and low back in addition to upper body muscles (see figure 11.5).

CUEING METHODS

Leadership skills are all-important in an indoor cycling class. In many other group modalities (e.g., step, high/low impact, kickboxing, slide), instructors must be concerned with getting all

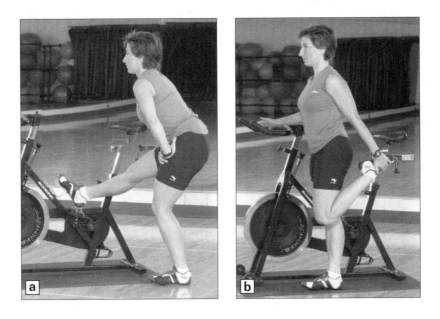

(continued)

Figure 11.5 Stretches for *(a)* hamstrings, *(b)* quadriceps,

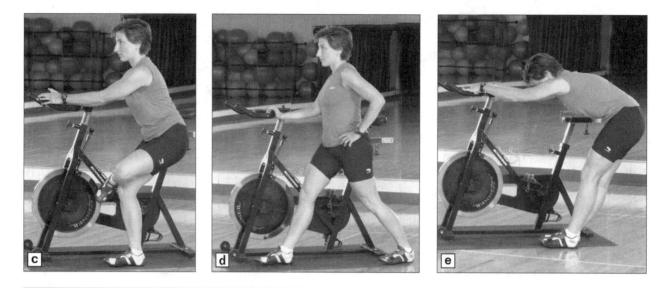

Figure 11.5 *(continued)*, stretches for *(c)* buttocks, *(d)* calves, and *(e)* low back.

participants to move together at the same time. Obviously, this is not necessary for group cycling. Instead, you'll need to focus more on motivating, coaxing, encouraging, and setting the mood with your voice and your cues. Use plenty of motivational cues such as, "You can do it!" "Altogether!" "Drive it forward!" Positive affirmations such as, "We are strong!" "We are committed!" "You can climb this mountain!" can help pull your class through more difficult segments.

Helping your students set goals for their workouts is another effective strategy: Ask them during the warm-up to create a focus or an intention for the class. Then remind them of their focus during the challenging segments. For example, "Hang onto that goal!"

Indoor cycling classes are perfect for promoting a sense of teamwork within the class. One popular method is to divide the class into two or three "pods" or small teams and then have the teams take turns sprinting or drafting in a race.

Remember to use visualizations during cycling class. Many instructors suggest that riders visualize following that yellow line straight down the highway, "feeling the wind in your face" or "smelling that clean ocean air." Some instructors create an entire trip within their class, taking them to Hawaii, to the beach, or through rolling hills.

Take advantage of the opportunity to teach off the bike. Walk through your class to check form and alignment and to support and encourage participants when the going gets tough. A simple "hang in there" to a fatigued class member can make all the difference.

Participants usually enjoy opportunities to make noise; you might try getting them to count the number of jumps, for example, or ask them to call out refrains to familiar songs you are playing. Theme classes are a great way to build camaraderie and fun; pick your music around a special event, theme, or holiday. Ideas include Halloween, Christmas, love songs on Valentine's day, patriotic music on Memorial Day or 4th of July, Motown music day, disco day, and beach music day. Encourage your students to relax and party!

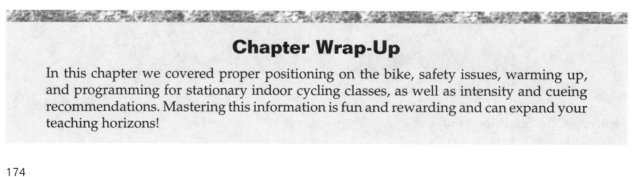

Chapter Wrap-Up

In this chapter we covered proper positioning on the bike, safety issues, warming up, and programming for stationary indoor cycling classes, as well as intensity and cueing recommendations. Mastering this information is fun and rewarding and can expand your teaching horizons!

Key Points From the Group Exercise Class Evaluation Form

- Gradually increase intensity. In a cycling class, this happens during the warm-up.
- Use a variety of cycling techniques such as flat road, standing run, and seated and standing climbs and minimize prolonged emphasis on any one technique.
- Demonstrate good form and alignment for indoor cycling. Be sure to help set up your participants properly on their bikes.
- Use music appropriately.
- Give clear cues and verbal directions, including intensity instructions, affirmations, visualizations, goal setting, and team building.
- Promote participant interaction and encourage fun.
- Help students to monitor their intensity during the cardio segment, either with heart rate checks or perceived exertion checks.
- Gradually decrease intensity during the postcardio cool-down and include some static stretches at the end of class.

Written Assignment

List 15 motivational cues and affirmations appropriate for cycling. List 10 examples of goals or workout intentions, and ideas for team building. Prepare a 45-min indoor cycling group exercise profile with music suggestions.

Practical Assignment

Prepare a 4-min indoor cycle class routine to present to a group of four or five students, using your favorite music. Use two different movement segments and at least two different cueing or coaching techniques.

Water Exercise

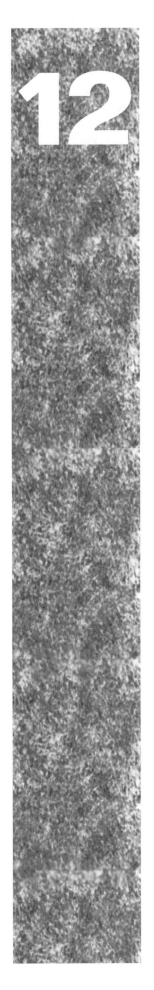

Chapter Objectives

By the end of this chapter, you will

- ■ know the benefits of water exercise,

- ■ understand the properties of water and Newton's laws of motion,

- ■ be able to give exercise examples using specificity of water training principles,

- ■ understand appropriate use of equipment specific to water exercise, and

- ■ be able to modify the group exercise evaluation form for water exercise.

As we strive to make the exercise experience more purposeful and fun for our participants, we need to consider using water exercise. This type of exercise is becoming more and more popular as our population ages and participants seek nonintimidating and nonimpact exercise. Also, pools are expensive to maintain when used only for lap swimming. A water exercise class can contain more than 25 participants in one area, all enjoying the benefits of the water's resistance. Water exercise could be the most effective form of group personal training if equipment is available to vary resistance. We need to think of our pools as giant resistance machines. Research tells us that pools have some similarities to our strength and conditioning areas. They both can provide overload to help train our muscles. The weight room variable-resistance machines overload by using weights that are designed to move against gravity. In a pool, we use the viscosity of the water and other properties of water to overload. Both weight training and water exercise improve muscular strength and endurance (see "Aquatic Exercise Research Findings").

In group exercise classes, we get a lot of newcomers seeking exercise instruction. Many participants who try water exercise for the first time find that the water environment allows them to set their own pace and intensity and to rest when necessary. The buoyancy of the water is particularly kind to women (Brown et al. 1997), since we contain more "stored energy" (body fat) because of our genetics. This stored energy assists us with buoyancy. When overweight participants enter a traditional group exercise class, they are often intimidated by the mirrors and the fact that people can see them. In a water exercise class, one's body is covered up and extra body fat actually makes the person more buoyant. Obesity is an epidemic in Western societies, which will continually increase the popularity of water as a mode for comfortable exercise. According to Mokdad et al. (2004) poor diet and physical inactivity may soon overtake tobacco as the leading cause of death in the United States. Finally, for those who need a more intense workout, the resistance that water provides acts in all directions on one's muscles, no matter what the movement. In some ways, water exercise is safer than land-based activity—falls don't carry the same threat of injury, and the stress of impact on joints

is lessened. Furthermore, water cools participants as they work out, so sweating is not a problem (Sanders et al. 1997).

As we move from aesthetic fitness to more functional fitness, use of the water for resistance exercise will increase because it is one of the best environments to accomplish functional, specific resistance training (Bravo et al. 1997, Simmons et al. 1996, Suomi and Koceja 2000). Sports experts know that to improve performance, muscles must be trained with movements as close as possible to the desired movements or skills in a specific sport. From a health perspective, what skills are needed for improved daily living? Skills that enhance proper posture are the answer! For example, does performing supine curl-ups on land prepare the abdominals to be strong in a functional, upright position? Not really. With curl-ups, the abdominals are strengthened in a forward flexed position. In the water, working the abdominals in an upright position by simply walking through the water and using its natural resistance can strengthen the abdominals specifically to improve daily functioning (Kennedy and Sanders 1995). Performing basic locomotor patterns (i.e., walking and running) using the water's resistance enhances functionality as the body stabilizes itself against resistance, plus there is little load on the body's lower extremity joints. Thus, another major benefit of water exercise is that it provides specific resistance in an upright, functional position while at the same time unloading the musculo-skeletal system (Norton et al. 1997). The main points on the group exercise class evaluation form for water exercise are found in figure 12.1.

✓ BACKGROUND CHECK

Before working your way through this chapter, you should do the following:

READ

- ❑ the chapter 4 warm-up segment and
- ❑ information about muscular strength and endurance actions from chapter 6.

PRACTICE

- ❑ cardiorespiratory skills (monitoring intensity using the RPE methods), movement options, and participant interaction as discussed in chapter 5.

Key Points for Warm-Up Segment

- Uses an appropriate amount of dynamic movement.
- Gives rehearsal moves for water exercise.
- Stretches major muscle groups in a biomechanically sound manner (dynamically).
- Gives clear cues and verbal directions.
- Uses music that fits the movement.

Key Points for Cardio Segment

- Gradually increases intensity.
- Uses a variety of water exercise techniques and minimizes prolonged emphasis on any one technique.
- Demonstrates good form and alignment for water exercise.
- Uses music appropriately.
- Gives clear cues and verbal directions.
- Promotes participant interaction and encourage fun.
- Gradually decreases intensity during postcardio cool-down.

Figure 12.1 Group exercise class evaluation form for water exercise.

AQUATIC EXERCISE RESEARCH FINDINGS

- When the chest cavity is immersed, heart rates decrease and it is not appropriate to apply land-based target heart rates to predict $\dot{V}O_2$ level (Craig and Dvorak 1968, D'Acquisto et al. 2001, Svedenhag and Seger 1992).

- Training from water exercise can carry over to improve function and health on land (Bushman et al. 1997, Davidson and McNaughton 2000, DeMaere and Ruby 1997, Eyestone et al. 1993, Frangolias et al. 2000, Gehring et al. 1997, Takeshima et al. 2002).

- Women perform deep water running with less physiologic stress than men (Brown et al. 1997).

- Pool exercises targeting activities of daily living (ADLs) can improve one's ability to perform ADLs on land (Sanders et al. 1997, Templeton et al. 1996).

- Interval training in the water is recommended for beginners to reduce local muscular fatigue, increase duration, and help them enjoy the workout more (Frangolias et al. 1996, Michaud et al. 1995, Quinn et al. 1994, Wilbur et al. 1995).

- Water exercise, in general, has a greater anaerobic demand (in untrained water exercise participants) and therefore provides muscular strength and endurance training throughout the entire session (Brown et al. 1997, Evans and Cureton 1998, Frangolias and Rhodes 1995, Michaud et al. 1995, Wilbur et al. 1996).

- Reducing the speed of movement between water and land activities is essential. With effort, speed in water is approximately one half to one third slower than land speed (39% slower) for equivalent energy expenditure (Frangolias and Rhodes 1995). Allow students to adjust their own speed based on RPE (Gehring et al. 1997, Hoeger et al. 1995).

- Once participants are trained, challenge them by increasing resistance just as you do in strength and conditioning programs. Equipment overload (usually surface area) needs to be applied progressively along with speed adjustments (Mayo 2000).

PROPERTIES OF WATER

Let's examine the properties of water that make water exercise different from exercise on land. We need to understand Newton's laws of motion to effectively exercise in the water. Applying these laws and principles will be important to have maximum success with this activity.

Viscosity

Viscosity, or the friction between molecules, causes resistance to motion. Water is more viscous than air, just as molasses is more viscous than water (Aquatic Exercise Association 1995). Because water is more viscous than air, water provides more resistance to motion than air. When you walk forward in the water for a few feet, the viscosity (cohesion and adhesion) of the water allows you to get a "block" of water to move with you. This block of water, often called a drag force, adds overload, which can increase energy expenditure.

Buoyancy

We have gravity on land, but in the water we have *buoyancy.* Buoyancy pushes the body upward and has the opposite effect of gravity. Buoyancy is closely related to density; the relative density of an object determines whether an object will float (Bates and Hanson 1996). Body composition also affects a participant's buoyancy. The more body fat a participant has, the more buoyant he or she will be. On the other hand, the less body fat a participant has, the more relative density he or she has and thus the more that participant will need assistance with buoyant devices during deep water exercise. Therefore, a very lean athlete who is running in deep water would need a different flotation device than a female with average body fat. When you are cueing specific exercises like the outer thigh abductor exercise, for example (figure 12.2), discuss range of motion because buoyancy will cause the leg to rise to the top. If the leg goes beyond the 45° range of motion of the hip abductors, the quadriceps and not the hip abductor will be the primary mover. You must cue to keep the movement to a 45° degree range of motion (figure 12.2).

Progressive Resistance

Progressive resistance is developed by variations in speed, surface area, travel, and work against

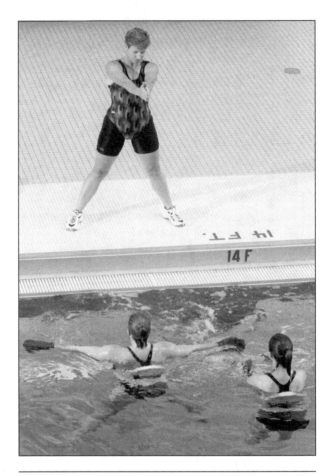

Figure 12.2 Cue hip abduction to 45° or buoyancy will cause hip flexion at 90° to occur.

buoyancy. Overload can be created by using the water's resistance and engaging it effectively against the body to achieve training effects. A water exercise intensity progression is outlined in figure 12.3. Varying the planes of movement during resistance training is one of the most important benefits of water exercise and is difficult to achieve in a traditional group exercise class. For example, when a participant is performing horizontal adduction (a basic pectoral press) standing on land holding a weight, gravity forces the deltoid muscle to be the prime mover; for this movement to be effective for the pectoral muscles, the participant has to lie in the supine position to perform a bench press. When the participant is standing in water, the pectorals are the prime mover because the deltoids are assisted by buoyancy. Because gravity does not affect the direction of resistance, you can vary movements and planes and also work in an upright functional position. In other words, water exercise

DESIGNING A WORKOUT USING SPECIFICITY OF WATER TRAINING PRINCIPLES

According to Weltman (1995), $\dot{V}O_2max$ is not the best predictor of endurance performance. He believes that blood lactate responses to submaximal exercise are better indicators of endurance. Studies (Brown et al. 1997, DeMaere and Ruby 1997) on water exercise have verified that there are higher blood lactate responses to an exercise in the water compared with the same exercise performed on land. The resistance of the water creates more of an anaerobic response to exercise, similar to what happens physiologically when one is resistance training. A big increase in blood lactate levels, especially in the deconditioned participant, can be uncomfortable and lead to adherence problems. Interval training has been recommended in the water, especially for beginners, because it is a resistant medium. One does not go into a weight room and continuously lift weights. There is a period of rest between muscle groups or sets to allow the blood lactate to be recycled within the body. The first resistant set marks the move and increases range of motion. The second set can then provide maximum muscular overload. Frangolias et al. (2000) determined that when participants are water trained, they begin to adapt to the environment and thus do not show an increase in blood lactate levels. In other words, once they gain the strength to overcome the resistance of the water, they won't see the big increases in blood lactate levels that they did when they first started. Progressive overload is important to the success of a water exercise class if one wants to keep improving. Progressive resistance is reviewed in figure 12.3.

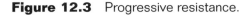

- Increase speed or force
- Increase surface area
- Increase speed more
- Travel against the current
- Increase speed of travel
- Use trunk stabilizers (suspend the move)

Figure 12.3 Progressive resistance.

allows you more options for upright overload. Let's take this same pectoral press movement through a progression.

Before starting progressive muscular strength and endurance exercise, you need to warm up. To warm up the pectoral muscles, stand in place and practice a pattern of horizontal adduction of the shoulder joint in a relaxed fashion, using functional range of motion. Then increase speed or force, which will push the body backward. Then increase surface area by putting on webbed gloves. Increase the speed again. Next begin to jog forward, traveling against the current while still performing horizontal adduction of the shoulder joint. Increase the speed of travel again. Finally, suspend the body by lifting the feet off the bottom to mimic deep water, thus dragging the surface area of the body through the water. It is important to contract the trunk stabilizers, thus adding more drag with the body and more core stability work to stabilize against the effects of buoyancy. This same progression can be applied for all muscle groups.

NEWTON'S LAWS OF MOTION

A general understanding of Newton's laws of motion is essential for providing safe and effective water exercise instruction. Lets take a moment to review these laws while applying them to water exercise movement design (see "Designing a Workout Using Specificity of Water Training Principles").

Inertia

Inertia is the first of Newton's laws of motion. Inertia is the tendency of a body to remain in a state of rest or of uniform motion in a straight line until acted on by a force to change that state. Inertia currents are created when we move in the water. The direction of the movement of the water currents will have an impact on how effective the exercise is. For example, running in circles in the water reduces the work, whereas turning around and running against the inertia currents increases the work. If one were to stand in place in the water, there would be little inertia to work against. Therefore, standing is place is less work. Using short travel moves like running 10 ft and turning around and running back for 10 ft is a good way to use the inertia currents for overload. Have beginners do most of their exercises in place to gain balance and skill without using the inertia currents.

Acceleration

Acceleration is mentioned in Newton's second law of motion, which states that force equals mass times acceleration. Speed (acceleration) can be used to create resistance overload. For example, when walking in the water, if you want to increase intensity then you should walk faster without changing your range of motion. You will be moving the same amount of water, but it will be harder because you are moving faster. Power is what you gain from including acceleration, because power is defined as resistance times speed. Be careful not to compromise range of motion when you include acceleration; shorter ranges of motion make the muscle movement more isometric in nature and result in more pain signals from lack of blood flow. Full range of motion exercise is the optimal way to train muscles.

Action and Reaction

The concept of *action and reaction* is explained in Newton's third law of motion, which states that for every action force, there is an equal and opposite reaction force. When we reach out in front with extended arms and push the water behind us, our body will move forward. The action is the arm movement and the reaction is the body movement. Use this concept to analyze what you want out of a movement so you can see if it is effective. For example, when you are performing shoulder adduction (a latissimus dorsi movement), the concept of action and reaction means that if you adduct the shoulder in deep water, the body will pull up slightly. If you want to use action and reaction to overload instead of allowing the body to come up, you could (in shallow water) bend your knees; you will be resisting the

action and reaction law and therefore performing more work. Determine the assisting direction of the action and then work against it for overload and with it for recovery.

LAND AND WATER DIFFERENCES

One of the reasons exercising in the water is comfortable and relatively pain free is because without equipment, there is very little eccentric muscle contraction. Eccentric muscle contractions are often associated with delayed onset muscle soreness (Byrnes 1985). The nonimpact nature of water activity coupled with the fact that it involves predominantly concentric muscle contractions makes it a very comfortable workout environment. You need to understand the different physiological implications of water exercise to become an effective instructor. Table 12.1 gives an overview of the difference in muscle contraction compared with land exercise for hip standing flexion and extension.

WARM-UP

Warming up for a water exercise class is slightly different than warming up for a land class. Dynamic range of motion exercises replace static stretching movements. For example, in a land class, the hamstrings are warmed up and then stretched statically. In the water, hip flexion and extension exercises both warm up and stretch the quads and hamstrings because there is not any eccentric muscle contraction due to the lack of gravity. If participants are in cool water (80-82°), a more vigorous warm-up may be appropriate to promote thermoregulation of the body. If the pool temperature is 86° or above, which is considered *thermoneutral*, it is not as necessary to move vigorously because the body is warmer. Full range of motion exercises are appropriate and encouraged in a water exercise warm-up.

Dynamic Movement and Rehearsal Moves

Following are some sample dynamic, rehearsal warm-up moves that target specific muscle groups. Have participants perform each of these

Table 12.1 Hip Flexion and Extension Muscle Contraction, Land Versus Water

Environment	Equipment	Joint action	Rectus femoris iliopsoas	Glutes/ hamstrings
Land	None	Hip flexion	Concentric	None
Land	None	Hip extension	Eccentric	None
Water	None or surface area devices	Hip flexion	Concentric	None
Water	None or surface area devices	Hip extension	None	Concentric
Water[a]	Buoyant cuff on ankle	Hip flexion	None	Eccentric
Water[a]	Buoyant cuff on ankle	Hip extension	None	Concentric

Note. Participant should stand upright, hands at the sides, with feet shoulder-width apart.

[a]Slow speed to resist buoyancy.

movements through the full range of motion with little increase in tempo. In figure 12.4, the participant progresses the pectorals by using a breaststroke move backward to assist the move (12.4*a*) and then jogging into the move (12.4*b*) to resist the move and overload it.

Figures 12.5 through 12.9 show total body movements that can be used to thermoregulate the body by increasing core temperature through energy expenditure. In these movements, participants can use inertia currents by traveling against and then with the current.

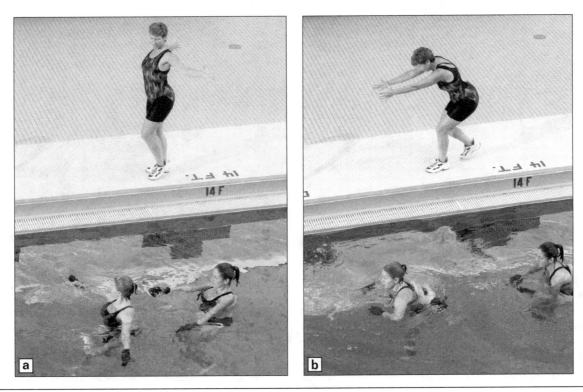

Figure 12.4 Pectoral progression: *(a)* assist and *(b)* resist.

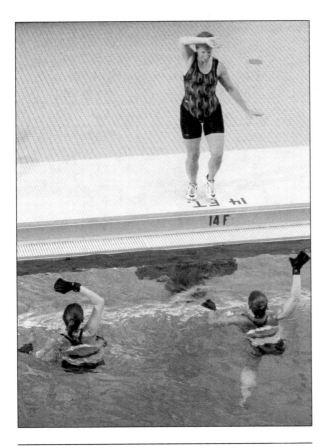

Figure 12.5 Parade wave with external resistance and arm out of water (aerobics and entertainment).

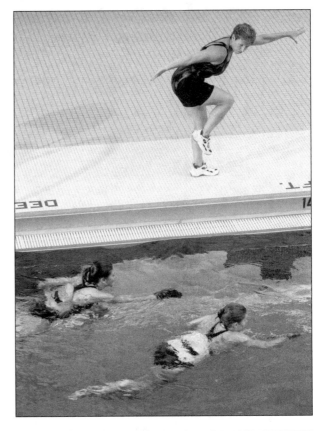

Figure 12.7 Rock climber: Resist by pushing hands down in the water (glutes and triceps).

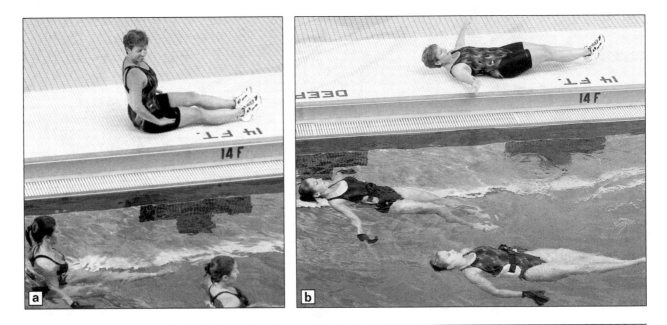

Figure 12.6 (a) Seated flutter kick with backward movement and (b) change in surface areas (quads and ab stabilizers).

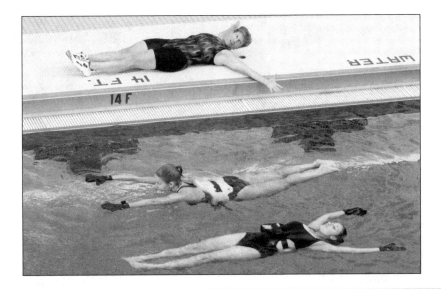

Figure 12.8 Abdominals: Lie supine, tuck knees, and stretch out in a prone Superman position.

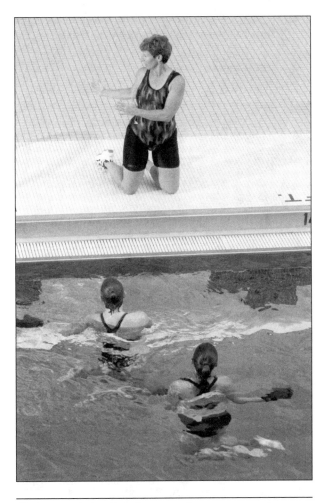

Figure 12.9 Washing machine move in deep water; use buoyant devices in shallow water (obliques and rotator cuff).

Stretching Major Muscle Groups

Taking the muscles through a full range of motion replaces static stretching in water exercise. Therefore, you do not use a stretching segment when teaching a water exercise class. There is not a force against gravity; therefore, the opposing muscle is automatically stretched.

Verbal Cues and Tempo

Teaching from the deck is very important in water exercise, because visual cues are as important as verbal cues. We recommend that you give a visual demonstration and allow participants to learn all moves before they get into the water. In terms of music, water exercise is a lot like indoor cycling: Use music to set the mood and not necessarily the tempo. If you move on the beat all the time, you will not progress participants properly. Use the tempo of the music as a gauge. For example, start with the beat and then ask participants to speed up faster than the beat for 15 s.

> ☑ **TECHNIQUE AND SAFETY CHECK**
>
> Here are some water exercise warm-up recommendations:
>
> ☐ Make sure the deck demonstration speed is appropriate for the movement.

185

- ❑ Emphasize full range of motion with each movement.
- ❑ Keep participants moving and check for water temperature comfort.
- ❑ Identify individual muscle groups and use total body movements to keep the body warm.
- ❑ Demonstrate use of music tempo by moving on the beat, moving faster than the beat, and then moving slower than the beat.

TECHNIQUE AND SAFETY

Before teaching a water exercise class, make sure a lifeguard is present so your only job will be to instruct the class. You cannot be responsible for both safety and instruction. However, do discuss safety issues, especially for those who are not comfortable in the water. Believe it or not, many people cannot swim. If you are teaching a deep water exercise class, make sure the participants have their flotation devices adjusted properly. Review how each piece of equipment should be worn before starting the class. For example, there are different levels of buoyancy belts in deep water exercise. A participant who is lean will need a device that provides more buoyancy, whereas a participant with more body fat will need a less buoyant belt. In fact, some participants who have a lot of "stored energy" may not even need a buoyancy belt for the class. Once the class has started, take a moment to remind participants of some safety skills, especially in deep water exercise. While in the water, some participants may fall forward with their face in the water or fall back and not be able to get their legs down; teach them some recovery skills and remind them throughout the workout to engage their abdominals to stay upright. Inform the lifeguard about any participants who are not comfortable in the water, so the lifeguard can watch them closely. Finally, if you are in a pool where there is a deep water drop-off, be sure the lane lines separate shallow and deep areas.

TECHNIQUE AND SAFETY CHECK

To help keep your classes safe, observe the following recommendations.

REMEMBER TO

- ❑ encourage full range of motion movements before speeding up,
- ❑ use different movement planes,
- ❑ encourage participants to maintain neutral spine and neck, with head and eyes up,
- ❑ encourage participants to keep abdominals lifted and contracted,
- ❑ review all major muscle groups and identify these for increased body awareness,
- ❑ make sure a lifeguard is on duty and water safety practices are introduced,
- ❑ demonstrate movements visually on deck so participants understand the movement, and
- ❑ encourage individuality and proper progression throughout the workout by allowing participants to work at their own levels.

AVOID

- ❑ following the tempo of the music for the entire class,
- ❑ speeding up your deck demonstrations to land speed, and
- ❑ getting in the water with participants before performing visual deck demonstrations.

BASIC MOVES

Understanding the basic water exercise movements will help you create an exercise routine in the water. Keep in mind there are different water depths to teach in:

1. Deep water using a flotation device
2. Transitional depth, where you are standing but the lungs are submerged
3. Shallow depth, where the water line is below the xiphoid process

In shallow depth there are three different ways to use the water:

1. Rebound a move and jump, which creates more impact and more intensity.

2. Stay neutral with the shoulders at the water surface and use the resistance of the water more with less impact.

3. Suspend the move, which is more difficult but has the least impact.

Understanding basic moves by muscle group will get you started on basic water movement combinations. We will review basic moves for total body movements seen in figures 12.10 through 12.13. These movements use large muscle groups to increase energy expenditure and are also very functional. For example, the "mall walk" move is a basic walking movement named after the most popular leisure activity—shopping! The cross-country skier move mimics the motion of cross-country skiing. Anytime functionality can be brought into this activity, it will benefit participants by making these same movements easier to perform on land.

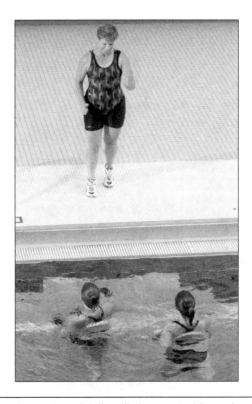

Figure 12.11 Mall walk (increased lever length, hip flexor strengthener).

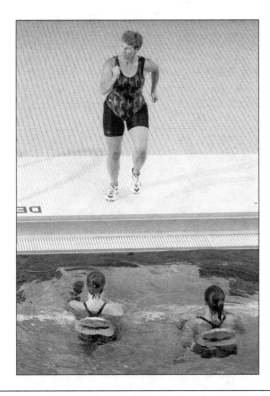

Figure 12.10 General jogging and walking (quads, hip flexors, hamstrings).

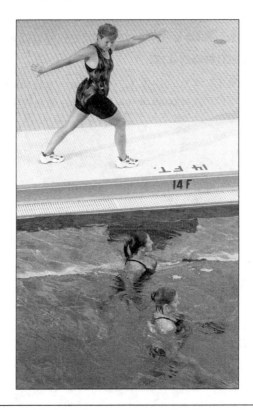

Figure 12.12 Cross-country skier legs and arms (hip flexor, glutes, hamstrings, deltoids, lats).

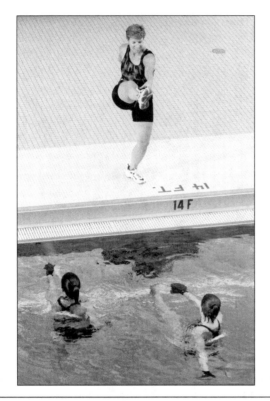

Figure 12.13 Straight leg raises with opposite hand and foot (hip flexor, lats, posterior deltoids).

Basic Moves for Total Body Conditioning

Figures 12.14 through 12.16 illustrate total body conditioning movements that involve both the upper and lower body. These movements fit well

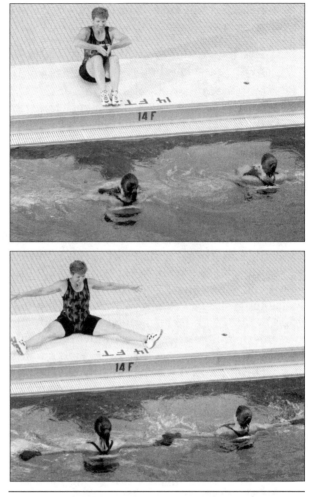

Figure 12.15 Seated V-position using pectorals and adductors (creates backward motion in deep water and suspension in shallow water).

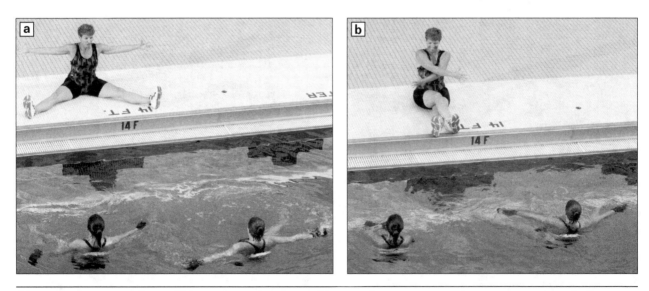

Figure 12.14 (a) Seated V-position with arms and legs in deep water or (b) a jumping jack in shallow water (pectorals, rhomboids, abductors, adductors).

in the muscular strengthening and cardio section of a water exercise workout. Use acceleration, inertia currents, and progressive resistance to challenge participants.

ments but also remain a part of the cardio segment because the body has to be supported while performing these isolation movements.

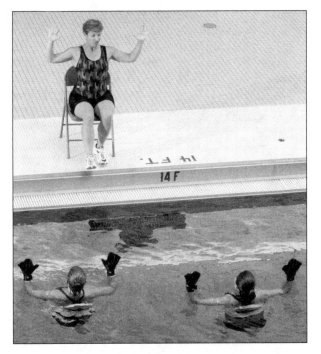

Figure 12.17 Sit kicks using knee flexion and extension in deep water and standing on one leg in shallow; repeat on the other leg (quads, hamstrings).

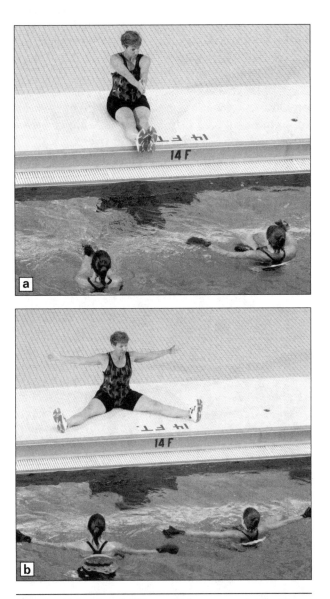

Figure 12.16 (a) Seated V-position using rhomboids and abductors (creates motion in deep water and suspension in shallow water). (b) Sitting, retract shoulder blades with long lever arm and abduct legs. You will travel forward (rhomboids, abductors).

Basic Moves for Lower Body Conditioning

Figures 12.17 through 12.20 demonstrate exercises that work the lower body muscle groups—quadriceps and hamstrings. They are isolation move-

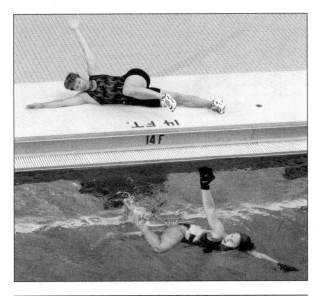

Figure 12.18 Bicycle in circle. In deep water keep arms out to the side, and in shallow water use a flotation device under the arms (hamstrings, glutes, quads, deltoids).

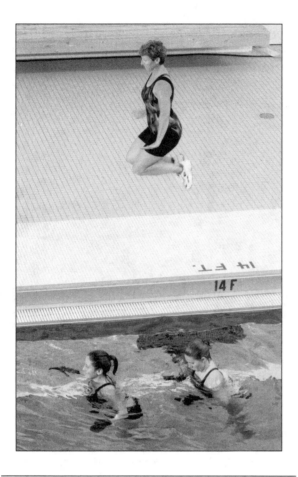

Figure 12.19 Frustrated dolphin—upright double-leg curls in deep, jog backward in shallow (hamstrings).

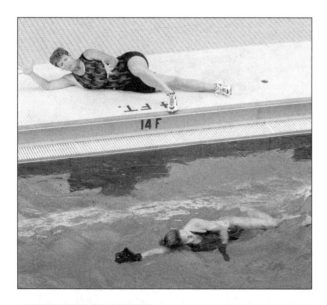

Figure 12.20 Bicycle in a circle—add overload by opening hand while circling (quadriceps, hamstrings).

Basic Moves for Upper Body Conditioning

Figure 12.21a works the rhomboid muscle group, with a reverse breaststroke moving the body forward to assist the movement followed by a flutter kick with the legs (figure 12.21b) to resist the movement. Participants should move the arms in different planes while working the pectorals or rhomboids, because this is one of the advantages of water exercise. The body moves in more natural patterns, and the direction of resistance is less important than with land-based exercises.

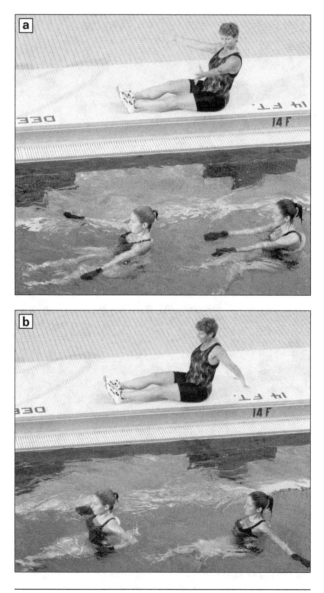

Figure 12.21 (a) Assist: reverse breaststroke, pull arms down and back, and use different planes and (b) resist: kick legs in front (rhomboids/traps).

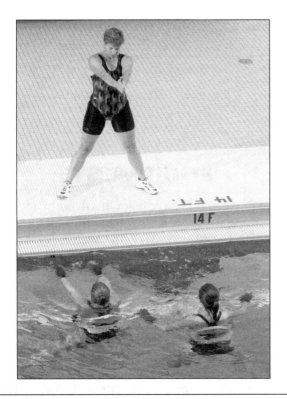

Figure 12.22 Jumping jacks—move legs in different planes (abductors, adductors, pecs, lats).

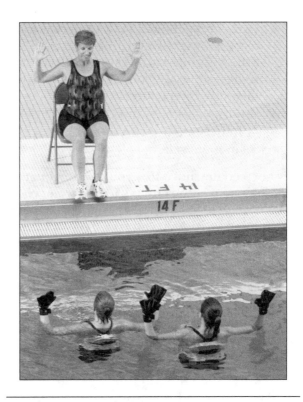

Figure 12.23 The professional sitter or walker exercise (ab stabilizers, deltoids).

Figure 12.22 shows one example of different warm-up movements using the abductors in the jumping jack movement pattern and the pecs and lats in the upper body movement patterns. Figure 12.23, along with figures 12.8 and 12.9 presented earlier in the chapter, emphasize core and stabilizer movement warm-up ideas. Figure 12.23 works the abdominals isometrically while the deltoids propel the body into motion. Figure 12.8 works the abs and low back muscles in a full range of motion. Finally, figure 12.9 isolates the oblique muscles in rotation. All of the exercise examples are excellent dynamic and rehearsal moves for a water exercise class. See appendix H for a sample water exercise routine.

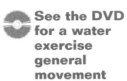 **See the DVD for a water exercise general movement overview.**

TRAINING SYSTEMS

Because untrained water exercise participants experience an initial increase in lactate that is higher than that experienced during the same movement on land, we can modify the workout plan by including some interval exercise coupled with continuous movement (Eyestone 1993). If we interval train in the water, we can help participants adapt to the eventual blood lactate change more easily and help them enjoy the activity more. The premise of interval training is that an individual can produce a greater amount of work if the work bouts are spaced between periods of rest (Kravitz 1994). For example, many people find the resistance of the water too difficult for continuous work. Following are some terms to help you understand interval training:

- Work interval: Time of the high-intensity work effort.

- Recovery interval: Time between work intervals. The recovery interval may consist of light activity (sculling only) or moderate activity (easy jogging).

- Work–recovery ratio: Time ratio of the work and recovery intervals. A work–recovery ratio of 1:3 means that the recovery interval is three times as long as the work interval, for example, jog 1 min and recover 3 min.

- Cycle or repetition: A work interval and a recovery interval represent one cycle. Since a recovery interval follows a work interval, some resources report the number of work intervals as repetitions.

- Set: The specific number of cycles. A series of four work–recovery cycles makes one set of four cycles.

It is not recommended that you perform interval training for an entire group exercise water class, but it is good to insert smaller segments of interval training when you can (see figure 12.24). A sample interval training water exercise series is outlined in table 12.2.

- Increased enjoyment due to added variety
- Potential for greater total work in a shorter period of time
- Improved anaerobic and aerobic power and capacity
- Potential for fewer injuries and less participant burn out
- Increased adherence to exercise in general

Figure 12.24 Benefits of interval training.

Table 12.2 Interval Water Exercise Series

3 min	3 cycles	40 s recovery and 20 s work
3 min	3 cycles	30 s recovery and 30 s work
3 min	3 cycles	20 s recovery and 40 s work

EQUIPMENT

Once participants have been involved in a water exercise class for 6 to 8 weeks, they likely will adapt to the resistance of the water; it eventually will be necessary to use some equipment for overload purposes. There are several different types of overload devices one can use; here we discuss surface area devices and buoyancy devices. Buoyancy devices used for long periods and used for full body support (without a belt) can be detrimental to the shoulders in deep water because of the effects of buoyancy pulling on the shoulder joint. These devices are best used in shallow water where they are less burdensome to the shoulder joint. Figure 12.25 shows some examples of buoyancy devices. Surface area devices are good in both deep and shallow water. Surface area devices predominantly use concentric muscle contractions of the agonist and antagonist muscle groups. They also overload the movement more as a greater amount of water is moved. Figure 12.26 shows some examples of surface area devices.

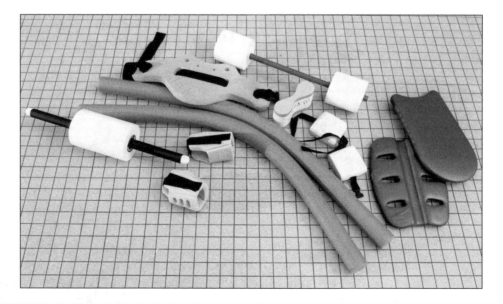

Figure 12.25 Buoyancy devices.

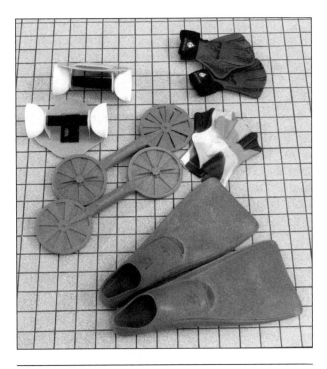

Figure 12.26 Surface area devices.

Encourage slow speeds to resist buoyancy or the equipment will bounce right out of the water, similar to how a dumbbell on land will fall to the ground if it is not lowered slowly. Buoyancy devices allow eccentric muscle contractions to occur in the water. Stabilizing the core is also crucial because the core serves as the base for many exercises. Water equipment companies are beginning to develop surface area and buoyancy devices for water exercise that can be individualized to the person, just like we have 5-, 10-, and 15-lb handheld weights in land classes. Check out the Water Exercise Resource List for water fitness products. We need to broaden our concept of resistance training and use as many different mediums as we can, especially as our population gets older and needs more nonimpact exercise choices. Water exercise is one medium you will want to know about.

WATER EXERCISE RESOURCE LIST

- www.sprintaquatics.com
- www.aquajogger.com
- www.waterfit.com
- www.aquatherapeutics.com
- www.fernoperformancepools.com
- www.aeawave.com

Chapter Wrap-Up

Water exercise is an effective form of group exercise. Plus, we all remember enjoying our leisure time outdoors on a warm day by the pool or beach. Connecting leisure and exercise helps enhance long-term adherence to exercise. Use the principles of Newton's laws of motion, use multiplanar movements, and make fun and enthusiasm a major component of your class.

Key Points From the Group Exercise Class Evaluation Form

- Use total body movements to get warmed up.
- Perform five to six repetitions of the major muscle groups you will focus on, and work on full range of motion exercises.
- In water exercise there is no static stretching in the warm-up because participants get cold.
- Dynamic full range of motion movements provide for muscle lengthening.
- Use at least one posture cue when introducing a new movement.
- Because water speed needs to be one half to one third of land speed, slow down all demonstrations of movements to correct water speed on the deck.

- Use the properties of water and Newton's laws to evaluate the effectiveness of movements.

- Use motivating music that fits the segment and mood. Following the beat the entire time does not allow for individualization of exercises.

- Active and dynamic movements can replace static stretching because of the loss of gravity. Some static stretching can be performed in shallow or in deep water with a ledge but is not required.

- Once you have relaxed and stretched, spend a few minutes in total body movements to rewarm before getting out of the pool if you are in cool water. If the water is warm, concentrate on relaxation and visualization.

Written Assignment

Attend a group water exercise class or view a water exercise class video. Using the group exercise class evaluation form, evaluate the class. Identify two properties of water and two of Newton's laws of motion you observed being used in the class.

Practical Assignment

Prepare a 4-min water exercise routine to present to a group of four or five students. Use two different movement segments and one cueing skill.

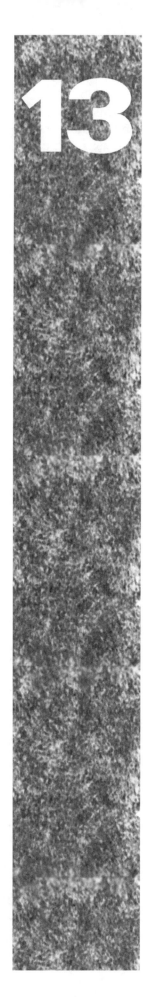

13

Other Group Exercise Modalities

Chapter Objectives

By the end of this chapter, you will have a basic understanding of other group exercise modalities, including

- equipment-based cardio training (e.g., treading, rowing),
- slide,
- rebounding,
- NIA,
- Latin, funk, hip-hop, and country,
- barre and dance,
- yoga,
- Pilates,
- t'ai chi,
- sport conditioning (e.g., skiing, golf, tennis),
- outdoor walking and in-line skating, and
- combination classes.

In this chapter we address some of the other modalities for group exercise that have become popular over the years. Group exercise is a diverse field with many teaching options for instructors. We recommend that you become skilled in teaching at least one of the more mainstream modalities covered earlier in this text: high/low impact, step, kickboxing, indoor cycling, and water exercise, plus muscle conditioning and flexibility training. After you have achieved a secure foundation teaching these types of classes, you may want to expand your employment opportunities and increase your marketability by developing the skills to teach additional exercise modes such as those included in this chapter. To teach many of the modes introduced here, you will need additional training, education, and certification (see the resources section at the end of the chapter). The main points on the group exercise class evaluation form for other modalities are found in figure 13.1.

☑ BACKGROUND CHECK

Before working your way through this chapter, you should do the following:

READ

☐ chapter 4 on warm-up,

☐ chapter 5 on cardiorespiratory training,

☐ chapter 6 on muscle conditioning, and

☐ chapter 7 on flexibility training.

EQUIPMENT-BASED CARDIO TRAINING

Group equipment-based cardio programming refers to classes that use traditional cardiorespiratory equipment such as treadmills, rowing machines, cross-country ski machines, and ellip-

---

Key Points for Warm-Up Segment

- Provides an appropriate amount of dynamic movement
- Gives rehearsal moves
- Stretches major muscle groups in an appropriate manner
- Gives clear cues and verbal directions
- Uses an appropriate music tempo

Key Points for Cardio Segment

- Gradually increases intensity
- Minimizes repetitive movements, using a variety of muscle groups
- Promotes participant interaction and encourages fun
- Demonstrates movement options
- Gives clear verbal cues and directions
- Checks participants' intensity levels and gives modifications based on results
- Gradually decreases intensity during postcardio cool-down
- Uses music appropriately

Key Points for Muscle Strength and Endurance Segment

- Gives cues for posture and alignment
- Encourages and demonstrates good body mechanics
- Observes participants' form and suggests modifications for injuries and special needs and progressions for advanced participants
- Gives clear verbal directions and uses appropriate music volume
- Uses music tempo appropriate for biomechanical movement

Key Points for Stretching and Relaxation Segment

- Chooses appropriate music
- Includes static stretching
- Appropriately emphasizes relaxation and visualization

Figure 13.1 Group exercise evaluation form for other modalities.

tical (cross-trainer) machines. Popular programs using one or more of these modalities have been developed by innovative instructors at several facilities (Nichols et al. 2000, Pillarella 1997). The steps involved in instructing an equipment-based cardio conditioning class are fairly simple:

1. Make certain you understand proper setup on your machines, including how to use the instrument panel (if any) and how to adjust the machine to each individual.

2. Be able to demonstrate and teach proper biomechanics, alignment, and technique on the machines.

3. Design a physiologically sound class format.

An appropriate class format adheres to the points outlined in the group exercise class evaluation form and includes a warm-up (usually on the machine itself at a low intensity), a cardio conditioning segment, and a postcardio cool-down. Some instructors then move the class into another room for muscle conditioning or stretching, although this is not necessary (see table 13.1). Many equipment-based classes use interval training, which can be adjusted for all levels of participants. Interval training involves repeated bouts of harder work interspersed with periods of easier work (or, occasionally, recovery periods). Participants will need instruction regarding the appropriate levels of intensity during these intervals. As a general rule, you can encourage your class to work at a 12 or 13 on the RPE scale during the easier interval and a 14 or 15 during the harder interval (see table 5.1 from chapter 5). In a treadmill (or treading) class, participants can walk or run, depending on their fitness level. Variables for increasing intensity on a treadmill include increasing the speed, elevation, or both. Motivating music can be played in the background, or you can try interspersing a song

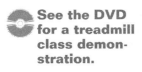
See the DVD for a treadmill class demonstration.

Table 13.1 Sample Equipment-Based Class Format (45 Min)

Workout segment	Duration (min)	Intensity
Warm-up	5	Light
Stretch	3	Light
Flat road or easy paddle	5	Moderate
Intervals	5	Moderate to hard
Recovery	2	Light
Steady work	5	Moderate
Intervals	5	Hard
Steady work	5	Moderate
Intervals	5	Moderate to hard
Cool-down and stretch	5	Light

with an appropriate beat, offering your class the option of walking, running, or rowing on the beat (see figure 13.2).

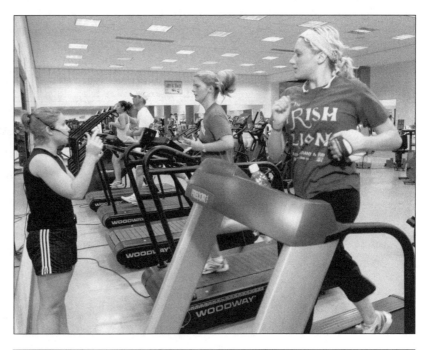

Figure 13.2 Group treadmill class.

SLIDE TRAINING

Another cardiorespiratory modality for group exercise is slide training, also known as lateral movement training. The slide workout has been shown to provide an aerobic workout comparable to other activities such as high/low impact, step, and cycling in terms of caloric expenditure (Frodge et al. 1993, Ludwig et al. 1994, Williford et al. 1993). Slide training involves lateral (side to side) motion and can train the body's systems in the frontal plane, which can be useful in many sports. Tennis, skating, skiing, basketball, and football all require the ability to move laterally and maintain lateral stability around the joints. Slide training is low impact, can enhance balance and agility, and can inject needed variety into group exercise.

Specially designed boards, known as slideboards, and special booties that fit over participants' shoes are required for slide training. Slideboards have end ramps, which stop the participant at each end of the board; most boards used in the fitness setting are 6 ft long. Workouts either can be given in the athletic training style (no music or offbeat) or can be taught to music, using choreography, combinations, and the 32-count phrase discussed in chapter 3. There are two basic stances: the upright stance and the athletic ready stance (which is more difficult and resembles the position of a speed skater). Several different moves are possible on the slideboard, including the basic slide, slide touch, knee lift, hamstring curl, fencing slide, lunge, cross-country skiing, slide squat, and speed skating, all of which can be accompanied by a variety of arm movements (see figure 13.3). Music speeds of approximately 124 to 140 beats/min allow most of these moves to be performed to the beat, if desired. A warm-up incorporating rehearsal moves on the slide should be performed before the workout, and a cool-down that includes appropriate stretching for the muscles used in lateral training (especially the hip abductors and adductors) is essential.

See the DVD for a slide demonstration.

REBOUNDING

Rebounding is a form of group exercise in which each participant performs moves on an individual device that looks like a minitrampoline. At least one study has shown comparable cardiorespiratory results between rebounding and treadmill exercise (McGlone et al. 2002), indicating that rebounding meets ACSM criteria for the achievement of aerobic fitness. Rebounding is classified as a low-impact activity and appears to place minimal stress on joints and connective tissue. Choreographed routines to music of approximately 126 beats/min can be created with a variety of moves such as jumping jacks, twists, and alternating strides (all double-leg moves with both feet contacting the rebounder at the same time) or jog-

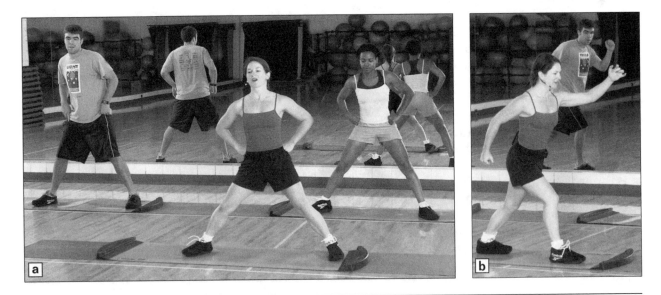

Figure 13.3   (a) Slide touch and (b) cross-country slide.

ging, knee lifts, and kicks (one-leg moves, where only one foot contacts the rebounder at a time). This modality is fun and playful and can provide a challenging workout (see figure 13.4).

NIA

NIA (neuromuscular integrative action) is a group exercise modality that incorporates the diverse elements of freestyle modern and ethnic dance, t'ai chi, martial arts, and yoga. It is intended to provide a cardiorespiratory stimulus coupled with increased mind–body awareness, blending elements of Eastern and Western philosophies. A typical NIA class is partly choreographed, with students following the instructor's lead, and partly freestyle, with participants dancing "as if no one were watching." Partners, lines, circles, and rows may be used to help vary the group dynamics. A variety of music styles are incorporated—New Age, funk, Latin, rock, rhythm and blues, and jazz—and the beats per minute vary from song to song, depending on the instructor's plan. Shoes are off, impact is reduced, and participants are encouraged to express themselves. A major objective of an NIA class is for participants to become more internally directed in their physical expressions, to "listen to their bodies" and move in ways that are holistic, pleasurable, and joyful (see figure 13.5).

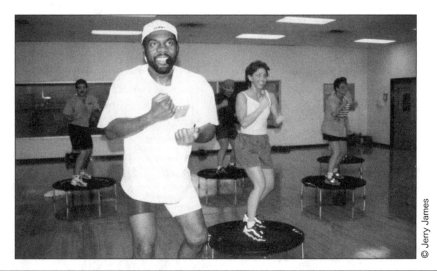

© Jerry James

Figure 13.4 A group rebounding class.

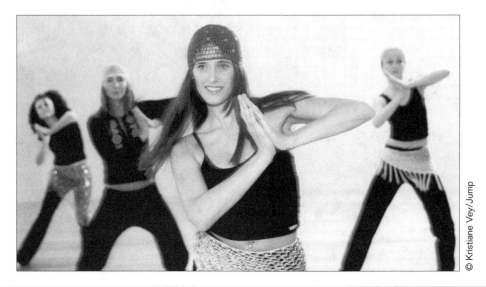

© Kristiane Vey/Jump

Figure 13.5 A group NIA class.

LATIN, FUNK, HIP-HOP, AND COUNTRY

Many clubs offer specialty classes in a particular movement style, such as Latin, funk, hip-hop, or country. This style is used in the warm-up, cardiorespiratory, and postcardio cool-down portions of class and is taught to Latin, funk, hip-hop, or country music.

Some of these modalities have moves that are specific to that style. Latin moves, for example, include the samba, rumba, merengue, cha-cha, lambada, salsa, calypso, and mambo (see figure 13.6). Country moves include swivels, hip bumps, the tush push, and the boot scoot; these moves are frequently arranged into line dances and can be readily adapted for fitness cardio classes (Lane 2000).

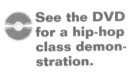 **See the DVD for a hip-hop class demonstration.**

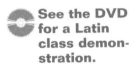 **See the DVD for a Latin class demonstration.**

Funk and hip-hop styles incorporate upper body isolations and many familiar dance moves (steptouch, march, jazz square, and plié) with African and street movement stylized accents, all to downbeat-centered music and complex rhythmic patterns.

BARRE AND DANCE-BASED CLASSES

A few clubs offer ballet barre or other dance-based classes fused with traditional fitness elements. This type of class depends on the instructor's background and skills and can include muscle conditioning exercises performed at the barre, traditional high/low impact or jazz-style dance in the center of the room, Pilates, and dance-based stretches. Barre work can consist of either traditional fitness style moves, such as standing hip abduction, hip adduction, extension work, lunges, and squats, or ballet moves such as plié, relevé, tendu, battement, frappé, rond de jambe, and port de bras. Center work could include traditional high/low impact moves or ballet work such as turns, pirouettes, jumps, and choreographed routines. Care should be taken in the fitness setting to modify some of the higher-risk dance moves for the general population. Moves such as full port de bras, grand pliés, and cervical hyperextensions in jazz pose risks for the neck, back, and knees that are not appropriate for deconditioned adults desiring health-related fitness. As always, a barre or dance-based class should have a proper warm-up and a sufficient cool-down, including flexibility work (see figure 13.7).

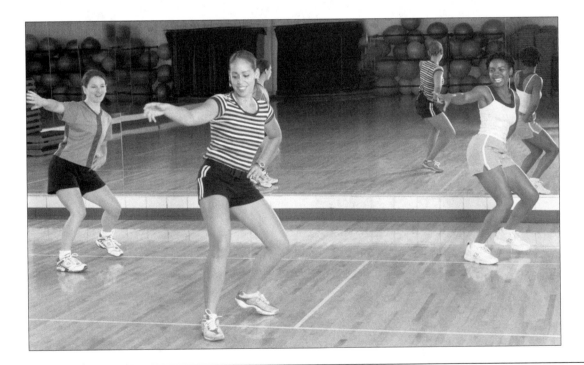

Figure 13.6 A Latin dancing class.

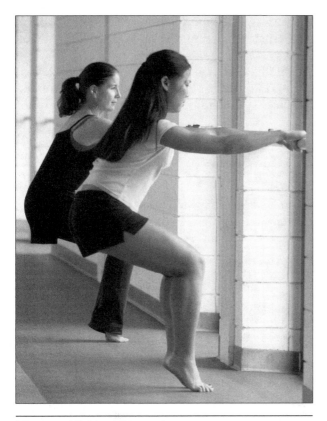

Figure 13.7 A barre class.

YOGA

Yoga or yoga–fitness fusion classes have become increasingly popular at most fitness facilities. Yoga is a 5,000-year-old discipline integrating and uniting mind, body, and spirit. It is intended to be a complete system for living, although many practitioners focus primarily on the physical aspect. The practice of yoga has many styles, such as Iyengar, Bikram, Astanga, Kripalu, Anusara, and Viniyoga, to name a few. In addition, yoga can run the gamut from a very easy, healing, and relaxing class focusing primarily on flexibility (appropriate for everyone) to an extremely vigorous, athletic, and strenuous workout focusing on strength, balance, and coordination as well as flexibility (appropriate for the advanced, very fit yoga practitioner). Yoga has many benefits and has been shown to increase muscle strength, endurance, flexibility, and balance; improve posture; and reduce stress, tension, pain, chronic fatigue, and asthma symptoms. It has also been shown to reduce coronary heart disease (Manchanda et al. 2000, Ornish et al. 1990). Prolonged repetitive sequences of dynamic postures in power-type classes may even provide a mild to moderate cardiorespiratory stimulus.

The physical practice of yoga has two main components: the poses, or asanas, and the breath work, or pranayama. Asanas are generally divided into forward bends, backbends, side bends, and twisting poses and can be performed in a variety of positions: supine, prone, side-lying, standing, all fours, and inverted. Some of the postures involve extreme flexibility or strength, but almost all can be modified; proper progression is as important in yoga as in other disciplines! Yoga instructors must understand common mechanisms of joint injury and know how to instruct their participants regarding proper range of motion and appropriate effort.

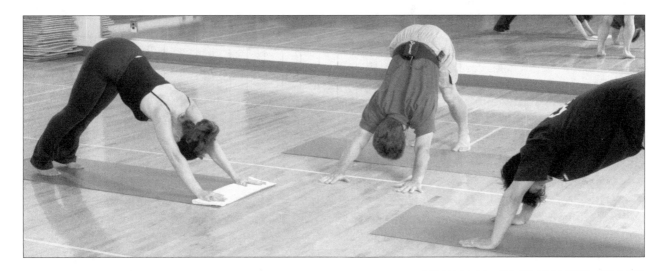

Figure 13.8 Yoga group exercise class.

Pranayama is the science of breathing as described in ancient texts. It involves controlling the prana, breath, or life force. Studies have shown that breath work can independently increase relaxation, reduce anxiety, and improve overall psychological well-being (Cappo and Homes 1984). The fundamental pranic breath in yoga is the basic abdominal or diaphragmatic breath—an excellent and healthful practice that can be incorporated into all types of fitness classes, especially during the final cool-down and relaxation segment.

Music varies in a yoga class, depending on the style or particular class segment. During the rigorous, repetitive sequences of a power-type class, world ethnic music (often

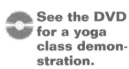

See the DVD for a yoga class demonstration.

with drums) is frequently used as background, although there is no movement "on the beat." During the more introspective opening and ending segments of class, music is soft, soothing, and meditative. Alternatively, some yoga instructors teach part or all of the class completely without music (see figure 13.8).

PILATES

Pilates is a system of muscular strength and flexibility conditioning named after its originator, Joseph H. Pilates. Special equipment is available for individual or small-group Pilates training, but the most common form of group exercise in health fitness settings is mat Pilates, which requires no equipment other than a mat (although blocks, bands, and fitness circles can also be used). A series of specific Pilates exercises are given that focus primarily on training the core muscles, which means the muscles controlling the stability of the pelvis, spine, scapulae, and neck. Joseph Pilates believed that without core stability and endurance, the body functions less efficiently and is much more prone to injuries. Therefore, Pilates exercises challenge the spine in flexion, extension, and, especially, in the neutral position, adding arm and leg movements to help overload the core (torso) muscles and stimulate improvement. Ideal body alignment, breathing, precision, concentration, flow, and increased body awareness are all very important in a Pilates class. Other central concepts include "hollowing" the abdominals (activating the transverse abdominis), lengthen-

ing through all joints (creating a sense of traction), and creating a spine that is supple (flexible) as well as strong.

Pilates exercises can be modified and progressed according to individual class members' needs. As in yoga, music is usually, though not

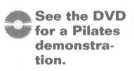

See the DVD for a Pilates demonstration.

always, used; when it is used, participants do not move on the beat but are encouraged to go at their own pace (see figure 13.9). See page 81 in chapter 6 for a description of some exercises used in mat Pilates.

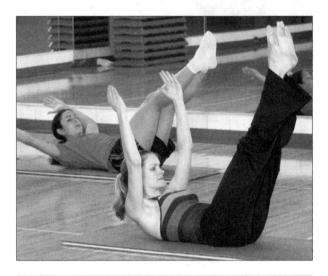

Figure 13.9 A group Pilates class.

T'AI CHI

Another mind–body discipline gaining in popularity is the 700-year-old Chinese system of martial arts exercise called t'ai chi. T'ai chi promotes flexibility, balance, muscle endurance, and coordination and has been advocated as an ideal exercise for lifelong well-being, with

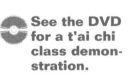

See the DVD for a t'ai chi class demonstration.

perhaps a special appeal to seniors due to its gentle, non-impact nature. Several different versions of t'ai chi exist, but the Yang style is

perhaps the most popular and accessible style, with 24 forms, or series of movements. These forms are meant to be practiced daily and can be practiced anywhere. T'ai chi encourages the integration of mind, body, and spirit, and, like yoga, t'ai chi focuses on bringing one's attention into the present moment without excessive mental chattering. This principle of mindfulness, as well as the focus on slow movement performed with complete awareness, is a concept that can be applied in other forms of group exercise (see figure 13.10).

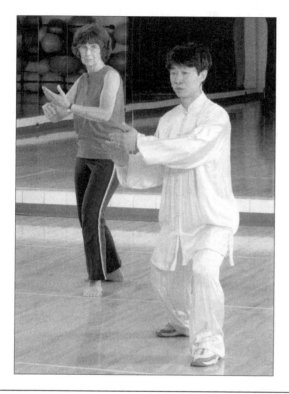

Figure 13.10 A group t'ai chi class.

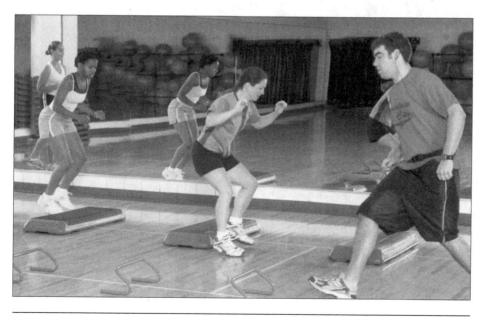

Figure 13.11 A sport conditioning class.

SPORT CONDITIONING

Sport conditioning classes can be formatted to address the demands of a specific sport, such as tennis, skiing, or golf, or they may be taught in a multisport format, designed to appeal to a variety of sport enthusiasts. Twist (2004) discusses how sports conditioning is on the fast track for professional athletes. Many recreational athletes in group exercise will also want to participate in this activity. The goal of most participants in such a class is to prepare for and improve performance in a particular sport. A sport conditioning class is often taught without music (or with music functioning as background only) and may be held in a traditional group exercise room, in a gymnasium, at a racquetball court, or even outside. Most classes emphasize the general athletic components of aerobic and anaerobic training, muscle strength and endurance, flexibility, balance, agility, coordination, visual acuity, lateral speed, and power. Intervals and various athletic drills form the basis of the workout, with the instructor functioning more as a coach than as a choreographer. Examples of exercises used in common athletic drills include shuttle runs (point A to point B and back again), lateral hopping, shuffles (cutting), relay runs, bounding and leaping, tuck jumps, rope jumping, and push-ups. Additionally, equipment such as steps, slides, medicine balls, tubing, hoops, floor ladders, cones, balance beams, balance boards, and low hurdles may all be incorporated. Follow safety guidelines whenever possible and modify strenuous drills for beginners. Above all, keep the class simple and fun (see figure 13.11).

> **See the DVD for a sport conditioning class demonstration.**

OUTDOOR WALKING AND IN-LINE SKATING

Walking is often ranked as the number one sport and recreational activity by many people, so leading a walking class can be a great way to expand your teaching options. A walking class should include a warm-up and cool-down with plenty of stretching. Many instructors also build drills such as backward and sideways walking into their classes or incorporate interval training. Some even provide circuit-type stations for muscle conditioning along the route. It's ideal to lead a walking class with two instructors, one as the leader in front and one as the "shepherd" in back. This way the class can accommodate participants of varying fitness levels and participants can walk at the speed that is appropriate for them.

See the DVD for a walking class demonstration.

Various walking adjuncts, or devices, may be added to help increase the intensity (Porcari 1999). These include weighted vests, hand weights or weighted gloves, walking poles, or power belts (a belt worn around the waist with attached resistance cords with handles). Encourage your class to walk with good technique: head and neck in neutral, eyes looking ahead, arms and hands relaxed, landing on heel of foot and rolling through, no hyperextended knees, pelvis in neutral. Power walking or power striding is a high-intensity version of walking that uses more vigorous upper body movements and some hip rotation (see figure 13.12).

In-line skating also has achieved popularity in recent years as an outdoor group exercise, and it is an appropriate form of exercise for improving cardiorespiratory fitness (Melanson et al. 1996). However, instructors must have the proper training, use appropriate locations (such as an empty parking lot), use proper equipment (skates, helmets, wrist guards, and elbow and knee pads), and, as always, promote safety and fun!

RAMPING

The newest trend to hit the fitness industry is ramping, which uses a new product called "the Ramp." The program is a cardiovascular workout that allows participants to vary the intensity of their workouts. Rather than stepping up onto a step, which requires participants to lift their body weight, participants perform more of a rocking movement in which they press or push off the

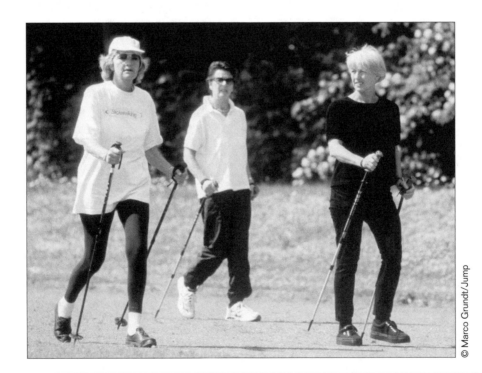

© Marco Grundt/Jump

Figure 13.12 An outdoor walking class.

ramp with their feet. Ramping is being touted as an activity that will work the glutes more than step, which predominantly works the quadri-ceps muscles. Some think of ramping as "incline walking." Because the Ramp is a relatively new product, we don't have a lot of information on participant response, but we like the concept because rarely is there a "cool" product invented for the beginner or less fit participant. Most new products have catered to the avid exerciser.

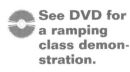
See DVD for a ramping class demonstration.

COMBINATION CLASSES AND OTHER OPTIONS

The number and types of combination classes are limited only by an instructor's imagination. Many popular fusions of the modalities covered in this text are currently popular. Yogilates (yoga plus Pilates), yoga t'ai chi, spinning plus yoga, ballet barre and Pilates, outdoor walking followed by muscle conditioning on a stability ball, step inter-vals interspersed with intervals of Latin dance, and rebounding followed by a 20-min stretch class are all ideas for combining various modali-ties. Circuit-type workouts are another great way to accomplish a lot of work in an hour: Set up muscle-conditioning stations around the room and have participants rotate through the sta-tions, either individually or in small groups (or pods). Some clubs offer a Jump and Pump class: intervals of jump rope interspersed with intervals of muscle conditioning. Be creative; you have an unlimited number of options!

Finally, yet another very significant type of group exercise exists that is population specific. Many facilities offer classes designed specifically for pregnant or postnatal women, seniors, people with arthritis, large exercisers, teens, and chil-dren. These specialty populations are out of the scope of this text, but many excellent resources exist. If you want to develop an area of expertise with a certain population, we encourage you to seek the appropriate training and certification for that group.

GROUP EXERCISE RESOURCE LIST

- The Indoor Rowing Institute, 800-245-5676, ext. 3022
- United States Rowing Association, 317-237-5656
- American Institute of Rebounding, www.healthbounce.com
- Urban Rebounding, www.urbanrebounding.com
- NIA, 800-762-5762, www.nia-nia.com
- Pilates Method Alliance, 866-573-4945, www.pilatesmethodalliance.org
- New York City Ballet Workout, 212-870-4068, www.nycballet.com
- Stott Pilates, 800-910-0001, www.stottpilates.com
- Balanced Body (Pilates method), www.balancedbody.com
- *Yoga Journal*, www.yogajournal.com
- Yoga Alliance, 877-964-2255, www.yogaalliance.org
- Yogafit training, 310-376-1036, www.yogafit.com
- T'ai chi, www.taichichih.org
- International In-Line Skating Association and certification, 407-368-9141
- Ramping, 800-900-7228, www.ramping.com

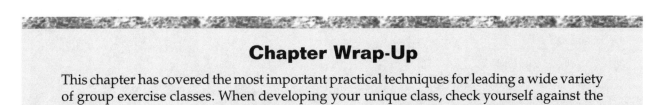

Chapter Wrap-Up

This chapter has covered the most important practical techniques for leading a wide variety of group exercise classes. When developing your unique class, check yourself against the group exercise class evaluation form to be sure you've met the basic criteria for leading each segment. You will find helpful contact information for specific formats in "Group Exercise Resource List."

Key Points From the Group Exercise Class Evaluation Form

- Gradually increase intensity in cardiorespiratory-oriented classes such as treadmill, rowing, slide, rebounding, and NIA.
- Use a variety of muscle groups and minimize repetitive movements. This is especially important in classes such as sport conditioning, NIA, ballet barre, Latin dance, hip-hop, and country line dancing.
- Demonstrate good form, alignment, and technique.
- Use music appropriately. Some classes may be highly choreographed (NIA, Latin, hip-hop, country dance), so an ability to teach to the beat and use the phrasing of the music is critical. Other classes such as sport conditioning, treadmill, and Pilates may only require the music as background, if at all.
- Give clear cues and verbal directions, including anticipatory cues, safety and alignment information, directional cues, and motivational cues.
- Promote participant interaction and encourage fun. This is important in most classes; however, some classes such as yoga, Pilates, and t'ai chi are more meditative in nature, and participants may be encouraged to cultivate an inner awareness.
- Gradually decrease intensity during cool-down in all classes.

Written Assignment

Evaluate a class or exercise video using the group exercise class evaluation form for any of the modalities mentioned in this chapter.

Practical Assignment

Participate in a class or exercise to a video using one or more of the modalities discussed in this chapter. Write a general overview of why you liked or disliked the class.

Group Exercise Class Evaluation Form

Name:_____

Evaluator: _____

Class: _____

Date: _____

Time:_____

PRECLASS ORGANIZATION

1. Knows participants and orients new participants ❑
2. Creates a positive atmosphere (attire, footwear, class format preview) ❑
3. Begins class on time with equipment ready for use ❑

Comments: _____

_____

Warm-Up Segment

1. Includes appropriate amount of dynamic movement ❑
2. Provides rehearsal moves ❑
3. Stretches major muscle groups in a biomechanically sound manner
   with appropriate instructions ❑

Muscle groups	Warm-up	Stretch
Quadriceps and hip flexors		
Hamstrings		
Calves		
Shoulder joint		
Low back		

4. Gives clear cues and verbal directions ❏

5. Uses an appropriate music tempo ❏

Comments: _____

_____

Cardiorespiratory Segment

1. Gradually increases intensity ❏
2. Uses a variety of muscle groups and minimizes repetitive movements ❏
3. Promotes participant interaction and encourages fun ❏
4. Demonstrates movement options and gives clear verbal cues and directions ❏
5. Gradually decreases intensity during postcardio cool-down ❏
6. Uses music appropriately ❏

Comments: _____

_____

Pulse Rate (PR) or Rate of Perceived Exertion (RPE) Application

1. Takes HR or RPE at middle of activity ❏
2. Keeps participants moving during HR counts ❏
3. Gives modifications based on HR and RPE results and encourages participants to work at individual levels and abilities ❏

Comments: _____

_____

Muscular Strength and Endurance Segment

Muscle group worked	Position or exercise for strengthening
Upper body	
Lower body	
Torso	

1. Gives verbal cues on posture and alignment ❏
2. Encourages and demonstrates good body mechanics ❏
3. Observes participants' form and suggests modifications for injuries or special needs and progressions for advanced participants ❏
4. Gives clear verbal directions and uses appropriate music volume ❏

From *Methods of Group Exercise Instruction* by Carol Kennedy and Mary Yoke, 2005, Champaign, IL: Human Kinetics.

5. Uses appropriate music tempo for
   biomechanical movement ❏

Comments: _____

_____

Flexibility Training and Cool-Down Segment

1. Chooses appropriate music ❏
2. Includes static stretching ❏
3. Appropriately emphasizes relaxation and visualization ❏

Poststretch muscle group	Position or exercise for stretching
Upper body	
Lower body	
Torso	

Comments: _____

_____

Overall evaluation: _____

_____

Short Health History Form

Name:_____ Date: _____

The following information will be kept strictly confidential and will be used only to enhance the safety of the exercise portions of this workshop or clinic. Please check any conditions that apply to you.

Have you ever been told by a physician that you have or have had any of the following?

- ❑ Heart attack
- ❑ Seizure
- ❑ Stroke
- ❑ High cholesterol levels (>200)
- ❑ High blood pressure
- ❑ Abnormal electrocardiogram

- ❑ Cancer
- ❑ Diabetes
- ❑ Lung problems
- ❑ Arthritis
- ❑ Osteoporosis
- ❑ Gout

If you are currently taking any prescription or over-the-counter medications, please list them:

_____

	YES	NO
1. Do you smoke?	❑	❑
2. Can you swim?	❑	❑
3. Do you exercise aerobically three to four times per week?	❑	❑

Do you have any past injuries to, or current problems with, any of the following areas?

- ❑ Irregular heart beat
- ❑ Chest pain
- ❑ Loss of coordination
- ❑ Heat intolerance
- ❑ Dizziness
- ❑ Fainting

- ❑ Cramping
- ❑ Shin splints
- ❑ Neck
- ❑ Hands
- ❑ Hips
- ❑ Calves

- ❑ Low back
- ❑ Middle back
- ❑ Shoulders
- ❑ Feet
- ❑ Ankles
- ❑ Knees

I realize that there are risks to all exercise, including injury and possible death, although every effort will be made to decrease any risk of injury. I take full responsibility for my participation in this class. Knowing that I may participate at my own pace, and that I am free to discontinue participation at any time, I will inform the instructor or workshop leader of any problems immediately.

Signature:_____ Date: _____

APPENDIX C

Long Health History Form

Name:_____

Street address:_____

City, state, zip code: _____

Home and work phone numbers: _____

Date of birth and age: _____

Physicians:_____

Date of last physical: _____

Date of last surgery:_____

Date of last electrocardiogram: _____

Please list any drugs, medication, or dietary supplements prescribed by a physician that you are taking now.

Drug: _____   Drug:_____

Dosage: _____   Dosage:_____

For: _____   For: _____

Reactions: _____   Reactions:_____

_____   _____

Please list any self-prescribed drugs, medication, or dietary supplements that you are taking now:

Drug: _____   Drug:_____

Dosage: _____   Dosage:_____

For: _____   For: _____

Reactions: _____   Reactions:_____

_____   _____

If necessary, please list other medications on the back of this page.

Please indicate a yes response to the following questions by placing a check in the space provided.

Have you ever been told by a doctor that you have or have had the following?

- ❏ Rheumatic fever
- ❏ Heart murmur
- ❏ Heart or vascular problems
- ❏ Heart attack
- ❏ Seizure/epilepsy
- ❏ Stroke
- ❏ High cholesterol levels (>200)
- ❏ High blood pressure
- ❏ High blood triglycerides
- ❏ Abnormal electrocardiogram
- ❏ Blood clots or thrombophlebitis
- ❏ Cancer

- ❏ Diabetes
- ❏ Lung or pulmonary conditions
- ❏ Arthritis
- ❏ Osteoporosis
- ❏ Gout or hyperuricemia
- ❏ Thyroid disorders
- ❏ Allergies
- ❏ Neck problems
- ❏ Middle back problems
- ❏ Low back problems
- ❏ Varicose veins

Has anyone in your immediate family (grandparents, parents, brothers, or sisters) had any of the following?

- ❏ Heart attack or stroke before the age of 55
- ❏ Heart surgery
- ❏ High cholesterol levels (>200)

- ❏ High blood pressure
- ❏ High blood triglycerides
- ❏ Diabetes

Do you smoke?

- ❏ Yes   ❏ No

If you smoke, how much?

- ❏ Half a pack or less a day   ❏ One pack a day   ❏ Two or more packs a day

If you smoke, for how long?

- ❏ Less than 5 years   ❏ Between 5 and 15 years   ❏ More than 15 years

Which type of exercise do you do regularly?

- ❏ None
- ❏ Walking
- ❏ Jogging
- ❏ Running
- ❏ Group exercise (step, kickboxing, indoor cycling)
- ❏ Stationary cycling
- ❏ Rebounding

- ❏ Competitive sports
- ❏ Outdoor cycling
- ❏ Weightlifting
- ❏ Dancing
- ❏ Swimming or water exercise
- ❏ Other _____

How many times per week do you participate in the previously listed activities?

- ❏ 1   ❏ 2   ❏ 3   ❏ 4   ❏ 5   ❏ 6   ❏ 7

From *Methods of Group Exercise Instruction* by Carol Kennedy and Mary Yoke, 2005, Champaign, IL: Human Kinetics.

How much time do you spend at each session?

- ❏ <15 min
- ❏ 15-20 min
- ❏ 20-30 min
- ❏ 30-45 min
- ❏ 45-60 min
- ❏ >60 min

What word best describes how hard your average workout is?

- ❏ Very light
- ❏ Light
- ❏ Moderate
- ❏ Hard
- ❏ Very hard
- ❏ Extremely hard

With exercising, with exertion, or after exercise, do you experience any of the following?

- ❏ Shortness of breath or wheezing
- ❏ Side aches or side stitches
- ❏ Extremely high heart rate
- ❏ Irregular heart beat
- ❏ Sharp chest pain
- ❏ Dull, aching chest pain
- ❏ Overall or one-sided weakness
- ❏ Loss of coordination
- ❏ Heat intolerance
- ❏ Dizziness
- ❏ Mental confusion
- ❏ Fainting
- ❏ Vomiting
- ❏ Swelling of ankles or hands
- ❏ Cramping
- ❏ Shin splints
- ❏ Arm or neck pain
- ❏ Hip pain
- ❏ Calf pain
- ❏ Low back pain
- ❏ Middle back pain
- ❏ Shoulder pain
- ❏ Foot or ankle pain
- ❏ Knee pain

What would you like to accomplish through exercise? _____

_____

I acknowledge that my answers to the questions are true and complete. I will immediately inform the exercise instructor of any changes in my health.

Signature:_____ Date: _____

APPENDIX D

Informed Consent Form

I desire to engage voluntarily in _____ (name of program, club, or agency) to improve my physical fitness.

I know that I am required to fill out a health and lifestyle questionnaire before I begin to exercise. The information obtained from the questionnaire will be used in the following ways:

1. To indicate any cardiac risk or other reason why I should not exercise based on the ACSM guidelines
2. To determine the need for a physician's evaluation and written approval before I enter the exercise program
3. To recommend the types of exercise I should concentrate on to reach my fitness goals and types of exercises I should avoid

I understand that my participation in the program may not benefit me directly in any way. I realize that the program may help me evaluate my lifestyle, choose those activities I may safely carry out, and increase my quality of life.

I also understand that the reaction of the body to activity cannot always be predicted with complete accuracy. The changes that may occur and are associated with physical activity include, but are not limited to, the following signs and symptoms:

- Abnormal blood pressure or heart rate responses
- Breathlessness
- Chest discomfort
- Muscular or skeletal injury
- Heart attack and death, in very rare instances

I realize my responsibility in recognizing these potential hazards; monitoring myself before, during, and after exercise; and seeking help in the event of injury, if possible. I will attend the orientation session and talk to my personal trainer or exercise instructor to learn how to minimize these potential hazards and what I should do in an emergency. I understand that I can take steps to minimize my risk during exercise by following these steps:

1. I will give priority to regular attendance.
2. I will not withhold any information pertinent to my health or condition to the instructor or supervisor in charge of the program, and will immediately update my health and lifestyle questionnaire if changes in medication or status occur.
3. I will report any unusual symptoms or problems that I experience before, during, or after exercise.

4. I will follow the amounts and types of activities recommended during the orientation session.
5. I will not exceed my target heart rate.
6. I will not exercise when not feeling well or for 2 hr after eating, after smoking a cigarette, after drinking alcohol, or after taking over-the-counter medications or street drugs.
7. I will cool down slowly after exercise and will not take an extremely hot shower after exercise.
8. I will not undertake isometric, straining, or any other exercise that I know by experience or my physician's or therapist's recommendation to be painful or detrimental to me.
9. I realize that unsupervised exercise done on my own is performed at my own risk, even though I may be following guidelines or recommendations established during this program.

The information obtained from this exercise program will be treated as privileged and confidential and will not be released to any person without my written consent. Information regarding my health and program may be shared with instructors involved in my instruction or physical training. The information obtained also may be used for statistical or scientific purposes, with my right to privacy retained.

I, the undersigned, waive and release _____(name of program, club, or agency) and its employees, officers, or directors against any and all claims in any way connected with my participation in this program. This agreement is binding on my heirs and executors.

I acknowledge that I have read or heard this document in its entirety and that I fully understand it. I have asked any questions that may have occurred to me and have been answered to my satisfaction.

Signature:_____ Date: _____

Witness: _____ Date: _____

From *Methods of Group Exercise Instruction* by Carol Kennedy and Mary Yoke, 2005, Champaign, IL: Human Kinetics.

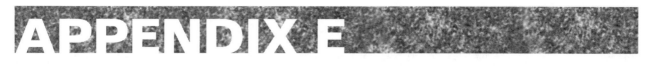

APPENDIX E

Physical Activity Readiness Questionnaire (PAR-Q)

Physical Activity Readiness
Questionnaire - PAR-Q
(revised 2002)

PAR-Q & YOU

(A Questionnaire for People Aged 15 to 69)

Regular physical activity is fun and healthy, and increasingly more people are starting to become more active every day. Being more active is very safe for most people. However, some people should check with their doctor before they start becoming much more physically active.

If you are planning to become much more physically active than you are now, start by answering the seven questions in the box below. If you are between the ages of 15 and 69, the PAR-Q will tell you if you should check with your doctor before you start. If you are over 69 years of age, and you are not used to being very active, check with your doctor.

Common sense is your best guide when you answer these questions. Please read the questions carefully and answer each one honestly: check YES or NO.

YES	NO		
☐	☐	1.	**Has your doctor ever said that you have a heart condition <u>and</u> that you should only do physical activity recommended by a doctor?**
☐	☐	2.	**Do you feel pain in your chest when you do physical activity?**
☐	☐	3.	**In the past month, have you had chest pain when you were not doing physical activity?**
☐	☐	4.	**Do you lose your balance because of dizziness or do you ever lose consciousness?**
☐	☐	5.	**Do you have a bone or joint problem (for example, back, knee or hip) that could be made worse by a change in your physical activity?**
☐	☐	6.	**Is your doctor currently prescribing drugs (for example, water pills) for your blood pressure or heart condition?**
☐	☐	7.	**Do you know of <u>any other reason</u> why you should not do physical activity?**

If

you

answered

YES to one or more questions

Talk with your doctor by phone or in person BEFORE you start becoming much more physically active or BEFORE you have a fitness appraisal. Tell your doctor about the PAR-Q and which questions you answered YES.

- You may be able to do any activity you want —— as long as you start slowly and build up gradually. Or, you may need to restrict your activities to those which are safe for you. Talk with your doctor about the kinds of activities you wish to participate in and follow his/her advice.
- Find out which community programs are safe and helpful for you.

NO to all questions

If you answered NO honestly to <u>all</u> PAR-Q questions, you can be reasonably sure that you can:
- start becoming much more physically active – begin slowly and build up gradually. This is the safest and easiest way to go.
- take part in a fitness appraisal – this is an excellent way to determine your basic fitness so that you can plan the best way for you to live actively. It is also highly recommended that you have your blood pressure evaluated. If your reading is over 144/94, talk with your doctor before you start becoming much more physically active.

DELAY BECOMING MUCH MORE ACTIVE:
- if you are not feeling well because of a temporary illness such as a cold or a fever – wait until you feel better; or
- if you are or may be pregnant – talk to your doctor before you start becoming more active.

PLEASE NOTE: If your health changes so that you then answer YES to any of the above questions, tell your fitness or health professional. Ask whether you should change your physical activity plan.

<u>Informed Use of the PAR-Q</u>: The Canadian Society for Exercise Physiology, Health Canada, and their agents assume no liability for persons who undertake physical activity, and if in doubt after completing this questionnaire, consult your doctor prior to physical activity.

No changes permitted. You are encouraged to photocopy the PAR-Q but only if you use the entire form.

NOTE: If the PAR-Q is being given to a person before he or she participates in a physical activity program or a fitness appraisal, this section may be used for legal or administrative purposes.

"I have read, understood and completed this questionnaire. Any questions I had were answered to my full satisfaction."

NAME _____

SIGNATURE _____   DATE _____

SIGNATURE OF PARENT _____   WITNESS _____
or GUARDIAN (for participants under the age of majority)

Note: This physical activity clearance is valid for a maximum of 12 months from the date it is completed and becomes invalid if your condition changes so that you would answer YES to any of the seven questions.

CSEP
SCPE © Canadian Society for Exercise Physiology   Supported by: [Canadian flag] Health Canada   Santé Canada   continued on other side...

Canada's Physical Activity Guide to Health Active Living, Health Canada, 1998, http://www.hc-sc.gc.ca./hppb/paguide/pdf/guideEng.pdf © Reproduced with permission from the Minister of Public Works and Government Services Canada, 2002. From *Methods of Group Exercise Instruction* by Carol Kennedy and Mary Yoke, 2005, Champaign, IL: Human Kinetics.

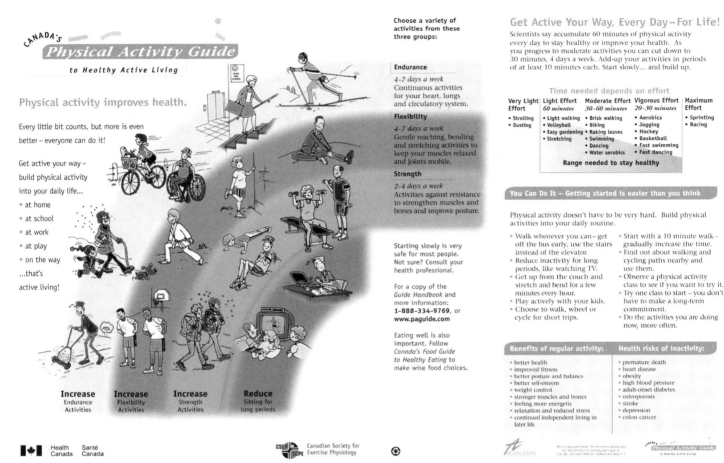

...continued from other side

PAR-Q & YOU

Physical Activity Readiness
Questionnaire - PAR-Q
(revised 2002)

FITNESS AND HEALTH PROFESSIONALS MAY BE INTERESTED IN THE INFORMATION BELOW:

The following companion forms are available for doctors' use by contacting the Canadian Society for Exercise Physiology (address below):

The **Physical Activity Readiness Medical Examination (PARmed-X)** — to be used by doctors with people who answer YES to one or more questions on the PAR-Q.

The **Physical Activity Readiness Medical Examination for Pregnancy (PARmed-X for Pregnancy)** — to be used by doctors with pregnant patients who wish to become more active.

References:

Arraix, G.A., Wigle, D.T., Mao, Y. (1992). Risk Assessment of Physical Activity and Physical Fitness in the Canada Health Survey
  Follow-Up Study. **J. Clin. Epidemiol.** 45:4 419-428.
Mottola, M., Wolfe, L.A. (1994). Active Living and Pregnancy, In: A. Quinney, L. Gauvin, T. Wall (eds.), **Toward Active Living: Proceedings of the International
  Conference on Physical Activity, Fitness and Health**. Champaign, IL: Human Kinetics.
PAR-Q Validation Report, British Columbia Ministry of Health, 1978.
Thomas, S., Reading, J., Shephard, R.J. (1992). Revision of the Physical Activity Readiness Questionnaire (PAR-Q). **Can. J. Spt. Sci.** 17:4 338-345.

To order multiple printed copies of the PAR-Q, please contact the:

Canadian Society for Exercise Physiology
202-185 Somerset Street West
Ottawa, ON K2P 0J2
Tel. 1-877-651-3755 • FAX (613) 234-3565
Online: www.csep.ca

The original PAR-Q was developed by the British Columbia Ministry of Health. It has been revised by an Expert Advisory Committee of the Canadian Society for Exercise Physiology chaired by Dr. N. Gledhill (2002).

Disponible en français sous le titre «Questionnaire sur l'aptitude à l'activité physique - Q-AAP (revisé 2002)».

© Canadian Society for Exercise Physiology   Supported by: Health Canada   Santé Canada

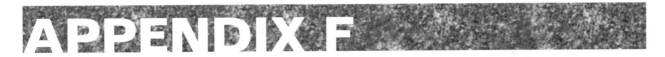

APPENDIX F
Muscles and Joint Actions

Table F.1 Shoulder Joint Muscles and Their Actions

Muscle	Flexion	Extension	Abduction	Adduction	Internal rotation	External rotation	Horizontal adduction	Horizontal abduction
Anterior deltoid	PM		Asst		Asst		PM	
Medial deltoid			PM					PM
Posterior deltoid		Asst				Asst		PM
Latissimus dorsi		PM		PM	Asst			Asst
Teres major		PM		PM	PM			Asst
Pectoralis major, clavicular	PM		Asst		Asst		PM	
Pectoralis major, sternal		PM		PM	Asst		PM	
Supraspinatus			PM					
Subscapularis	Asst		Asst	Asst	PM		Asst	
Infraspinatus						PM		PM
Teres minor						PM		PM
Biceps, long head			Asst					
Biceps, short head	Asst			Asst	Asst		Asst	
Triceps, long head		Asst		Asst				

Note. PM = prime mover; Asst = assistant mover.

Adapted, by permission, from P.J. Rasch and R.K. Burke, *Kinesiology and applied anatomy*, 7th edition (Philadelphia, PA: Lippincott, Williams and Wilkins), 172.

Table F.2 Shoulder Girdle (Scapulothoracic) Muscles and Their Actions

Muscle	Elevation	Depression	Protraction	Retraction	Upward rotation	Downward rotation
Trapezius I	PM					
Trapezius II	PM			Asst	PM	
Trapezius III				PM		
Trapezius IV		PM		Asst	PM	
Rhomboids	PM			PM		PM
Levator scapulae	PM					
Pectoralis minor		PM	PM			PM
Serratus anterior			PM		PM	

Note. PM = prime mover; Asst = assistant mover.

Adapted, by permission, from P.J. Rasch and R.K. Burke, *Kinesiology and applied anatomy,* 7th edition (Philadelphia, PA: Lippincott, Williams and Wilkins), 158.

Table F.3 Elbow and Radioulnar Joint Muscles and Their Actions

Muscle	Flexion	Extension	Pronation	Supination
Biceps brachii	PM			Asst
Brachialis	PM			
Brachioradialis	PM		Asst	Asst
Pronator teres	Asst		Asst	
Pronator quadratus			PM	
Triceps brachii		PM		
Anconeus		Asst		
Supinator				PM
Flexor carpi radialis	Asst		Asst	
Flexor carpi ulnaris	Asst			
Extensor carpi radialis longus		Asst		Asst
Extensor carpi ulnaris		Asst		

Note. PM = prime mover; Asst = assistant mover.

Adapted, by permission, from P.J. Rasch and R.K. Burke, *Kinesiology and applied anatomy,* 7th edition (Philadelphia, PA: Lippincott, Williams and Wilkins), 190.

Table F.4   Spinal Joint Muscles and Their Actions

Muscle	Flexion	Extension	Lateral flexion	Rotation to the same side	Rotation to the opposite side
Sternocleidomastoid	PM		PM		
Erector spinae group (iliocostalis, longissimus, spinalis)		PM	PM	PM	
Multifidus		PM	PM		PM
Rectus abdominis	PM		Asst		
Internal obliques	PM		PM	PM	
External obliques	PM		PM		PM
Quadratus lumborum			PM		

Note. PM = prime mover; Asst = assistant mover. Traverse abdominis: no joint actions, responsible for abdominal compression, vigorous exhalation and expulsion.

Adapted from P.J. Rasch and R.K. Burke, *Kinesiology and applied anatomy,* 7th edition (Philadelphia, PA: Lippincott, Williams and Wilkins).

Table F.5 Hip Joint Muscles and Their Actions

Muscle	Flexion	Extension	Abduction	Adduction	Inward rotation	Outward rotation
Psoas	PM		Asst			Asst
Iliacus	PM		Asst			Asst
Rectus femoris	PM		Asst			
Sartorius	Asst		Asst			Asst
Gluteus maximus		PM	Asst[a]	Asst[b]		PM
Biceps femoris		PM				Asst
Semitendinosus		PM			Asst	
Semimembranosus		PM			Asst	
Gluteus medius	Asst[c]	Asst[a]	PM		Asst[c]	Asst[a]
Gluteus minimus	Asst[c]	Asst[a]	Asst		PM	Asst[a]
Tensor fasciae latae	Asst		Asst		Asst	
Pectineus	PM			PM	Asst	
Gracilis	Asst			PM	Asst	
Adductor longus	Asst			PM	Asst	
Adductor brevis	Asst			PM	Asst	
Adductor magnus	Asst[a]	Asst[b]		PM	Asst	
Six outward rotators						PM

Note. PM = prime mover; Asst = assistant mover. The six outward rotators are the piriformis, obturator internus, obturator externus, quadratus femoris, gemellus superior, and gemellus inferior.

[a]Upper fibers; [b]lower fibers; [c]anterior fibers.

Adapted, by permission, from P.J. Rasch and R.K. Burke, *Kinesiology and applied anatomy,* 7th edition (Philadelphia, PA: Lippincott, Williams and Wilkins), 282.

Table F.6 Knee Joint Muscles and Their Actions

Muscle	Flexion	Extension	Inward rotation	Outward rotation
Biceps femoris	PM		PM	
Semitendinosus	PM		PM	
Semimembranosus	PM			PM
Rectus femoris		PM		
Vastus lateralis		PM		
Vastus intermedius		PM		
Vastus medialis		PM		
Sartorius	Asst		Asst	
Gracilis	Asst		Asst	
Popliteus[a]	Asst		PM	
Gastrocnemius	Asst			
Plantaris	Asst			

Note. PM = prime mover; Asst = assistant mover.

[a]Unlocks the knee at the start of knee flexion.

Adapted, by permission, from P.J. Rasch and R.K. Burke, *Kinesiology and applied anatomy,* 7th edition (Philadelphia, PA: Lippincott, Williams and Wilkins), 309.

Table F.7   Ankle Joint Muscles and Their Actions

Muscle	Dorsiflexion	Plantar flexion	Inversion	Eversion
Tibialis anterior	PM		PM	
Extensor digitorum longus	PM			PM
Peroneus tertius	PM			PM
Gastrocnemius		PM		
Soleus		PM		
Peroneus longus		Asst		PM
Peroneus brevis		Asst		PM
Flexor digitorum longus		Asst	Asst	
Tibialis posterior		Asst	PM	

Note. PM = prime mover; Asst = assistant mover.

Adapted, by permission, from P.J. Rasch and R.K. Burke, *Kinesiology and applied anatomy,* 7th edition (Philadelphia, PA: Lippincott, Williams and Wilkins), 330.

APPENDIX G

Sample Step Routine

This is the sample warm-up routine found in chapter 9 of the DVD that demonstrates

- the appropriate amount of dynamic movement,
- rehearsal moves for step, and
- methods to limber and statically stretch the erector spinae, hamstring, calf, hip flexor, and chest and anterior shoulder muscles by using the step.

Table G.1   Teach Block 1

Move	Foot pattern	No. of counts
Grapevine	R, L, R, tap	4
Tap-up, tap-down	Up, tap, down, tap[a]	4
Grapevine	L, R, L, tap	4
Tap-up, tap-down	Up, tap, down, tap[b]	4
Repeat combination		16

Note. R = right; L = left. Keep drilling the combination as necessary until participants know it.
[a]Lead L off R end of step; [b]lead R off L end of step.

Table G.2   Teach Block 2

Move	Foot pattern	No. of counts
March on floor	R, L, R, L	4
March on step	R, L, R, L	4
March on floor	R, L, R, L	4
March on step	R, L, R, L	4

Note. R = right; L = left. Repeat, adding arms: pump or shake hands down when marching on floor, pump hands up shaking R, L, R, L when marching on step. Keep drilling this combination as necessary until participants know it.

Table G.3 Teach Block 3

Move	Foot pattern	No. of counts
Step-touch on floor	R, L tap, L, R tap (repeat)	8
Step-touch on step	R, L tap, L, R tap (repeat)	8
Step-touch on floor	R, L tap, L, R tap (repeat)	8
Step-touch on step	R, L tap, L, R tap (repeat)	8

Note. R = right; L = left. Keep drilling this combination as necessary.

Table G.4 Combine Elements of the Blocks to Create a Total Combination

Move	Foot pattern	No. of counts
March on floor	R, L, R, L	4
March on step	R, L, R, L	4
March on floor	R, L, R, L	4
March on step	R, L, R, L	4
Step-touch on floor	R, tap, L, tap	4
Step-touch on floor	R, tap, L, tap	4
Grapevine R	R, L, R, tap	4
Tap-up, tap-down on step	L, tap, R, tap	4

Note. R = right; L = left.

Table G.5 Repeat All Leading Left

Move	Foot pattern	No. of counts
March on floor	L, R, L, R	4
March on step	L, R, L, R	4
March on floor	L, R, L, R	4
March on step	L, R, L, R	4
Step-touch on floor	L, tap, R, tap	4
Step-touch on floor	L, tap, R, tap	4
Grapevine L	L, R, L, tap	4
Tap-up, tap-down on step	R, tap, L, tap	4

Note. R = right; L = left. Entire combination can be repeated with arms.

Table G.6 Begin to Incorporate Joint-Specific Limbering and Static Stretches Near L Corner

Move	Foot pattern	No. of counts
Tap-up, tap-down on step	R, tap, L, tap	4
Wide squat on floor, hands on thighs	Wide for 2, together for 2	4
Tap-up, tap-down on step	R, tap, L, tap	4
Wide squat on floor, hands on thighs	Wide for 2, together for 2	4
Stay in squat position with hands on thighs and rhythmically move in and out of spinal flexion (e.g., neutral spine, spinal flexion, neutral spine, spinal flexion).		16+
Hold in spinal flexion for erector spinae static stretch.		8+
Move to L corner of bench; place R heel on bench and hip-hinge for R hamstring stretch. Perform ankle dorsiflexion and plantar flexion.		8+
Hold static R hamstring stretch.		8+
Place R foot completely on step and move into calf stretch position. Perform L ankle limbering with dorsiflexion and plantar flexion (add arms reaching up and down).		8
Hold L calf stretch.		8+
Bending L knee, roll L heel up and down, adding rhythmic pelvic tilting (add biceps curls).		8+
Hold L hip flexor stretch (pelvis is posteriorly tilted). Simultaneously perform a static chest stretch.		8+

Note. R = right; L = left.

Table G.7 Transition to Other Side by Performing Initial Combo One Time

Move	Foot pattern	No. of counts
March on floor	R, L, R, L	4
March on step	R, L, R, L	4
March on floor	R, L, R, L	4
March on step	R, L, R, L	4
Step-touch on floor	R, tap, L, tap	4
Step-touch on floor	R, tap, L, tap	4
Grapevine R	R, L, R, tap	4
Tap-up, tap-down on step	L, tap, R, tap	4

Note. R = right; L = left.

Table G.8   Begin to Incorporate Joint-Specific Limbering and Static Stretches Near R Corner

Move	Foot pattern	No. of counts
Tap-up, tap-down on step	L, tap, R, tap	4
Wide squat on floor, hands on thighs	Wide for 2, together for 2	4
Tap-up, tap-down on step	L, tap, R, tap	4
Wide squat on floor, hands on thighs	Wide for 2, together for 2	4
Stay in squat position, alternately press shoulders down toward floor, rotating the upper spine.		16
Hold R shoulder down for static stretch, turn head to L.		8
Hold L shoulder down for static stretch, turn head to R.		8
Move to R corner of bench; place L heel on bench and hip hinge for L hamstring stretch. Perform ankle dorsiflexion and plantar flexion.		8+
Hold static L hamstring stretch.		8+
Place L foot completely on step and move into calf stretch position. Perform R ankle limbering with dorsiflexion and plantar flexion (add arms reaching up and down).		8
Move to R corner of bench; place L heel on bench and hip-hinge for L hamstring stretch. Perform ankle dorsiflexion and plantar flexion.		8+
Hold R calf stretch.		8+
Bending R knee, roll R heel up and down, adding rhythmic pelvic tilting (add biceps curls).		8+
Hold R hip flexor stretch (pelvis is posteriorly tilted). Simultaneously perform a static chest stretch.		8+

Note. R = right; L = left.

APPENDIX H

Sample Water Workout Plan

WARM-UP

- Songs: "Brilliant Disguise" and "Sneaker Pumps"—8 min.
- Teach proper posture for using buoyancy belts.
- Review basic total body movements: jogging, mall walk, cross-country skier, and mountain climber.
- Review muscle groups and perform movements through full range of motion:
  - Upper back—hands in front, thumbs up
  - Chest—hands out to the side, horizontally adduct toward the front, use different planes
  - Abdominals—side to side and superman or lie in the sun
  - Lats—arms out to the side, adduct toward the body, action and reaction, move up
  - Biceps/triceps—review movement
  - Abductors and adductors—jumping jacks with full range of motion
  - Hamstrings/quads—sit kicks and opposite hand or foot exercise for hip flexion or extension

HIP JOINT

- Total body conditioning: Afroceltic—7 to 5 min
- Seated V-position with arms and legs; power the move (pectorals/adductors)
- Seated V-position with arms and legs together (rhomboids/abductors)
- Seated V-position using pectorals and abductors (little traveling)
- Seated V-position using rhomboids and adductors (little traveling)
- Sitting, scissor arms, legs starting with arms, legs in front (rhomboids/abductors)
- Legs straight, crisscross legs with a small ROM (adductors/abdominal stabilizers)

UPPER BODY SEGMENT

- "I Can See Clearly Now" and "Mixica"—7 min
- Pectorals—mark the movement, move backward, run against the resistance
- Upper back—mark the movement, move forward, flutter kick against the resistance
- Lats—action and reaction and then overload by not moving the legs at all

QUAD AND HAMSTRING KNEE FLEXION AND EXTENSION EXERCISES

- "Beautiful Life" and "Born to Run"—8 min
- Sit kicks using knee flexion and extension (quads, hamstrings)
- Frustrated dolphin—upright double leg curls
- Bicycle in a circle, right—sliced arms out to the side (hamstrings, glutes)
- Bicycle in a circle, add overload by opening hand while circling
- Sitting-legs in V-position, flex heel to seat (hamstrings, deltoids)

INTERVAL TRAINING SEGMENT USING MOSTLY TOTAL BODY MOVEMENTS AND AB WORK—6 TO 8 MIN

- 30 s work, 30 s rest—watch big clock.
- Six to eight different segments based on participants' feedback.
- Suggested movements: all ab movements first, then jogging, mall walk, cross-country, mountain climber, lats leap frog movement, opposite hand and foot, jumping jacks.

USING INERTIA CURRENTS

- "Turn Turn Turn"—4 min.
- Form a circle and jog into the circle.
- Turn around and run against the inertia current.
- Use all four corners to move and change the movement to mountain climber.

WALL MOVEMENTS TO COOL DOWN

- "Secret Garden"—4 min.
- Perform some standing hip rotation exercises.
- Perform some standing stretches—total body.
- Put feet on the wall for hamstring and calf stretch.
- Hold legs in V-shape and walk side to side on the wall.
- Face into pool and stretch the shoulders (Titanic move).

THERMAL REWARMING SEGMENT

- "Streets of Philadelphia"—3 min.
- Perform flutter kick using belts on stomach and in front.
- Stand on the belt for balance training.
- Perform your favorite move and then put equipment away.

From *Methods of Group Exercise Instruction* by Carol Kennedy and Mary Yoke, 2005, Champaign, IL: Human Kinetics.

BIBLIOGRAPHY

Adams, K.J., N.B. Allen, J.E. Schumm, and A.M. Swank. 1997. Oxygen cost of boxing exercise utilizing a heavy bag (abstract). *Med. Sci. Sports Exerc.* 29(5):S1067.

Aerobics and Fitness Association of America (AFAA). 2002. *Fitness Theory and Practice, Fourth Edition.* L. Gladwin (ed.) Sherman Oaks, CA: AFAA.

Ahmed, C., W. Hilton, and K. Pituch. 2002. Relations of strength training to body image among a sample of female university students. *J. Strength and Cond. Res.* 16(4):645-8.

Alan, K. 2003. Building socialization into choreography. *IDEA Fitness Edge,* Sept: 1-5.

Albano, C., and D.J. Terbizan. 2001. Heart rate and RPE difference between aerobic dance and cardio-kickboxing (abstract). *Med. Sci. Sports Exerc.* 33(5):S604.

Alter, M.J. 1996. *The science of flexibility.* Champaign, IL: Human Kinetics.

American College of Sports Medicine. 1978. The recommended quantity and quality of exercise for developing and maintaining fitness in healthy adults. *Med. Sci. Sports Exerc.* 10:vii-x.

American College of Sports Medicine. 1990. The recommended quantity and quality of exercise for developing and maintaining fitness in healthy adults. *Med. Sci. Sports Exerc.* 22, 265-274.

American College of Sports Medicine. 1998. The recommended quantity and quality of exercise for developing and maintaining cardiorespiratory and muscular fitness, and flexibility in healthy adults. *Med. Sci. Sports Exerc.* 30(6):975-91.

American College of Sports Medicine. 2001. Exercise recommendations for flexibility and range of motion. In *ACSM's Resource Manual for Guidelines for Exercise Testing and Prescription, 4th ed.,* p. 468. New York: Lippincott, Williams & Wilkins.

American College of Sports Medicine. 2006. *ACSM's resource manual for guidelines for exercise testing and prescription,* 7th ed. Philadelphia: Lippincott, Williams & Wilkins.

American Council on Exercise. 2000. *Group exercise instructor manual.* San Diego, CA: American Council on Exercise.

Anderson, P. 2000. The active range warm-up: Getting hotter with time. *IDEA Fitness Edge* April: 6-10.

Anning, J.H., C. Armstrong, E. Mylona, S. Norkus, R. Sterner, and F. Andres. 1999. Physiological responses during cardiovascular kickboxing: A pilot study (abstract). *Med. Sci. Sports Exerc.* 31(5):S403.

Aquatic Exercise Association. 1995. *Aquatic fitness professional manual.* Nokomis, FL: Aquatic Exercise Association.

Ariyoshi, M., K. Sonoda, K. Nagata, T. Mashima, M. Zenmyo, C. Paku, Y. Takamiya, H. Yoshimatsu, Y. Hirai, H. Yasunaga, H. Akashi, H. Imayama, T. Shimokobe, A. Inoue, Y. Mutoh. 1999. Efficacy of aquatic exercise for patients with low-back pain. *Kurume Med. J.* 46(2):91-6.

Åstrand, O. 1992. Why exercise? *Med. Sci. Sports Exerc.* 24(2):153-62.

Åstrand, P., and K. Rodahl. 1977. *Textbook of work physiology.* New York: McGraw-Hill.

Baechle, T., and T. Earle. 2003. *Essentials of strength training and conditioning,* 3rd ed. Champaign, IL: Human Kinetics.

Bain, L., T. Wilson, and E. Chaikind. 1989. Participant perceptions of exercise programs for overweight women. *Res. Q.* 60(2):134-43.

Baker, A. 1998. *Bicycling medicine: Cycling nutrition, physiology, and injury prevention and treatment for riders of all levels.* New York: Fireside.

Bandy, W.D., and J.M. Irion. 1994. The effect of time of static stretch on the flexibility of the hamstring muscles. *Phys. Ther.* 74:845-52.

Bates, A., and N. Hanson. 1996. *Aquatic exercise therapy.* Philadelphia: Saunders.

Beals, K. 2003. Mirror, mirror on the wall, Who is the most muscular one of all? *ACSM's Health and Fitness Journal,* March/April: 6-11.

Bednarski, K. 1993. Convincing male managers to target women customers. *Working Woman* June:23-8.

Bellinger, B., G.A. St. Clair, A. Oelofse, and M. Lambert. 1997. Energy expenditure of a noncontact boxing training session compared with submaximal treadmill running. *Med. Sci. Sports Exerc.* 29(12):1653-6.

Benson, H. 1980. *The relaxation response.* New York: Avon.

Bissonette, D., N. Guzman, L. McMillan, S. Catalano, M. Giroux, K. Greenlaw, S. Vivolo, R.M. Otto, and J. Wygand. 1994. The energy requirements of karate aerobic exercise versus low impact aerobic dance (abstract). *Med. Sci. Sports Exerc.* 26(5):S58.

Blahnik, J., and P. Anderson. 1996. Wake up your warm up. *IDEA Today* June:46-52.

Blessing, D., G. Wilson, J. Puckett, and H. Ford. 1987. The physiologic effects of 8 weeks of aerobic dance with and without hand-held weights. *Am. J. Sports Med.* 15(5): 508-10.

Borg, G. 1982. Psychophysical bases of perceived exertion. *Med. Sci. Sports Exerc.* 14:377-81.

Bortz, W. 2003. Prevention: A solution to combat rising health care costs. *ACSM's Health and Fitness Journal,* Nov/Dec: 6-8.

Bottomley, J. 1997. *T'ai-Chi: Choreography of body and mind. Complementary therapies in rehabilitation: Holistic approaches for prevention and wellness.* Thorofare, NY: Slack.

Bradford, A., M. Scharff-Olson, H.N. Williford, S. Walker, and S. Crumpton. 1999. Cardiorespiratory responses to traditional and advanced group cycling techniques (abstract). *Med. Sci. Sports Exerc.* 31(5):S422.

Bravo, G., P. Gauthier, P.M. Roy, H. Payette, and P. Gaulin. 1997. A weight bearing, water-based exercise program for orthopedic women: Its impact on bone, functional fitness, and well being. *Arch. Phys. Med. Rehabil.* 78(12): 1375-80.

Brooks, D. 1995. *Resist-a-Ball, programming guide for professionals.* Mammoth Lakes, CA: Moves International.

Brown, P., and M. O'Neill. 1990. A retrospective survey of the incidence and pattern of aerobics-related injuries in Victoria, 1987-1988. *Aust. J. Sci. Med. Sport* 22(3):77-81.

Brown, S., L. Chitwood, K. Beason, and D. McLemore. 1997. Male and female physiologic responses to treadmill and deep water running at matched running cadences. *J. Strength Cond.* 11(2):107-14.

Burke, E.R. 1994. Proper fit of the bicycle. *Clin. Sports Med.* 13:1-14.

Burnette, K., K. Johnson, and P. Kolber. 1999. *Reebok martial arts training: Trainer manual.* Canton, MA: Reebok.

Buschbacher, R.M., and T. Shay. 1999. Martial arts. *Phys. Med. Rehabil. Clin. North Am.* 10(1):35-47.

Bushman, B., M. Flynn, F. Andres, C. Lambert, M. Taylor, and W. Braunl. 1997. Effect of 4 weeks of deep water run training on running performance. *Med. Sci. Sports Exerc.* 29(5):694-9.

Byrnes, W. 1985. Muscle soreness following resistance exercise with and without eccentric contractions. *Res. Q. Sport* 56:283.

Calarco, L., R. Otto, J. Wygand, J. Kramer, M. Yoke, and F. D'Zamko. 1991. The metabolic cost of six common movement patterns of bench-step aerobic dance (abstract). *Med. Sci. Sports Exerc.* 23(4):S839.

Cappo, B.M., and D.S. Homes. 1984. The utility of prolonged respiratory exhalation for reducing physiological and psychological arousal in non-threatening and threatening situations. *J. Psychosom. Res.* 28:263-73.

Capra, F. 1982. *The turning point.* New York: Bantam Books.

Carriere, B. 1998. *The Swiss Ball: Theory, basic exercises and clinical application.* Berlin, Germany: Springer-Verlag.

Carron, A., H. Hausenblas, and D. Mack. 1996. Social influence and exercise: A meta-analysis. *J. Sport Exerc. Psychol.* 18:1-16.

Carron, A., W. Widmeyer, and L. Brawley. 1988. Group cohesion and individual adherence to physical activity. *J. Sport Exerc. Psychol.* 10:127-38.

Chen, W. 1989. *Body mechanics of t'ai chi ch'uan.* New York: Chen.

Chinsky, A., J. DeFrancisco, K. Flanagan, R.M. Otto, and J. Wygand. 1998. A comparison of two types of spin exercise classes (abstract). *Med. Sci. Sports Exerc.* 30(5): S954.

Choi, P., J. Van Horn, D. Picker, and H. Roberts. 1993. Mood changes in women after an aerobics class: A preliminary study. *Health Care Women Int.* 14(2):167-77.

Chu, D.A. 1992. *Jumping into plyometrics.* Champaign, IL: Human Kinetics.

Cinque, C. 1989. Back pain prescription: Out of bed and into the gym. *Phys. Sportsmed.* 17(9):185-8.

Clapp, J., and K. Little. 1994. The physiological response of instructors and participants to three aerobics regimens. *Med. Sci. Sports Exerc.* 26(8):1041-6.

Claxton, C., and A. Lacy. 1991. Pedagogy: The missing link in aerobic dance. *J. Phys. Educ. Recreation Dance* August:49-52.

Copeland-Brooks, C., and D. Brooks. 1995. Guide to slide. *IDEA Today* 13(3):33-40.

Cosio-Lima, L.M., M.T. Jones, V.J. Paolone, and C.R. Winter. 2001. Effects of a physioball training program on trunk and abdominal strength and static balance measures (abstract). *Med. Sci. Sports Exerc.* 33(5):S1825.

Craig, A.B., and A.M Dvorak. 1968. Thermal regulation of man exercising during water immersion. *J. Appl. Physiol.* 25:23-35.

Crumpton, S., M. Scharff-Olson, H.N. Williford, A. Bradford, and S. Walker. 1999. The effects of a commercially-produced "spinning" video: Aerobic responses and caloric expenditure (abstract). *Med. Sci. Sports Exerc.* 31(5):S415.

D'Acquisto, L. D. D'Acquisto, D. Renne. (2001). Metabolic and cardiovascular responses in older women during shallow water exercise. *J Strength Cond. Res.* 15(1):12-9.

Darby, LA., K.D. Browder, and B.D. Reeves. 1995. The effects of cadence, impact, and step on physiological responses to aerobic dance exercise. *Res. Q. Exerc. Sport* 66:231-8.

Darby, L.A., W.A. Skelly, B. Durbin, R.P. Heitkamp, C.J. Hansen, and A.C. Stillman. 2002. Physiological responses to bench stepping on three different landing surfaces (abstract). *Med. Sci. Sports Exerc.* 34(5):S1651.

Davidson K. & L. McNaughton. 2000. Deep water running training and road running training improve VO₂ max in untrained women. *J. Strength Cond.* 14(2): 191-5.

Davis, C. 1994. The role of physical activity in the development and maintenance of eating disorders. *Psychol. Med.* 24:957-67.

Davis, S.E., L.J. Romaine, K. Casebolt, and K. Harrison. 2002. Incidence of injury in kickboxing (abstract). *Med. Sci. Sports Exerc.* 34(5):S1438.

DeMaere, J.M., and B.C. Ruby. 1997. Effects of deep water and treadmill running on oxygen uptake and energy expenditure in seasonally trained cross country runners. *J. Sports Med. Phys. Fitness* 37(3):175-81.

DiCarlo, L.J., P.B. Sparling, B.T. Hinson, T. Snow, and L. Rosskopf. 1995. Cardiovascular, metabolic and perceptual responses to hatha yoga standing poses. *Med. Exerc. Nutr. Health* 4:107-12.

Dunbar, C., R. Robertson, R. Baun, M. Blandin, K. Metz, R. Burdett, and R. Goss. 1992. The validity of regulating exercise intensity by ratings of perceived exertion. *Med. Sci. Sports Exerc.* 24(1):94-9.

Dwyer, J. 1995. Effect of perceived choice of music on exercise intrinsic motivation. *J. Health Behav. Educ. Promotion* 19(2):18-26.

Eklund, R., and S. Crawford. 1994. Social physique anxiety, reasons for exercise, and attitudes toward exercise settings. *J. Sport Exerc. Psychol.* 16:70-82.

Eller, D. 1996. News + views: Is aerobics dead? *Women's Sports and Fitness* Jan/Feb:19-20.

Estabrooks, P. 2000. Sustaining exercise participation through group cohesion. *Exerc. Sport Sci. Rev.* April 28: 2, 63-67.

Estabrooks, P., and A. Carron. 1999. The influence of the group with elderly exercisers. *Small Group Research* 30(4):438-52.

Estivill, M. 1995. Therapeutic aspects of aerobic dance participation. *Health Care Women Int.* 16(4):341-50.

Evans, E. 1993. Body image: Programming for a healthy perspective. *NIRSA Journal* Fall:46-51.

Evans, E., and P. Connor. 1995. Body image of water aerobic instructors (abstract). *Med. Sci. Sports Exerc.* 27(5):852.

Evans, E., and K. Cureton. 1998. Metabolic, circulatory and perceptual responses to bench stepping in water. *J. Strength Cond. Res.* 12(2):95-100.

Evans, E., and C. Kennedy. 1993. The body image problem in the fitness industry. *IDEA Today* May:50-6.

Eyestone, E., G. Fellingham, J. George, and G. Fisher. 1993. Effect of water running and cycling on maximum oxygen consumption and 2-mile run performance. *Am. J. Sports Med.* 21(1):41-4.

Falsetti, H., S. Blau, E. Burke, and K. Smith. 1995. Heart rate response and caloric expenditure during a Spinning class. *In Johnny G Spinning Instructor Manual*, pp. 4.15-4.18. Venice, CA: Johnny Goldberg Publications.

Feigenbaum, M., and M. Pollock. 1997. Strength training. *Phys. Sportsmed.* 25(2):44-64.

Feland, J.B. 2000. The effect of stretch duration on hamstring flexibility in an elderly population (abstract). *Med. Sci. Sports Exerc.* 32(5):S354.

Fischer, M.E., B.W. Evans, J.E. Edwards, and J.S. Kuhlman. 1998. Changes in fitness after a twelve week step aerobic program in women 50 to 65 years (abstract). *Med. Sci. Sports Exerc.* 30(5):S951.

Flanagan, K., J. DeFrancisco, A. Chinsky, J. Wygand, and R.M. Otto. 1998. The metabolic and cardiovascular response to select positions and resistances during spinning exercise (abstract). *Med. Sci. Sports Exerc.* 30(5): S944.

Flegal, K., M. Carroll, C. Ogden, and C. Johnson. 2002. Prevalence and trends in obesity among US adults, 1999-2000. *JAMA* 288(14):1723-7.

Fonda, J. 1981. *Jane Fonda's workout book.* New York: Simon & Schuster.

Fox, L., J. Rejeski, and L. Gauvin. 2000. Effects of leadership style and group dynamics on enjoyment of physical activity. *Am. J. Health Promot.* 15(5):277-83.

Francis, L. 1991. Improving aerobic dance programs: The key role of colleges and universities. *J. Phys. Educ. Recreation Dance* Sept:59-62.

Francis, P. 1990. In step with science. *Fitness Management* 6(6):37-8.

Francis, P., and L. Francis. 1988. *If it hurts, don't do it.* Rocklin, CA: Prima.

Francis, P.R., A.S. Witucki, and M.J. Buono. 1999. Physiological response to a typical studio cycling session. *ACSM's Health & Fitness Journal* 3(1):30-6.

Francis, P.R., L. Francis, G. Miller, K. Tichenor, and B. Rich. 1994. *Introduction to Step Reebok.* San Diegor, CA: San Diego University.

Francis, P.R., J. Poliner, M.J. Buono, and L.L. Francis. 1992. Effects of choreography, step height, fatigue and gender on metabolic cost of step training (abstract). *Med. Sci. Sports Exerc.* 24(5):S69.

Frangolias, D., and E. Rhodes. 1995. Maximal and ventilatory threshold responses to treadmill and water immersion running. *Med. Sci. Sports Exerc.* 27(7): 1007-13.

Frangolias, D., E. Rhodes, and J. Taunton. 1996. The effects of familiarity with deep water running on maximal oxygen consumption. *J. Strength Cond. Res.* 10(4):215-9.

Frangolias, D.D., E.C. Rhodes, J.E. Taunton, A.N. Belcastro, and K. Dcoutts. 2000. Metabolic responses to prolonged work during treadmill and water immersion running. *J. Sci. Med. Sports* 3(4):476-92.

Franzese, P., T. Taglione, C. Flynn, J. Wygand, and R.M. Otto. 2000. The metabolic cost of specific Taebo ™ exercise movements (abstract). *Med. Sci. Sports Exerc.* 32(5):S150.

Freeman, R. 1988. *Bodylove: Learning to like our looks and ourselves.* New York: Harper-Collins.

Frodge, S., A. Kunz, R. Liebman, J. Wygand, A. VanGelder, and R.M. Otto. 1993. A metabolic comparison of treadmill walking versus slideboard exercise (abstract). *Med. Sci. Sports Exerc.* 25(5):S622.

Frymoyer, J.W., and W.L. Cats-Baril. 1991. An overview of the incidences and costs of low back pain. *Orthop. Clin. North Am.* 22:263.

Gaesser, G. 1999. Thinness and weight loss: Beneficial or detrimental to longevity? *Med. Sci. Sports Exerc.* 31(8): 1118-28.

Gallegaher, S.P., and R. Kryzanowska. 1999. *The Pilates method of body conditioning.* Philadelphia: Trans-Atlantic.

Garber, C.E., J.S. McKinney, and R.A. Carleton. 1992. Is aerobic dance an effective alternative to walk–jog exercise training? *J. Sports Med. Phys. Fitness* 32(2):136-41.

Gehring, M., B. Keller, and B. Brehm. 1997. Water running with and without a flotation vest in competitive and recreational runners. *Med. Sci. Sports Exerc.* 29(10): 1374-8.

Ginis, M., M. Jung, and L. Gauvin. 2003. To see or not to see: Effects of exercising in mirrored environments on sedentary women's feeling states and self-efficacy. *Health Psychol.* 22(4):354-61.

Girouard, C., and B. Hurley. 1995. Does strength training inhibit gains in range of motion from flexibility training in older adults? *Med. Sci. Sports Exerc.* 27(10):1444-9.

Goldenberg, L., and P. Twist. 2002. *Strength ball training.* Champaign, IL: Human Kinetics.

Goleman, D. 1998. *Working with emotional intelligence.* New York: Bantam Books.

Goodman, S. 1997. The care and feeding of your sound system. *IDEA Today* June:43-50.

Goss, F.L., R.J. Robertson, R.J. Spina, T.E. Auble, D.A. Cassinelli, R.M. Silberman, R.W. Galbreath, and K.F. Metz. 1989. Energy cost of bench stepping and pumping light handweights in trained subjects. *Res. Q. Exerc. Sport.* 60(4):369-72.

Grant, S., K. Todd, T. Aitchison, P. Kelly, and D. Stoddart. 2004. The effects of a 12-week group exercise programme on physiological and psychological variables and function in overweight women. *Public Health* 118(1): 31-42.

Greene, L., L. Kravitz, J. Wongsathikun, and T. Kemerly. 1999. Metabolic effect of punching tempo (abstract). *Med. Sci. Sports Exerc.* 31(5):S674.

Greenlaw, K., L. McMillan, S. Catalano, S. Vivolo, M. Giroux, J. Wygand, and R.M. Otto. 1995. The energy cost of traditional versus power bench step exercise at heights of 4, 6, and 8 inches (abstract). *Med. Sci. Sports Exerc.* 27(5): S1343.

Grier, T.D., L.K. Lloyd, J.L. Walker, and T.D. Murray. 2001. Metabolic cost of aerobic dance bench stepping at varying cadences and bench heights (abstract). *Med. Sci. Sports Exerc.* 33(5):S123.

Hahn, S., D. Stanforth, P.R. Stanforth, and A. Phillips. 1998. A 10 week training study comparing Resistaball® and traditional trunk training. *Med. Sci. Sports Exerc.* 30(5): S1128.

Hale, B.S., and J.S. Raglin. 2002. State anxiety responses to acute resistance training and step aerobic exercise across eight weeks of training. *J. Sports Med. Phys. Fitness* 42(1):108-12.

Heidel, S., and J. Torgerson. 1993. Vocal problems among aerobic instructors and aerobic participants. *J. Commun. Disord.* 26(3):179-91.

Heinzelmann, F., and P. Bagley. 1970. Response to physical activity programs and their effects on health behavior. *Public Health Rep.* 86:905-11.

Hoeger, W., J. Warner, and G. Fahleson. 1995. Physiologic responses to self-paced water aerobics and treadmill running (abstract). *Med. Sci. Sports Exerc.* 27(5):83.

Hooker, S. 2003. The exercise/fitness professional's expanding role in promoting physical activity and the public's health. *ACSM's Health and Fitness Journal.* May/June: 7-11.

Hostler, D., C.I. Schwirian, F.C. Hagerman, R.S. Staron, G. Campos, K. Toma, M.T. Crill, and G. Hagerman. 1999. Skeletal muscle adaptations in elastic resistance trained young men and women (abstract). *Med. Sci. Sports Exerc.* 31(5):S1632.

Hutton, R.S. 1992. Neuromuscular basis of stretching exercises. In *Strength and power in sports,* ed. P.V. Komi, 29-38. Boston: Blackwell Scientific.

Ibbetson, J. 1996. Body image and self-esteem: Factors that affect each and recommendations for fitness professionals. *NIRSA Journal* Fall:22-27.

Immel, D.D., T. Tripplett-McBride, D.C.W. Fater, and C. Foster. 2000. Physiological responses to cardio kickboxing in females (abstract). *Med. Sci. Sports Exerc.* 32(5): S1557.

Iyengar, B.K.S. 1996. *Light on yoga.* New York: Schocken Books.

Jakicic, J.M., B.H. Marcus, K.I. Gallagher, M. Napolitano, and W. Lang. 2003. Effect of exercise duration and intensity on weight loss in overweight, sedentary women. *JAMA* 290(10):1323-30.

John, D.H., and P. Schuler. 1999. Accuracy of using RPE to monitor intensity of group indoor stationary cycling (abstract). *Med. Sci. Sports Exerc.* 31(5):S643.

Johnson, B.F., K.D. Johnston, and S.A. Winnier. 1993. Bench-step aerobic ground forces for two steps at variable bench heights (abstract). *Med. Sci. Sports Exerc.* 25(5):S1100.

Kahlkoetter, J. 2002. Respect your body. *Triathlete* Feb: 48-9.

Kellett, K., D. Kellett, and L. Nordholm. 1991. Effects of an exercise program on sick leave due to back pain. *Phys. Ther.* 71:283-93.

Kennedy, C. 1997. Exercise analysis. *IDEA Today* Jan:70-3.

Kennedy, C. 2003. Functional exercise progression. *IDEA Personal Trainer* Feb: 36-43.

Kennedy, C. 2004. Making a real difference. *IDEA Health and Fitness Source* Jan:40-4.

Kennedy, C., and D. Legel. 1992. *Anatomy of an exercise class: An exercise educators' handbook.* Champaign, IL: Sagamore.

Kennedy, C., and M. Sanders. 1995. Strength training gets wet. *IDEA Today* May:25-30.

Kennedy, M.M., and M. Newton. 1997. Effect of exercise intensity on mood in step aerobics. *J. Sports Med. Phys. Fitness* 37:3.

Kernodle, R. 1992. Space: The unexplored frontier of aerobic dance. *J. Phys. Educ. Recreation Dance* May/ June:65-9.

Kiesling, S. 1990. *The complete recreational rower and racer: From indoor rowing machines to outdoor shells.* New York: Crown.

Kin Isler, A., S.N. Kosar, and F. Korkusuz. 2001. Effects of step aerobics and aerobic dancing on serum lipids and lipoproteins. *J. Sports Med. Phys. Fitness* 41(3):380-5.

Kory, K., and T. Seabourne. 1999. *Power pacing for indoor cycling.* Champaign, IL: Human Kinetics

Koszuta, L. 1986. Low-impact aerobics: Better than traditional aerobic dance? *Phys. Sportsmed.* 14(7):156-61.

Kraemer, W.J., M. Keuning, N.A. Ratamess, J.S. Volek, M. McCormick, J.A. Bush, B.C. Nindl, S.W. Gordon, S.A. Mazzetti, R.U. Newton, A.L. Gomez, R.B. Wickham, M.R. Rubin, and K. Hakkinen. 2001. Resistance training combined with bench step aerobics enhances women's health profile. *Med. Sci. Sports Exerc.* 33(2):259-69.

Kraftsow, G. 1999. *Yoga for wellness: Healing with the timeless teachings of viniyoga.* New York: Penguin Books.

Krane, V., S. Shipley, J. Waldron, and J. Michalenok. 2001. Relationships among body satisfaction, social physique anxiety, and eating behaviors in female athletes and exercisers. *J. Sport Behav.* 24(3):247-64.

Kravitz, L. 1994. The effects of music on exercise. *IDEA Today* Oct:56-61.

Kravitz, L., L. Greene, and J. Wongsathikun. 2000. The physiological responses to kick-boxing exercise (abstract). *Med. Sci. Sports Exerc.* 32(5):S148.

Kravitz, L., V.H. Heyward, L.M. Stolarczyk, and M.V. Wilmerding. 1995. Effects of step training with and without handweights on physiological and lipid profiles of women (abstract). *Med. Sci. Sports Exerc.* 27(5):S1012.

Kravitz, L., V. Heyward, L. Stolarczyk, and V. Wilmerding. 1997. Does step exercise with handweights enhance training effects? *J. Strength Cond.* 11(3):194-9.

Kunz, A., R. Liebman, J.W. Wygand, R.M. Otto, A. VanGelder, J. Meegan, and J. Ludwig. 1993. The effects of body position and slide technique on the metabolic response of slideboard exercise (abstract). *Med. Sci. Sports Exerc.* 25(5):S623.

Lally, D. 1994. Stretching and injury in distance runners. *Med. Sci. Sports Exerc.* 26(5):S84.

Lane, C. 2000. *Christy Lane's complete book of line dancing,* 2nd ed. Champaign, IL: Human Kinetics.

Liemohn, W., and G. Pariser. 2002. Core strength: Implications for fitness and low back pain. *ACSM's Health and Fitness Journal* 6:5, 10-16.

Liggett, C.S. 1999. The Swiss ball: An overview of applications in sports medicine. *J. Man. Manipulative Ther.* 7(4):190-6.

Lofshult, D. 2002. Group fitness trend watch 2002. *IDEA Health and Fitness Source* July/Aug:69-76.

Long, J., H. Williford, M. Olson, and V. Wolfe V. 1998. Voice problems and risk factors among aerobics instructors. *J. Voice* 12(2):197-207.

Ludwig, J., A. VanGelder, J.W. Wygand, and R.M. Otto. 1994. The metabolic cost of fixed slideboard exercise at two different board lengths (abstract). *Med. Sci. Sports Exerc.* 26(5):S55.

MacAuley, D. 1995. *A guide to cycling injuries: Prevention and treatment.* San Francisco: Bicycle Books.

Malek, M., D. Nalbone, D. Berger, and J. Coburn. 2002. Importance of health science education for personal fitness trainers. *J. Strength Cond. Res.* 16(1):19-24.

Manchanda, S.C., R. Narang, K.D. Reddy, U. Sachdeva, D. Prabhakaran, S. Dharmanand, M. Rajani, and R. Bijlani. 2000. Retardation of coronary atherosclerosis with yoga lifestyle intervention. *J. Assoc. Phys. India* 48:687.

Massie, J., and R. Sheperd. 1971. Physiological and psychological effects of training: A comparison of individual and gymnasium programs, with a characterization of the exercise "drop-out." *Med. Sci. Sports* 3:110-7.

Mayo, J. 2000. Practical guidelines for the use of deep water running. *J. Strength and Conditioning,* 22(1): 26-29.

McArdle, W.D., F.I. Katch, and V.L. Katch. 2001. *Exercise physiology: Energy, nutrition, and human performance,* 5th ed. Philadelphia: Lippincott Williams & Wilkins.

McGlone, C., L. Kravitz, and J. Janot. 2002. Rebounding: A low-impact exercise alternative. *ACSM's Health and Fitness Journal* 6(2):11-5.

McKinney-Vialpando, K. 1999. *CARDIO TKO: Aerobic kickboxing for the fitness professional,* 2nd ed. Idaho Falls, ID: SAFAX Fitness Training.

Melanson, E.L., P.S. Freedson, R. Webb, S. Jungbluth, and N. Kozlowski. 1996. Exercise responses to running and in-line skating at self-selected paces. *Med. Sci. Sports Exerc.* 28(2):247-50.

Menezes, A. 1998. *The complete guide to Joseph H. Pilates' techniques of physical conditioning.* Alameda, CA: Hunter House.

Meyers, C. 1992. *Walking: A complete guide to a complete exercise.* New York: Random House.

Michaud, T., D. Brennan, R. Wilder, and N. Sherman. (1995). Aquarunning and gains in cardiorespiratory fitness. *J. Strength Cond.* 9(2):78-84.

Michaud, T., J. Rodriguez-Zayas, F. Andres, M. Flynn, and C. Lambert. 1995. Comparative exercise responses of deep-water and treadmill running. *J. Strength Cond.* 9(2):104-9.

Miller, J.M., M.D. Rossi, H. Schurr, L.E. Brown, and M. Whitehurst. 2001. Force production in healthy males during a horizontal press that uses elastics for resistance (abstract). *Med. Sci. Sports Exerc.* 33(5):S139.

Miller, W. 1999. How effective are traditional dietary and exercise interventions for weight loss? *Med. Sci. Sports Exerc.* 31(8):1129-34.

Mokdad, A.H., J. Marks, D. Stroup, and J. Gerberding. 2004. Actual causes of death in the US, 2000. *JAMA* 291(10):1238-1245.

Monroe, M. 1999. And the beat goes on. *IDEA Health and Fitness Source* October:31-7.

Monroe, R., R. Nagarathma, and H.R. Nagendra. 1990. *Yoga for common ailments.* New York: Simon & Schuster.

Moses, R.D. 1993. Ground reaction forces in bench aerobics (abstract 49). Presented at 22nd Annual Meeting, Southeast Regional Chapter of the American College of Sports Medicine, Greensboro, NC.

Mutoh, Y., S. Sawai, Y. Takanashi, and L. Skurko. 1988. Aerobic dance injuries among instructors and students. *Phys. Sportsmed.* 16(12):81-6.

Myers, M.J., and P. Boyd. 2001. Metabolic cost of stepping: Effects of cadence and load (abstract). *Med. Sci. Sports Exerc.* 33(5):S501.

Nardini, M., J. Raglin, and C. Kennedy. 1999. Body image, disordered eating, obligatory exercise and body composition among women fitness instructors (abstract 1472). *Med. Sci. Sports Exerc. Suppl.* 31(5):S297.

Neiman, D. 2003. *Exercise testing and prescription,* 5th ed. New York: McGraw-Hill.

Nichols, J.F., C.L. Sherman, and E. Abbott. 2000. Treading is new and hot. *ACSM's Health and Fitness Journal* 4(2):12-7.

Nogawa-Wasman, D. 2002. How to make group fitness profitable with fee-based programming. *IDEA Health and Fitness Source* May:29-35.

Norton, C., K. Hoobler, A. Welding, and G.M. Jensen. 1997. Effectiveness of aquatic exercise in the treatment of women with osteoarthritis. *J. Phys. Ther.* 5(3):8-15.

O'Driscoll, E., J. Steele, H.R. Perez, S. Yreys, N. Snowkroft, and F. Locasio. 1999. The metabolic cost of two trials of boxing exercise utilizing a heavy bag (abstract). *Med. Sci. Sports Exerc.* 31(5):S676.

Ogden, C., K. Flegal, M. Carroll, and C. Johnson. 2002. Prevalence and trends in overweight among US children and adolescents, 1999-2000. *JAMA* 288:14, 1728-1732.

Olson, M., H. Williford, D. Blessing, and R. Greathouse. 1991. The cardiovascular and metabolic effects of bench-stepping exercise in females. *Med. Sci. Sports Exerc.* 23(11):1311-8.

Olson, M., L. Williford, R. Brown, and S. Pugh. 1996. Self-reports on the Eating Disorder Inventory by female aerobic instructors. *Percept. Mot. Skills* 82:1051-8.

Ornish, D. 1998. *Love and survival.* New York: Harper Collins.

Ornish, D., S.E. Brown, L.W. Scherwitz, J.H. Billings, W.T. Armstrong, T.A. Ports, S.M. McLanahan, R.L. Kirkeeide, R.J. Brand, and K.L. Gould. 1990. Lifestyle heart trial. *Lancet* 336:129-33.

Otto, R., C. Parker, T. Smith, J. Wygand, and H. Perez. 1986. The energy cost of low impact and high impact aerobic exercise (abstract). *Med. Sci. Sports Exerc.* 18: S523.

Otto, R., M. Yoke, J. Wygand, and P. Larsen. 1988. The metabolic cost of multidirectional low impact and high impact aerobic dance (abstract). *Med. Sci. Sports Exerc.* 20(2):S525.

Page, P., and T. Ellenbecker, eds. 2003. *The scientific and clinical application of elastic resistance.* Champaign, IL: Human Kinetics.

Parker, S., B. Hurley, D. Hanlon, and P. Vaccaro. 1989. Failure of target heart rate to accurately monitor intensity during aerobic dance. *Med. Sci. Sports Exerc.* 21(2): 230-4.

Pate, R.R., M. Pratt, S.N. Blair, W.L. Haskell, C.A. Macera, C. Bouchard, D. Buchner, W. Ettinger, G.W. Heath, A.C. King, et al. 1995. Physical activity and public health: A recommendation from the Centers for Disease Control and Prevention and the American College of Sports Medicine. *JAMA* 273(5):402-7.

Pearson, D., A. Faigenbaum, M. Conley, and W. Kraemer. 2000. The National Strength and Conditioning Association's basic guidelines for resistance training of athletes. *Strength Cond. J.* 22(4):14-27.

Perez, H.R., E. O'Driscoll, J. Steele, S. Yreys, N. Snowkroft, C. Steizinger, and F. Locasio. 1999. Physiological responses to two forms of boxing aerobics exercise (abstract). *Med. Sci. Sports Exerc.* 31(5):S673.

Peterson, T., D. Verstraete, W. Schultz, and J. Stray-Gundersen. 1993. Metabolic demands of step aerobics (abstract). *Med. Sci. Sports Exerc.* 25(5):S448.

Pilates, J.H. 1945. *Pilates' return to life through contrology.* Available from Balanced Body: (800)-PILATES

Pilates, J.H., W.J. Miller, S.P. Gallagher, and R. Kryzanowska, eds. 2000. *The complete writings of Joseph H. Pilates: Return to life through contrology and your health—the authorized editions.* Philadelphia: Bainbridge Books.

Pillarella, D. 1997. Ready, set, row! *IDEA Today* 15(8): 36-43.

Porcari, J.P. 1999. Pump up your walk. *ACSM's Health and Fitness Journal* 3(1):25-9.

Posner-Mayer, J. 1995. *Swiss Ball applications for orthopedic and sports medicine.* Denver: Ball Dynamics International.

Prins, J., and D. Cutner. 1999. Aquatic therapy in the rehabilitation of athletic injuries. *Clin. Sports Med.* 18(2):427-35.

Public Health Service, U.S. Department of Health and Human Services. 2004. *Healthy people 2010: National health promotion and disease prevention objectives.* Washington, DC: U.S. Printing Office. 2:22, 1-7-2004.

Quinn, T., D. Sedory, and B. Fisher. 1994. Physiological effects of deep water running following a land-based training program. *Res. Q. Exerc. Sport* 65:386-9.

Reebok University. 1993. *Reebok training manuals: Slide Reebok basic training and slide Reebok endurance training.* Canton, MA: Reebok University Press.

Reese, S. 1991. Slideboards: A conditioning and rehabilitative tool. *National Strength and Conditioning Association Journal* 13(5):22-4.

Richey, R.M., R.M. Zabik, and M.L. Dawson. 1999. Effect of bicycle spinning on heart rate, oxygen consumption, respiratory exchange ratio, and caloric expenditure (abstract). *Med. Sci. Sports Exerc.* 31(5):S692.

Richie, D., S. Kelso, and P. Bellucci. 1985. Aerobic dance injuries: A retrospective study of instructors and participants. *Phys. Sportsmed.* 13(2):130-40.

Riker, H.A., R.M. Zabik, M.L. Dawson, and P.A. Frye. 1998. The effect of step height and upper body involvement on oxygen consumption and energy expenditure during step aerobics (abstract). *Med. Sci. Sports Exerc.* 30(5):S945.

Roach, B., P. Croisant, and J. Emmett. 1994. The appropriateness of heart rate and RPE measures of intensity during three variations of aerobic dance (abstract). *Med. Sci. Sports Exerc. Suppl.* 26(5):24.

Robertson, R., F. Goss, T. Auble, D. Cassinelli, R. Spina, E. Glickman, R. Galbreath, R. Silberman, and K. Metz. 1990. Cross-modal exercise prescription at absolute and relative oxygen uptake using perceived exertion. *Med. Sci. Sports Exerc.* 22(5):653-9.

Rodgers, C.D., C.E. Bjorkquist-Bearding, L.C. Forsblom, and M.E. Ewing. 1994. Comparison of high impact and controlled eccentric aerobic dance routines on cardio-

respiratory parameters during exercise and recovery in college-aged women (abstract). *Med. Sci. Sports Exerc.* 26(5):S585.

Rupp, J.C., B.F. Johnson, and D.A. Rupp. 1992. Bench step activity: Effects of bench height and hand held weights (abstract). *Med. Sci. Sports Exerc.* 24(5):S12.

Ryan, P. 2003. Fitness trends report. *IDEA Fitness Manager* Oct: 1-13.

Sanders, M.E., N. Constantino, and N. Rippee. 1997. A comparison of results of functional water training on field and laboratory measures in older women. *Med. Sci. Sports Exerc.* 29(5):ixx-ixx.

Santana, J. 2002. The four pillars of human movement. *IDEA Personal Trainer* Feb:22-8.

Schaller, K. 1996. Tai chi chih: An exercise option for older adults. *J. Gerontol. Nurs.* 22(10):12-7.

Scharff-Olson, M., and H.N. Williford. 1996. The energy cost associated with selected step training exercise techniques. *Res. Q. Exerc. Sport* 67:465-8.

Scharff-Olson, M., H.N. Williford, A. Bradford, S. Walker, and S. Crumpton. 1999. Physiological and subjective psychological responses to group cycling exercise (abstract). *Med. Sci. Sports Exerc.* 31(5):S418.

Scharff-Olson, M., H.N. Williford, D.L. Blessing, R. Moses, and T. Wang. 1997. Vertical impact forces during bench-step aerobics: Exercise rate and experience. *Percept. Mot. Skills* 84(1):267-74.

Scharff-Olson, M., H.N. Williford, W.J. Duey, J. Barber, and S. Baldwin. 1997. Physiological responses of males and females to bench step exercise at two different rates (abstract). *Med. Sci. Sports Exerc.* 29(5):S160.

Scharff-Olson, M., H.N. Williford, W.J. Duey, S. Walker, S. Crumpton, and J. Sanders. 2000. The energy cost of martial arts aerobic exercise (abstract). *Med. Sci. Sports Exerc.* 32(5):S149.

Shrier, I. 1999. Stretching before exercise does not reduce the risk of local muscle injury: A critical review of the clinical and basic science literature. *Clinical Journal of Sports Medicine,* 9:221-227.

Schuster, K. 1979. Aerobic dance: A step to fitness. *Phys. Sportsmed.* 7(8):98-103.

Shrier, I., and K. Gossal. 2000. Myths and truths of stretching. *Phys. Sportsmed.* 28(8):57-63.

Shyba, L. 1990. Finding the elusive downbeat. *IDEA Today* June:23-30.

Silberstein, L., R. Striegel-Moore, and J. Rodin. 1987. Feeling fat: A woman's shame. Hillsdale, NJ: Erlbaum.

Siler, B. 2000. *The Pilates body.* New York: Broadway Books.

Simmons, V., and P. Hansen. 1996. Effectiveness of water exercise on postural mobility in the well elderly: An experimental study on balance enhancement. *J. Gerontol. Med. Sci.* 51A(5):M233-8.

Sovik, R. 2000. The science of breathing—the yogic view. *Prog. Brain Res.* 122:491-505.

Spink, K., and A. Carron. 1992. Group cohesion and adherence in exercise classes. *J. Sport Exerc. Psychol.* 14:78-86.

Spink, K., and A. Carron. 1993. The effects of team building on the adherence patterns of female exercise participants. *J. Sport Exerc. Psychol.* 15:39-49.

Spink, K., and A. Carron. 1994. Group cohesion effects in exercise classes. *Small Group Res.* 25(1):26-42.

Stanforth, D., and P. Stanforth. 1993. The effect of adding external weight on the aerobic requirements of bench stepping (abstract). *Med. Sci. Sports Exerc.* 25(5):S470.

Stanforth, D., P.R. Stanforth, and K.S. Velasquez. 1993. Aerobic requirement of bench stepping. *Int. J. Sports Med.* 14(3):129-33.

Stanforth, D., K. Velasquez, and P. Stanforth. 1991. The effect of bench height and rate of stepping on the metabolic cost of bench stepping (abstract). *Med. Sci. Sports Exerc.* 23(4):S143.

Stanforth, P.R., and D. Stanforth. 1996. The effect of adding external weight on the aerobic requirement of bench stepping. *Res. Q. Exerc. Sport* 67:469-72.

Step Reebok. 1997. *1997 revised guidelines for step Reebok.* Canton, MA: Reebok University.

Stephens, T., and S. Craig. 1990. *The well-being of Canadians: Highlights of the 1988 Campbell's survey.* Ottawa, ON: Canadian Fitness and Lifestyle Research Institute.

Sullivan, M.G., J.J. Dejulia, and T.W. Worrell. 1992. Effect of pelvic position and stretching method on hamstring muscle flexibility. *Med. Sci. Sports Exerc.* 24(12):1383-9.

Suomi, R., and D.M. Koceja. 2000. Postural sway characteristics in women with lower extremity arthritis before and after an aquatic exercise intervention. *Arch. Phys. Med. Rehabil.* 8(6):780-5.

Sutherland, R., J. Wilson, T. Aitchison, and S. Grant. 1999. Physiological responses and perceptions of exertion in a step aerobics session. *J. Sports Sci.* 17(6):495-503.

Svedenhag, J., and J. Seger. 1992. Running on land and in water: Comparative exercise physiology. *Med. Sci. Sports Exerc.* 24:1155-60.

Takeshima, N., M. Rogers, E. Watanabe, W. Brechue, A. Okada, T. Yamada, M. Islam, and J. Hayano. 2002. Water-based exercise improves health-related aspects of fitness in older women. *Med. Sci. Sports Exerc.* 33(3):544-51.

Taylor, D., J. Dalton, A. Seaber, and W. Garrett. 1990. Viscoelastic properties of muscle-tendon units: The biomechanical effects of stretching. *Am. J. Sports Med.* 18:300-9.

Telles, S., R.S. Kumar, and H.R. Nagendra. 2000. Oxygen consumption and respiration following two yoga relaxation techniques. *Appl. Psychophysiol. Biofeedback* 25(4):221-7.

Templeton, M.S., D.L. Booth, and W.D. O'Kelly. 1996. Effects of aquatic therapy on joint flexibility and functional ability in subjects with rheumatic disease. *J. of Orthopedic and Sports Therapy* 23:6, 376-381.

Tuosto, C.W., and R.P. Tobin. 1997. The effect of board length and cadence on cardiorespiratory and metabolic responses to Slideboard exercise (abstract). *Med. Sci. Sports Exerc.* 29(5):S1064.

Twist, P. 2004. Sports conditioning fast track, *IDEA Personal Trainer,* Jan: 21-26.

U.S. Department of Health and Human Resources. January 2000. *Healthy People 2010.* Washington, DC. Available at: www.healthy.gov/healthy-people/

VanMechelen, W., H. Hlobil, C. Kemper, W. Voorn, and H. deJongh. 1993. Prevention of running injuries by warm-up, cool-down, and stretching exercises. *American J. of Sports Medicine* 21:711-719.

Velasquez, K., and J.H. Wilmore. 1992. Changes in cardiorespiratory fitness and body composition after a 12 week bench step training program (abstract). *Med. Sci. Sports Exerc.* 24(5):S464.

Walker, M. 1989. *Jumping for health.* Garden City, NY: Avery.

Wallace, A. 2002. True thighs. *More* Sept:90-5.

Wallin, D., B. Ekblom, R. Grahn, and T. Nordenborg. 1985. Improvement of muscle flexibility. A comparison between two techniques. *Am. J. Sports Med.* 13(4): 263-8.

Walter, J., F. Figoni, and F. Andres. 1995. Effect of stretching intensity and duration on hamstring flexibility (abstract). *Med. Sci. Sports Exerc.* 27(5):S240.

Wang, N., M. Scharff-Olson, and H.N. Williford. 1993. Energy cost and fuel utilization during step aerobics exercise (abstract). *Med. Sci. Sports Exerc.* 25(5):S630.

Watts, J.H. 1996. Sport-specific conditioning for anaerobic athletes. *Strength Cond. J.* 18(4):33-5.

Webb, T. 1989. Aerobic Q signs. *IDEA Today* 10:30-1.

Weltman, A. 1995. *The blood lactate response to exercise.* Champaign, IL: Human Kinetics.

Westcott, W. 1991. Role-model instructors. *Fitness Management* March:48-50.

Westcott, W. 2000. Strength training frequency. *Fitness Management* Nov: 50-54.

Whaley, M. 2003. ACSM credentialing: The more towards formal education. *Health and Fitness Journal* July/Aug: 31-2.

Whitney, C., J.P. Porcari, W. Floyd, and L.A. Chase. 1993. Step aerobics: The influence of different arm movements and step heights (abstract). *Med. Sci. Sports Exerc.* 25(5): S453.

Wilbur, R., R. Moffatt, B. Scott, K. Biggerstaff, and K. Hayes. 1995. Comparison of physiological responses during submaximal deep water and treadmill running (abstract). *Med. Sci. Sports Exerc.* 27(5):1352.

Wilbur, R., R. Moffatt, B. Scott, D. Lee, and N. Cucuzzo. 1996. Influence of water run training on the maintenance of aerobic performance. *Med. Sci. Sports Exerc.* 28(8):1056-62.

Williford, H., D. Blessing, M. Olson, and F. Smith. 1989. Is low impact aerobic dance an effective cardiovascular workout? *Phys. Sportsmed.* 17(3):95-109.

Williford, H.N., M. Scharff-Olson, and D.L. Blessing. 1989. The physiological effects of aerobic dance, a review. *Sports Med.* 8(6):335-45.

Williford, H.N., M. Scharff-Olson, A. Bradford, S. Walker, and S. Crumpton. 1999. Maximum cycle ergometry and group cycle exercise: A comparison of physiological responses (abstract). *Med. Sci. Sports Exerc.* 31(5): S423.

Williford, H.N., N. Wang, M. Scharff-Olson, D.L. Blessing, and J. Buzbee. 1993. Energy expenditure of Slideboard exercise training (abstract). *Med. Sci. Sports Exerc.* 25(5): S621.

Wilmore, J.H., and D.L. Costill. 1999. *Physiology of sports and exercise.* Champaign, IL: Human Kinetics.

Wininger, S. 2002. Instructors' and classroom characteristics associated with exercise enjoyment by females. *Percept. Mot. Skills* 94(2):395-8.

Wolf, C. 2001. Moving the body. *IDEA Personal Trainer* June:23-31.

Woodby-Brown, S., K. Berg, and R.W. Latin. 1993. Oxygen cost of aerobic dance bench stepping at three heights. *J. Strength Cond. Res.* 7(3):163-7.

Workman, D., D. Kern, and C. Earnest. 1993. Cardiorespiratory responses of isolated arm movements and hand weighting during bench stepping aerobic dance in women (abstract). *Med. Sci. Sports Exerc.* 25(5):S466.

YMCA water fitness for health. 2001. Champaign, IL: Human Kinetics.

Yoke, M. 2001. *A Guide to Personal Fitness Training.* Sherman Oaks, CA:AFAA.

Yoke, M., and C. Kennedy. 2004. *Functional exercise progressions.* Monterey, CA: Healthy Learning.

Yoke, M., R. Otto, P. Larsen, C. Kamimukai, and J. Wygand. 1989. The metabolic cost of instructors' low impact and high impact aerobic dance sequences. In *IDEA 1989 Research Symposium Manual.* San Diego, CA: IDEA.

Yoke, M., R. Otto, J. Wygand, and C. Kamimukai. 1988. The metabolic cost of two differing low impact aerobic dance exercise modes (abstract). *Med. Sci. Sports Exerc.* 20(2):S527.

Zabukovec, R., and P.M. Tiidus. 1998. Physiological and anthropometric profile of elite kickboxers. *J. Strength Cond. Res.* 9(4):240-2.

Zeni, A., M.D. Hoffman, and P.S. Clifford.. 1996. Energy expenditure with indoor exercise machines. *JAMA* 275(18):1424-7.

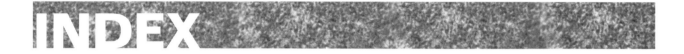
INDEX

NOTE: The italicized *f* and *t* following page numbers refer to figures and tables, respectively. The italicized *ff* and *tt* following page numbers refer to multiple figures and tables, respectively.

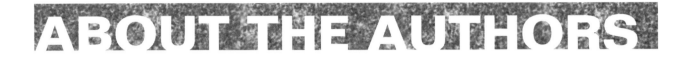

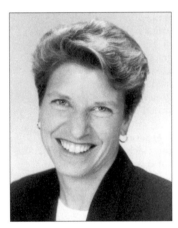

Carol A. Kennedy, MS, is a lecturer in the fitness specialist program within the department of kinesiology at Indiana University, Bloomington. During her more than 25 years of teaching and training fitness leaders, she has served on the American Council on Exercise (ACE) and the American College of Sports Medicine (ACSM) credentialing committees, and she chaired the IDEA Water Fitness Committee.

Certified through ACE as a group fitness instructor and ACSM as a health fitness instructor, Kennedy is a regular presenter at fitness conferences and has produced videos on exercise progression and water exercise. At Indiana University, she created and managed the Recreational Sports Fitness/Wellness Program, which included more than 100 group exercise sessions per week before moving to the department of kinesiology to assist with the creation of the fitness specialist undergraduate major.

Kennedy earned her bachelor's degree in leisure studies from the University of Illinois, and her master's degree in exercise and sport science from Colorado State University. She has created and taught a methods of group leadership class at three major universities and continues to teach group exercise classes on a regular basis.

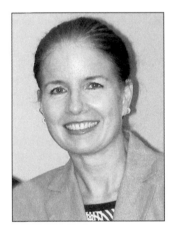

Mary Yoke, MA, MM, has more than 21 years of experience teaching and training group exercise leaders. In addition to leading group exercise classes on a regular basis, she is an adjunct professor at Adelphi University in New York, where she teaches a graduate course in exercise leadership. She is an adjunct board member and master trainer for the Aerobics and Fitness Association of America (AFAA) and served on the American College of Sports Medicine (ACSM) credentialing committee for six years.

Yoke has led seminars for fitness professionals in Europe, Asia, Africa, and South America. She gives numerous presentations throughout the United States to both fitness professionals and the general public. She is the author of two other books on fitness, as well as three videos.

Holding over 19 certifications from organizations such as the ACSM, AFAA, American Council on Exercise (ACE), National Academy of Sports Medicine (NASM), and Stott Pilates, Yoke received her bachelor's and master's degrees in music from Indiana and Florida State Universities, respectively. She then earned a master's degree in exercise physiology from Adelphi University, where she has authored several research studies on group exercise.

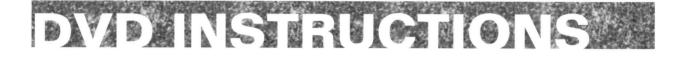

DVD INSTRUCTIONS

The enclosed DVD includes group exercise demonstrations. You can view the video content either on a television set with a DVD player or on a computer with a DVD-ROM drive.

The DVD includes a chapter selections menu. When you select a chapter, you'll be taken to a menu with a list of the specific video clips for that chapter. After you have viewed one video clip, the DVD will automatically return to the list of video clips for that chapter, where you can select the next video clip or choose any other video clip.

To use the DVD, place it in your DVD player or DVD-ROM drive. A title screen will welcome you to the program. Then the main menu will appear. To view the video clips, select the "Chapter Selections" button.

Select the HK Running Man logo on the main menu to access information on contacting Human Kinetics to order other products and production credits.